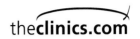

# INFECTIOUS DISEASE CLINICS OF NORTH AMERICA

## Fever of Unknown Origin

GUEST EDITOR
Burke A. Cunha, MD

CONSULTING EDITOR
Robert C. Moellering, Jr, MD

December 2007 • Volume 21 • Number 4

**SAUNDERS**

An Imprint of Elsevier, Inc.
PHILADELPHIA   LONDON   TORONTO   MONTREAL   SYDNEY   TOKYO

**W.B. SAUNDERS COMPANY**
*A Division of Elsevier Inc.*

Elsevier, Inc., 1600 John F. Kennedy Blvd., Suite 1800, Philadelphia, PA 19103-2899.

http://www.theclinics.com

INFECTIOUS DISEASE CLINICS
OF NORTH AMERICA
December 2007
Editor: Barbara Cohen-Kligerman

Volume 21, Number 4
ISSN 0891–5520
ISBN-10: 1-4160-5562-2
ISBN-13: 978-1-4160-5562-4

The ideas and opinions expressed in *Infectious Disease Clinics of North America* do not necessarily reflect those of the Publisher. The Publisher does not assume any responsibility for any injury and/or damage to persons or property arising out of or related to any use of the material contained in this periodical. The reader is advised to check the appropriate medical literature and the product information currently provided by the manufacturer of each drug to be administered to verify the dosage, the method and duration of administration, or contraindications. It is the responsibility of the treating physician or other health care professional, relying on independent experience and knowledge of the patient, to determine drug dosages and the best treatment for the patient. Mention of any product in this issue should not be construed as endorsement by the contributors, editors, or the Publisher of the product or manufacturers' claims.

*Infectious Disease Clinics of North America* (ISSN 0891–5520) is published in March, June, September, and December (For Post Office use only: volume 20 issue 4 of 4) by Elsevier Inc., 360 Park Avenue South, New York, NY 10010-1710. Business and Editorial Offices: 1600 John F. Kennedy Blvd., Suite 1800, Philadelphia, PA 19103-2899. Customer Service Office: 6277 Sea Harbor Drive, Orlando, FL 32887-4800. Periodicals postage paid at New York, NY and additional mailing offices. Subscription prices are $202.00 per year for US individuals, $339.00 per year for US institutions, $101.00 per year for US students, $238.00 per year for Canadian individuals, $410.00 per year for Canadian institutions, $267.00 per year for international individuals, $410.00 per year for international institutions, and $131.00 per year for Canadian and foreign students. To receive student rate, orders must be accompanied by name of affiliated institution, date of term, and the *signature* of program/residency coordinator on institution letterhead. Orders will be billed at individual rate until proof of status is received. Foreign air speed delivery is included in all *Clinics* subscription prices. All prices are subject to change without notice. **POSTMASTER:** Send address changes to *Infectious Disease Clinics of North America*, Elsevier Periodicals Customer Service, 6277 Sea Harbor Drive, Orlando, FL 32887-4800. **Customer Service: 1-800-654-2452 (US). From outside of the US, call 1-407-345-4000. E-mail: elspcs@elsevier.com.**

*Infectious Disease Clinics of North America* is also published in Spanish by Editorial Inter-Médica, Junin 917, 1$^{er}$ A 1113, Buenos Aires, Argentina.

Reprints. For copies of 100 or more, of articles in this publication, please contact the Commercial Reprints Department, Elsevier Inc., 360 Park Avenue South, New York, New York 10010-1710. Tel. (212) 633-3813, Fax: (212) 462-1935, email: reprints@elsevier.com.

*Infectious Disease Clinics of North America* is covered in *Index Medicus, Current Contents/Clinical Medicine, Science Citation Alert, SCISEARCH,* and *Research Alert.*

Printed in the United States of America.

# GUEST EDITOR

**BURKE A. CUNHA, MD, MACP,** Chief, Infectious Disease Division, Winthrop-University Hospital, Mineola, Long Island; Professor of Medicine, State University of New York School of Medicine, Stony Brook, New York

# CONTRIBUTORS

**ALYS ADAMSKI, BS,** Division of Infectious Diseases, Department of Internal Medicine and Medical Microbiology/Immunology, Southern Illinois School of Medicine, Springfield, Illinois

**DIVYA AHUJA, MD,** Assistant Professor of Medicine, Department of Medicine, University of South Carolina School of Medicine, Columbia, South Carolina

**ANASTASIA ANTONIADOU, MD,** Senior Lecturer, University General Hospital ATTIKON, Fourth Department of Internal Medicine, Athens, Greece

**JASON J. BOFINGER, MD,** Fellow, Section of Infectious Diseases, Temple University Hospital, Philadelphia, Pennsylvania

**ELISABETH BOTELHO-NEVERS, MD,** Unité des Rickettsies, Faculté de Médecine, Université de la Méditerranée, Marseille, France

**EMILIO BOUZA, MD, PhD,** Professor of Medicine, and Chief, Division of Clinical Microbiology and Infectious Diseases, Universidad Complutense de Madrid, Hospital General Universitario Gregorio Marañón, Madrid, Spain

**CHARLES S. BRYAN, MD,** Heyward Gibbes Distinguished Professor of Internal Medicine, Department of Medicine, University of South Carolina School of Medicine, Columbia, South Carolina

**DENNIS J. CLERI, MD,** Program Director, Internal Medicine Residency, St. Francis Medical Center, Trenton; Professor of Medicine, Seton Hall University, School of Graduate Medical Education, South Orange, New Jersey

**BURKE A. CUNHA, MD, MACP,** Chief, Infectious Disease Division, Winthrop-University Hospital, Mineola, Long Island; Professor of Medicine, State University of New York School of Medicine, Stony Brook, New York

**CHESTON B. CUNHA,** Pennsylvania State University College of Medicine, Hershey, Pennsylvania

**HELEN GIAMARELLOU, MD, PhD,** Professor, University General Hospital ATTIKON, Fourth Department of Internal Medicine, Athens, Greece

**ARNAUD HOT, MD,** Université Paris V, Service des Maladies Infectieuses et Tropicales, Centre d'Infectiologie Necker-Pasteur, Hôpital Necker-Enfants Malades, Paris, France

**NANCY KHARDORI, MD, PhD,** Professor of Medicine and Microbiology/Immunology; and Chief, Division of Infectious Diseases, Department of Internal Medicine and Medical Microbiology/Immunology, Southern Illinois School of Medicine, Springfield, Illinois

**DANIEL C. KNOCKAERT, MD, PhD,** Professor of Medicine, Division of General Internal Medicine, Gasthuisberg University Hospital, Leuven, Belgium

**BELÉN LOECHES, MD,** Fellow in Infections Disease and Microbiology, Division of Clinical Microbiology and Infectious Diseases, Hospital General Universitario Gregorio Marañón, Madrid, Spain

**OLIVIER LORTHOLARY, MD, PhD,** Université Paris V, Service des Maladies Infectieuses et Tropicales, Centre d'Infectiologie Necker-Pasteur, Hôpital Necker-Enfants Malades, Paris; and Centre National de Référence Mycologie et Antifongiques, Institut Pasteur, Paris, France

**PATRICIA MUÑOZ, MD, PhD,** Professor of Medicine, Division of Clinical Microbiology and Infectious Diseases, Universidad Complutense de Madrid, Hospital General Universitario Gregorio Marañón, Madrid, Spain

**ADNAN MUSHTAQ, MD,** Division of Infectious Diseases, Department of Internal Medicine and Medical Microbiology/Immunology, Southern Illinois School of Medicine, Springfield, Illinois

**DEAN C. NORMAN, MD,** Adjunct Professor of Medicine, University of California, Los Angeles David Geffen School of Medicine; Chief of Staff, VA Greater Los Angeles Healthcare System, Los Angeles, California

**DIDIER RAOULT, MD, PhD,** Unité des Rickettsies, Faculté de Médecine, Université de la Méditerranée, Marseille, France

**ANTHONY J. RICKETTI, MD,** Chairman, Department of Medicine, St. Francis Medical Center, Trenton; Associate Professor of Medicine, Seton Hall University, School of Graduate Medical Education, South Orange, New Jersey

**DAVID SCHLOSSBERG, MD, FACP,** Professor of Medicine, Section of Infectious Diseases, Temple University School of Medicine; Medical Director, Tuberculosis Control Program, Philadelphia Department of Public Health, Philadelphia, Pennsylvania

**LAURA SCHMULEWITZ, BSc, MB, ChB,** Université Paris V, Service des Maladies Infectieuses et Tropicales, Centre d'Infectiologie Necker-Pasteur, Hôpital Necker-Enfants Malades, Paris, France

**LEON G. SMITH, MD,** Chairman of Medicine, Department of Infectious Diseases, St. Michael's Medical Center, Newark, New Jersey

**CRISTIAN SPEIL, MD,** Division of Infectious Diseases, Department of Internal Medicine and Medical Microbiology/Immunology, Southern Illinois School of Medicine, Springfield, Illinois

**JILL TOLIA, MD,** Staten Island University Hospital, Staten Island, New York; Formerly, Fellow, Department of Infectious Diseases, St. Michael's Medical Center, Newark, New Jersey

**JOHN R. VERNALEO, MD,** Chief, Division of Infectious Diseases, Wyckoff Heights Medical Center, Brooklyn, New York

**JEAN-PAUL VIARD, MD,** Université Paris V, Service des Maladies Infectieuses et Tropicales, Centre d'Infectiologie Necker-Pasteur, Hôpital Necker-Enfants Malades, Paris, France

**MEGAN BERNADETTE WONG, BS,** VA Greater Los Angeles Healthcare System, Los Angeles, California

**THOMAS T. YOSHIKAWA, MD,** Professor of Medicine, University of California, Los Angeles David Geffen School of Medicine; Director of the Geriatric Research, Education and Clinical Center, VA Greater Los Angeles Healthcare System, Los Angeles, California

**THIERRY ZENONE, MD,** Department of Medicine, Unit of Internal Medicine, Centre Hospitalier, Valence, France

# CONTENTS

Fever of unknown origin is a topic that has enduring interest to physicians. Prolonged fevers of infectious etiology were of particular concern to the ancient physician. This overview of prolonged fevers in antiquity focuses on malaria and typhoid fever as the primary infectious causes. By studying texts from Mesopotamian, Greek, and Roman physicians and observers of disease, it is possible to determine the likely etiology of many of these ancient plagues. The historical import of these diseases should not be overlooked, and it is for this reason that the prolonged fevers of antiquity have profound significance and enduring interest.

Fever of unknown origin (FUO) refers to disorders that present with prolonged and perplexing fevers that are difficult to diagnose. This article presents a clinical overview of classic and current causes of FUOs, which may be due to infectious, rheumatic/inflammatory, neoplastic, or miscellaneous disorders. Comprehensive but nonfocused diagnostic testing is ineffective and should be avoided. The FUO workup should be directed by the key history, physical, and laboratory findings in clinical presentation. The clinical syndromic approach in the differential diagnosis of FUOs is emphasized, and the diagnostic importance and significance of fever patterns are discussed.

This article describes both common and unusual zoonoses causing fevers of unknown origin. Simian immune virus is considered as a possible emerging infection. For special populations (the homeless, zoophiliacs, those whose occupation or leisure brings them in close contact with oceans or lakes, and veterinarians), zoonotic infection potentials are discussed.

examination, and to the epidemiological antecedents. This article examines an approach that considers different syndromes, followed by an etiologically oriented differential diagnosis.

## Fever of Unknown Origin in Febrile Leukopenia
Anastasia Antoniadou and Helen Giamarellou

Febrile neutropenia is a syndrome commonly anticipated in patients receiving treatment for cancer. Its management for the last three decades has included the prompt administration of empiric antibacterial therapy, which resulted in a reduction in mortality. Challenges remain the administration of the most appropriate empiric treatment regimen adapted to evolving and changing epidemiology of infections in neutropenic patients and resistance rates; the development of markers of early diagnosis of severe bacterial or fungal infections; the risk stratification of patients; the establishment of targeted empiric (preemptive) antifungal therapy criteria; and the containment of antimicrobial resistance that compromises effective treatment efforts, through effective antibiotic policies and implementation of infection control measures, especially hand hygiene. The need for targeted antimicrobial or antifungal prophylaxis and supportive strategies like the use of growth factors awaits further clarification.

## Fever of Unknown Origin in the Returning Traveler
Cristian Speil, Adnan Mushtaq, Alys Adamski, and Nancy Khardori

The returning traveler with fever presents a diagnostic challenge for the health care provider. When evaluating such a patient, the highest priority should be given to diseases that are potentially fatal or may represent public health threats. A good history is paramount and needs to include destination, time and duration of travel, type of activity, onset of fever in relation to travel, associated comorbidities, and any associated symptoms. Pretravel immunizations and chemoprophylaxis may alter the natural course of disease and should be inquired about specifically. The fever pattern, presence of a rash or eschar, organomegaly, or neurologic findings are helpful physical findings. Laboratory abnormalities are nonspecific but when corroborated with clinical and epidemiologic data may offer a clue to diagnosis.

## Fever of Unknown Origin in Rheumatic Diseases
Thierry Zenone

Noninfectious inflammatory diseases (connective tissue diseases, vasculitis syndromes, granulomatous diseases) emerged as the most frequent cause of fever of unknown origin in western countries. Among these diseases, giant cell arteritis and polymyalgia rheumatica are the most frequent specific diagnosis in the elderly and adult-onset Still's disease the most frequent in younger patients. This article focuses on noninfectious inflammatory diseases as a cause of classic fever of unknown origin (mainly rheumatic diseases, such as vasculitis and connective tissue diseases).

The causes of fevers of unknown origin (FUOs) are diverse and may be the result of infectious rheumatic or inflammatory, neoplastic, or miscellaneous disorders. This article reviews the focused diagnostic approach to FUOs, emphasizing relevant history, physical examination, and selected laboratory tests using a clinical syndrome approach. Laboratory tests should be guided by the most likely diagnoses based on the presenting clinical syndrome. Considered in concert, nonspecific laboratory tests may provide important diagnostic clues. Using a sequential diagnostic approach, a focused evaluation diagnoses all but the rarest or most obscure causes of FUO.

Recurrent fever of unknown origin is mostly caused by rather rare diseases and many cases remain unexplained. The very limited literature data do not allow one to construct a diagnostic algorithm. A number of general principles should be kept in mind before starting the investigation for this rare subtype of fever of unknown origin.

Empiric therapy has little or no role to play in cases of classic fever of unknown origin with three important exceptions: cases that meet criteria for culture-negative endocarditis; cases in which findings or the clinical setting suggests cryptic disseminated tuberculosis (or, occasionally, other granulomatous infections); and cases in which temporal arteritis with vision loss is suspected. Several studies indicate that patients with prolonged, undiagnosed fever of unknown origin generally have a favorable prognosis. A small and largely anecdotal literature suggests a small role for symptomatic use of corticosteroids or nonsteroidal anti-inflammatory agents in highly selected cases.

# FORTHCOMING ISSUES

# RECENT ISSUES

## The Clinics are now available online!

Access your subscription at:
**www.theclinics.com**

INFECTIOUS
DISEASE CLINICS
OF NORTH AMERICA

Infect Dis Clin N Am 21 (2007) xiii–xv

# Preface

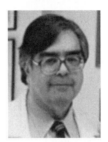

Burke A. Cunha, MD, MACP
*Guest Editor*

The hallmark of a master clinician is his or her diagnostic approach to fever of unknown origin (FUO). By definition, FUOs are undiagnosed and prolonged fevers with an unusually broad differential diagnosis that demands a focused diagnostic approach. FUOs represent one of the most common diagnostic problems encountered by physicians. Once the cause of the FUO is determined, it is relatively straightforward to determine appropriate therapy. Because infectious disease clinicians routinely assess a wide variety of infectious and noninfectious disorders, we are the most experienced in the focused diagnostic approach to FUO patients, although we routinely deal with acute fevers, which are diagnosed more readily than prolonged fevers.

The febrile response in humans to various microorganisms, and noninfectious disorders, remains intriguing and unexplained. The temperature range expressed by the majority of microorganisms is between 102°F and 106°F. This relatively narrow range orchestrates and optimizes the host's febrile response to microorganisms. Temperatures above 106°F are rarely, if ever, associated with an infectious etiology. Most noninfectious febrile disorders are associated with temperatures of 102°F or less. As with acute fevers, FUOs are caused by noninfectious and infectious disorders that have a range of febrile response. Most causes of noninfectious and infectious FUOs present with temperatures of 102°F or less (eg, subacute bacterial endocarditis). Relatively few causes of FUOs have temperatures greater than 102°F (eg, abscesses, lymphomas).

0891-5520/07/$ - see front matter © 2007 Elsevier Inc. All rights reserved.
doi:10.1016/j.idc.2007.08.012                                    *id.theclinics.com*

Prolonged and unexplained fevers have been a diagnostic problem since antiquity. In ancient Greece and Rome, clinicians appreciated differences between infectious fevers. In antiquity, physicians had only fever patterns to distinguish febrile disorders. Over time, fever patterns have been helpful diagnostically in several infectious diseases. It is not surprising that most infectious and noninfectious FUOs are associated with low-grade fevers (102°F or less). Temperatures greater than 102°F receive more diagnostic attention than easily overlooked, prolonged, and perplexing low-grade fevers of 102°F or less.

This issue of *Infectious Disease Clinics of North America* is devoted to the important topic of FUOs. Throughout the issue, the emphasis is on the diagnostic approach. The articles were written by experts in their respective fields. "Prolonged and Perplexing Fevers in Antiquity: Malaria and Typhoid Fever" was written by Cheston Cunha. His article includes translations from the original ancient Greek and Latin descriptions of malaria and typhoid fever. I contributed "Clinical Overview of Classic and Current Concepts" and an article on the focused diagnostic approach to FUOs.

Physical findings remain important in the diagnostic approach to FUOs, and Drs. Smith and Tolia from Newark, New Jersey reviewed this topic. FUO is common in elderly patients, and Drs. Yoshikawa and Norman from Los Angeles, California contributed the article on FUOs in the elderly. Given the rate of international travel today, physicians frequently encounter FUOs in returning travelers. This interesting article was written by Drs. Khardori and Speil from Springfield, Illinois. Drs. Lotholary and Hot from Paris, France wrote the in-depth article on FUOs in patients who have HIV.

Over the past decades, there has been an increase in rheumatic inflammatory FUOs. This key article was written by Dr. Zenone from Valence, France. Organ transplants are common, and various opportunistic infections in transplant patients have the potential to present as FUOs. Dr. Bouza from Madrid, Spain comprehensively reviewed FUO in transplant patients. Patients who have febrile neutropenia have always been a diagnostic challenge, and FUOs remain a difficult diagnostic problem in this patient population. The excellent overview of FUOs in febrile neutropenia was contributed by Drs. Giamarellou and Antoniadou from Athens, Greece. Drs. Raoult and Botelho-Nevers of Marseilles, France, internationally known for expertise in rickettsial diseases, have written the article on the rickettsial causes of FUOs. A comprehensive review of zoonoses and FUOs was contributed by Dr. Cleri from Trenton, New Jersey, who is an authority in this area. Tuberculosis remains an important cause of FUO. This article was ably written by Drs. Schlossberg and Bofinger from Philadelphia, Pennsylvania. Dr. Knockaert from Leuven, Belgium, who has contributed extensively to the FUO literature, reports on his experiences with recurrent FUOs.

Fevers of unknown origin remain, on the whole, a diagnostic problem. Most patients who have FUOs are diagnosed and then treated. However, empiric therapy for certain FUOs is important. Drs. Bryan and Ahuja from Columbia, South Carolina review this important topic to conclude this issue on FUOs.

This issue of *Infectious Disease Clinics of North America* should serve as a companion volume to an earlier (March 1996) *Infectious Disease Clinics of North America* issue entitled "Fever". This FUO issue is a reference source that is both current and clinically relevant for infectious disease consultants, who are faced daily with the continuing diagnostic challenge of FUOs.

Burke A. Cunha, MD, MACP
*Infectious Disease Division*
*Winthrop-University Hospital*
*259 First Street*
*Mineola, Long Island, NY 11501, USA*
*and*
*State University of New York School of Medicine*
*Stony Brook, NY, USA*

## Suggested Readings

Brusch JL, Weinstein L. Fever of unknown origin. Med Clin North Am 1998;72:1247–61.

Cabot R. Differential diagnosis. Philadelphia: W.B. Saunders; 1911.

Cunha BA. Fever of unknown origin. In: Gorbach SL, Bartlett JG, Blacklow NE, editors. Infectious Diseases. 3rd edition. Philadelphia: Lippincott Williams & Wilkins; 2004. p. 1568–77.

Cunha BA, editor. Fever of unknown origin (FUO). New York: Informa Healthcare; 2007.

Keefer CS, Leard SE. Prolonged and perplexing fevers. Boston: Little Brown & Co; 1955.

Louria DB. Fever of unknown etiology. Del Med J 1971;43:343–8.

FUO. Fever of undetermined origin. In: Murray HW, editor. Mount Kisco: Futura Publishing; 1983.

Petersdorf RG, Beeson PB. Fever of unexplained origin: report on 100 cases. Medicine 1961;40: 1–30.

Tumulty PA. Topics in clinical medicine. The patient with fever of undetermined origin. John Hopkins Med J 1967;120:95–106.

Weinstein L. Clinically benign fever of unknown origin: a personal retrospective. Rev Infect Dis 1985;7:692–9.

Wolf SM, Fauci AS, Dale DC. Unusual etiologies of fever and their evaluation. Annual Rev Med 1975;26:277–81.

ELSEVIER
SAUNDERS

Infect Dis Clin N Am 21 (2007) 857–866

INFECTIOUS
DISEASE CLINICS
OF NORTH AMERICA

# Prolonged and Perplexing Fevers in Antiquity: Malaria and Typhoid Fever

### Cheston B. Cunha

*Pennsylvania State University College of Medicine, Pennsylvania, USA*

If fever afflicts a person and then it releases him and then, on the third day, it afflicts him and pursues him, he continually has burning fever, severe fever, and lots of sweat, his illness has been prolonged and has knocked him down...

–Babylonian medical text.

Fever of unknown origin is a topic that has enduring interest to physicians. The sheer variety of potential etiologies can make it difficult to differentiate a primary cause (eg, infection, tumor, and so forth). Even today, with the great panoply of powerful diagnostic tools at a physician's disposal, fever of unknown origin can prove to be a challenging medical puzzle. Although this is often the case with the modern clinician, it was even more so with physicians of the Classical world. Within the overarching theme of fever of unknown origin, the prolonged fevers of infectious etiology must have been of particular concern to the ancient physician.

As texts of the period reveal, infection was widespread throughout the ancient world; but most of these diseases leave telltale signs of their identity. For example, the classic exanthems, such as smallpox, a likely cause of the second and third century AD Antonine plague, ran a relatively short course, displayed a characteristic set of signs and symptoms, and then resulted in death or complete recovery. Similarly, infection by an organism like *Bacillus anthracis*, which is well described in Virgil's Georgics Book III, was easily recognized by ancient physicians. Other diseases, such as measles, endemic typhus, or bubonic plague, the disease responsible for the Justiniac plague of the sixth century AD, elicited specific identifiable symptoms that eventually resolved with cure or death. Malaria or typhoid fever, however, could have presented as a prolonged fever, lasting several weeks or more, with

---

*E-mail address:* ccunha@hmc.psu.edu

few other distinguishing features to the ancient physician. Undoubtedly other conditions, such as occult malignancy, syphilis, and tuberculosis, were responsible for many of these fevers; nevertheless, this study of prolonged fever in antiquity focuses on malaria and typhoid fever as primary infectious causes [1,2].

Although the best way to obtain a definitive diagnosis of an ancient disease is by genetic analysis of surviving tissue, this is not always possible. The difficulty inherent to obtaining such samples from victims of ancient plagues often makes it impossible to use the technique of paleomicrobiology to determine the cause of ancient infection. It is frequently necessary to study literary descriptions of the disease written by the eminent physicians of the era to investigate the pandemics of the ancient world. Indeed, these descriptions are the most available and helpful to the modern investigator. The ancient physicians' lack of diagnostic and therapeutic tools made them keen observers of the natural course of the diseases they encountered, a fact that works in the modern investigator's favor when studying the ancient plagues. Essentially having only a history or present illness on which to base a diagnosis, the modern clinician can sharpen their diagnostic skills by attempting to identify these ancient plagues. Despite this often being the best evidence available, however, working with these sorts of documents can prove difficult. The difficulties encountered when translating any foreign text are compounded by the fact that so many words in the Classical languages have a variety of meanings. Additionally, because of the precision required for medical descriptions, words or phrases that are interpreted in ways other than what the original author intended can skew a description toward or away from an accurate diagnosis [3].

## Malaria

> He must not go into the lowlands by the river or an infectious disease will infect him.
>
> –Babylonian medical text

Malaria, caused by the *Plasmodium* organism, has affected humans since ancient times. Originally evolving in Africa, it was only a matter of time before the parasite made its way to the temperate climate of the Mediterranean to plague the early civilizations of that region. Carried by the *Anopheles* mosquito, the malarial parasite is transmitted to humans by the bite of the female mosquito. Breeding in standing water, malaria was of particular concern in areas with a high concentration of swamps and marshes and demonstrates an increased incidence during the warmer, wet seasons of the year. Once the human host is infected, the organism replicates during an asymptomatic period of 1 to 2 weeks inside the host's liver before entering the bloodstream. Once in the blood, the parasite infects the red blood cells and as a result of the destruction of blood cells, an intense febrile reaction occurs. Characteristically, patients with malarial infection note alternating periods of fever and chills along with periods of profuse sweating, particularly during the night. This can continue, depending on the species of malaria and the health of the host, for several weeks or even months.

Of the many species of malarial parasites that infect humans, it is important to differentiate them based on the locations in which they are typically endemic. *Plasmodium ovale* is seen almost exclusively in West Africa, whereas *Plasmodium falciparum*, *Plasmodium vivax*, and *Plasmodium malariae* all are principally found in the Mediterranean. It is these last three species of malaria that were of eminent concern to the ancient Greek, Roman, and Near Eastern cultures. Infection involving *P malariae*, the least malignant, but most chronic of the malarial species, produces fever peaks every 72 hours (a quartan fever) and would have presented as a prolonged fever. Although death from this form of malaria is uncommon, fatal nephrotic syndrome, characterized by extreme edema, can develop in some cases. *P vivax* is another relatively benign species of malaria, producing fevers peaking every 48 hours, causing it to be labeled a "benign tertian fever." The disease course associated with *P vivax* commonly lasts for several months and is often complicated by relapse following apparent cure, making it a frequent cause of prolonged fevers in antiquity. The more virulent form, *P falciparum*, is characterized by a tertian fever, occurring every 48 hours for a period of weeks to months. This form has the potential to cause severe complications, such as renal failure (known as "blackwater fever"); cerebral malaria; and potentially death. It is important to note that although primary infection with *P falciparum* frequently causes the characteristic tertian fever, a low-grade fever can persist between peaks in a subtertian fashion. Additionally, concurrent infection with multiple *P falciparum* subtypes can result in daily fever peaks, mimicking other infectious causes of a quotidian fever [4,5].

Because of the nature of the disease, which leaves no specific pathognomonic findings in the remains of its victims, evidence for the historical presence of malaria lies almost exclusively in the written reports of ancient physicians. References to potential malarial infections are seen in medical texts from the Mesopotamian, Chinese, and Indian civilizations and are usually described as a period of relapsing and remitting fever that is a punishment of the gods. It is, of course, possible that these texts describe infections that can mimic the relapsing nature of malarial fever, such as *Borrelia recurrentis*, but the meticulousness of the descriptions by these ancient authors is often so precise as to leave little doubt as to malaria being the causative agent.

Mesopotamian texts describe an illness that affects those who live near marshland during the summer months. "If he is sick for six days and on the seventh he gets well, on the eighth day he is sick and on the ninth he gets well, on the tenth day he is sick and on the eleventh he gets well (and) his illness has a turn for the worse, the [*asipu*] shall not make a prognosis as to his recovery." This classic description of a tertian fever is highly suggestive of infection by either *P vivax* or *P ovale*. There are even potential descriptions of a serious complication of *P falciparum* infection, cerebral malaria. The following sections of Babylonian text suggest the potential presence of nystagmus, lethargy, confusion, seizure, and cranial nerve involvement that can characterize cerebral malaria in those afflicted by prolonged fevers [6].

> If his face seems continuously to be spinning (and) his head, his hands, and his feet tremble...
>
> If...his limbs tremble and twist
>
> If when it comes over him, his left/right eye (makes bobbing movements similar to what) a spindle (does) when it spins (and) his right/left eye is full of blood, he continually opens his mouth and he bites [his] tongue...
>
> If his right cheek is pale (and) the left one is flushed [...] gives him a piercing pain, he is not [in full] possession of his faculties and [he...] sweat [...] LU-GAL.GIR.RA afflicts him.
>
> If when it comes over him, his right hand [and] the [left] side of his face [...] he growls like a \dog, [he grinds?] his teeth, [and] his eyes jerk, LUGAL.GIR.RA afflicts him...
>
> LUGAL.GIR.RA is an associate of Nergal, the god of pestilence.

Just as the Assyrians and Babylonians before them, the Greeks too struggled with, and chronicled in their writings, the impact of malaria on their culture. Herodotus describes the annual flooding of the Nile River, which would be highly conducive to mosquito breeding. He also describes the ancient Egyptians' methods to prevent malarial infection, such as living in elevated houses and sleeping with protective netting. This was not always sufficient, however, and Egyptian mummies provide some of the rare instances where genetic testing has proved the presence of malaria in the population living around the Nile delta around 3200 BC. Even the great poet Homer references malarial infection in Book II of his *Iliad*, describing times of illness during the "dog days" of summer, a typical time for malarial infection, when Sirius rises in the night sky [5].

Brief descriptions of seasonal fevers that occur near swamps and marshes are found throughout the writings of various other Greek authors, but it is not until Hippocrates that a fully detailed description of acute malaria is documented. His description of the tertian, semitertian, and quartan fevers is found in his Epidemics, Book I [7]:

> When the paroxysms fall on even days, the crises will be on even days; and when the paroxysms fall on odd days, the crises will be on odd days. Thus the first interval of those with crises on even days is on the fourth day, the sixth day, the eighth day, the tenth day, the fourteenth day, the twentieth day, the twenty-fourth day, the thirtieth day, the fortieth day, the sixtieth day, the eightieth day, and the one hundred and twentieth day. While those with crises on odd days, the first interval is on the third day, the fifth day, the seventh day, the ninth day, the eleventh day, the seventeenth day, the twenty-first day, the twenty-seventh day, and the thirty-first day.

Furthermore, it is necessary that one know that if the crises fall on days other than those mentioned above, there will be a relapse, and this may be deadly. But it is essential to pay attention and know in which times the crises will lead to death and in which to recovery, or during which is there tendency to fair better or worse. The intervals when crises occur in irregular fevers, quartans, quintans, septans and nonans, should also be considered.

–Hippocrates, epidemics, book I, XXVI (translation by Cheston Cunha).

Other texts in the Hippocratic corpus discuss those who live in or near marshland and drink stagnant marsh water developing weight loss, obtunded bellies, and splenomegaly; symptoms that may suggest chronic malaria. These individuals were noted to suffer prolonged, relapsing fevers along with profuse sweating during the course of their disease. It is impossible to say conclusively that this could only be a sign of chronic malaria, because such conditions as schistosomiasis (bilharzia), visceral leishmaniasis (kala-azar), or other parasitic infection could also present in this fashion.

By studying these descriptions in isolation, it is not always possible truly to understand the impact malaria and other infections had on the Ancient Greeks. There are numerous instances where disease has directly impacted the course of Greek history, however, the most obvious of which was the Peloponnesian War, lasting from 431 to 404 BC. In 430 BC, the city of Athens was decimated by plague, likely caused by epidemic typhus, greatly hindering their ability to wage war, and depriving them of the great leader Pericles. As ancient authors have described, when the Athenians under Alcibiades chose to open a second front in Sicily in the summer of 413 BC, the Syracusan forces were able to confine the Athenians to marshy areas that had long been known to be rampant with prolonged fevers. It is highly likely that malaria played a key role in the eventual Athenian defeat in Sicily. These texts clearly show that not only was malaria a recognizable condition in ancient Greece, but that the disease itself had a significant impact on Greek civilization [5].

Although Greece was certainly affected by malaria, it was the Romans who truly had to contend with malaria as a constant influencing force. It was the Roman author Frontinus who first referenced the "bad air" for which malaria gets its name, in his first century AD text. Beginning with Rome's founding, malaria and other infections played a critical role in the city's history and development. Arguably, the most important factor that determines the placement of cities and the nature of their development is water. The quantity of, and proximity to, this critical element can often decide whether a city thrives or perishes. Indeed, the ancient Romans went to great lengths to ensure that ample amounts of fresh water were brought to their capital and that a sufficient distribution network was constructed to allow most, if not all, of its citizens' access to this water supply. In the 10th century BC, when settlements first appeared on the hills overlooking what would later become the forum, the land between the Capitaline and

Palatine hills and throughout areas of Rome was primarily marshland. It was only after the Etruscan king Tarquinius Priscus installed a system of drainage canals in the sixth century BC, the most notable of which was the large *Cloaca Maxima*, that the first manmade water-related structures were constructed. The Romans covered this drain during the second century BC and it remains in use to this day, feeding into the Tiber River. Until this drainage system was complete, the local population was unable to travel far from their protected houses in the, as Livy describes them, "very healthy hills" of Rome without risk of contracting a prolonged fever. Indeed, throughout Italy, areas of marsh and swampland frequently interfered with urban development, as was chronicled by many Roman authors. The author Pausanius describes one instance where the city of Myous actually had to be abandoned because of the malaria spread by mosquitoes from nearby swamps. Columella's writings advise against building houses in areas near marshes, whereas Varo describes the transmission of prolonged fevers by small insects from "unhealthy marshes." It is interesting to note that, although Varo was never actually able to make the direct connection between the mosquito vector and the disease (he and his contemporaries believed it was the air from the marshes itself that caused fever) this was the closest the Classical world would come to determining the etiology of any of the prolonged fevers [8,9].

Perhaps the clearest and most meticulous of the Roman descriptions of the prolonged fevers that affected those living near marshland in the summer and fall months is that of Celsus. His classic description, found next, from the first century AD is highly suggestive of the course of malarial infection [10].

> But quartans are simpler. The fevers begin with shivering, then a heat erupts, and then, the fever having ended, the next two days are free of it. On the fourth day it returns.
>
> However, tertian fevers surely have two types. The one type beginning and ending in the same manner as a quartan, the other with only this difference; that it allows one day to be free of it, and returns on the third. The other type is far more insidious, for it always returns on the third day, and out of forty-eight hours, thirty-six of them (although sometimes less or more) are occupied by the paroxysm. Neither does it completely halt during remission, but only takes a lighter course. This type most physicians call semitertian.
>
> Quotidians, on the other hand, are surely varied and have many parts.
>
> For some begin immediately with a heat, others with a coldness, and still others with shivering. I call it coldness when the extremities of the body are cold; I call it shivering when the entire body trembles. Again, some end with that, and a period free of symptoms follows; others end thusly, so that the fever diminishes somewhat, but nevertheless, some remnants of disease remain, until another paroxysm occurs; and some often have no remission, and continue on. I say again, some have an intense fever, others a more tolerable one: some are the same everyday, other are different and, alternating,

the fever is milder one day, more severe the next. Some return at the same time the next day, others either later or sooner; some take a day and a night to have paroxysm and remission, some take less time, others more. Some, when they remit, cause a sweat, others do not; and from the sweat some are free of their disease, but in others the body is only made weaker by it. And the paroxysms sometimes occur only once during a single day, sometimes two or more times. Thus it often happens that everyday there are multiple paroxysms and remissions, as though each of the two answers its predecessor.

> –Celsus, de medicina, liber III (translation by Cheston Cunha).

Additionally, the great physician Galen clearly describes the characteristic fevers of malaria in many of his writings. Stating that Rome and the area surrounding it demonstrated a high prevalence of prolonged fever, he noted that, in some cases, these episodic fevers would resolve and return repeatedly for as many as 2 years, ultimately resulting in nephrotic syndrome and death. Other Roman authors provide very detailed descriptions of individual cases of malarial infection, the most notable of which is Cicero's writing concerning the infection of Atticus. He chronicles the course of the disease from the original high fever in the fall, through periods of recurrence after intervals when Atticus was free of fever, ultimately resulting in complete resolution after many months. Martial also provides a somewhat briefer example of epistle writings involving what is almost certainly malaria [5,11].

> But, Maximus, nothing more scandalous was ever done by Carus than his dying of fever, for it too committed an outrage. The cruel, deadly fever should have, at least, been a quartan! At least that disease should have been reserved for its own physician. (Carus was a physician who specialized in the diagnosis and treatment of quartan fevers)
> –Martial, epigrams X LXXVII.
> For his old friend, Maro, sick with a severe, burning, semi-tertian fever, vowed, and he did this aloud, that if the sick man were not sent down to the Stygian shades, a victim, welcome to mighty Jove, should die. The physicians begin to promise a definite recovery. Maro now makes vows not to pay his vow.
> –Martial, epigrams X XII XC (translation and parenthetical by Cheston Cunha).

The historical impact of malaria on ancient Roman civilization is not completely understood but is potentially underestimated. Although efforts to drain marshland and provide freshwater to cities and towns were largely successful, much of the Roman and Mediterranean region continued to be plagued by malaria well into the medieval and Renaissance periods. This ultimately meant that much of the Roman population constantly had to deal with chronic malarial infection. There are reports from ancient writers that Julius Caesar, while on campaign against Pompey, contracted a quartan fever for a time from which he recovered fully. Although other infections, such as bubonic plague or smallpox, inflicted enormous damage on the Roman Empire during the Antonine and Justiniac plagues, the constant presence of prolonged fevers of malarial infection must have been a force acting against Roman society.

## Typhoid fever

> If [setu] burns him and sometimes he is hot, sometimes he is cold, he has [li'bu] but he does not have a sweat, that person has been sick for a month...
>
> –Babylonian medical text.

Typhoid fever, caused by the organism *Salmonella typhi*, is the other potentially undiagnosed, prolonged fever that affected the classical world. Because of its nature, it is often difficult to differentiate from malaria using history alone as a diagnostic tool. Indeed, until Sir William Osler analyzed the precise fever patterns of each disease, malaria and typhoid fever were often misdiagnosed as one another or as a combined entity. Although certain cardinal features stand out in each disease (eg, chills are nearly always present in malaria, but are rare in typhoid) it is, nevertheless, often difficult to distinguish between the two, particularly when using ancient texts as a primary source, which may not include findings helpful to a clinician in discriminating between the two diseases [12].

There is relatively few classical descriptions that can be specifically ascribed to typhoid fever. Indeed, without precise ways of measuring the exact temperatures of patients, ancient physicians may not have been aware of the classic stepwise progression of fever so characteristic of typhoid. Instead, typhoid would likely present to them as an insidious, prolonged fever, very similar in nature to the daily fevers seen with some malarial infections. Only in cases where a distinguishing feature presents itself, such as the intestinal bleeding or peritonitis of typhoid, is it possible to differentiate the ancient descriptions of persistent, lingering fever. In several sources, Babylonian medical writings allude to potential typhoid infection with intestinal bleeding. "If he has been sick for a long time and red liquid flows from his anus, his illness will let up. He burns with fever, he will get well. His days will be long..." [6].

It has been suggested that Alexander the Great ultimately died as a result of infection from typhoid fever, and this remains one of the great historical and medical mysteries. The descriptions of Alexander's last days, provided by Arrian and Plutarch, are fairly detailed, and clearly indicate a prolonged fever was responsible for Alexander's death, but, unfortunately, they do not provide an obvious diagnosis. Depending on how certain elements of the description are translated, a diagnosis of malaria or typhoid could be supported. Immediately after returning to Babylon in 324 BC, Alexander decided to inspect the swampy marshland surrounding the city, despite the advice of seers and priests to stay out of Babylon. It is likely that at this point he became infected with the organism (either typhoid or malaria) that was endemic to the swamps of Mesopotamia, and which ultimately killed him. Several days later, as the royal diaries relate, he became severely ill [13]:

On the 29th May he slept in the bathroom because he was feverish. Next day, after taking a bath, he moved into the bedchamber and spent the day playing dice with Medius. He took a bath late in the evening, offered sacrifice to the gods, dined, and remained feverish throughout the night. On the 31st of May, he again bathed and sacrificed as usual and while he was lying down in the bathroom he was entertained by listening to Nearchus' account of his voyage and his exploration of the great sea. On June 1st, the fever grew more intense: He had a bad night and all through the next day his fever was very high. He had his bed moved and lay in it by the side of the great plunge bath; there he discussed with his commanders the vacant posts in the army and how to fill them with top caliber officers. On the 4th of June his fever was still worse and he had to be turned on his side to perform the sacrifice. He then gave orders to his senior commanders to spend the night outside. On June 5th he was moved to the palace on the other side of the Euphrates, and there slept a little, but the fever did not abate. When his commanders entered the room he was speechless and remained so through June 6th. The Macedonians now believed he was dead and crowded the doors of the palace; they began to shout and threaten the Companions, who at length were forced to let them in. When the doors had been thrown open they all slowly filed past his bedside one by one, wearing neither cloak nor armor. Nothing could keep them from seeing him one last time and they were moved, in almost every heart was grief and a sort of helpless bewilderment at the thought of losing their king. Lying speechless as the men filed by, he struggled to raise his head, and in his eye there was a look of recognition for each individual as he passed. Python and Seleucus were sent to the temple of Serapis to ask whether Alexander should be moved there. The god replied that they should leave him where he was. On the 28th day of the month of Daisios (10 June, 323 BC) toward evening he died. Alexander was not yet thirty-three.

Based on this description, it seems as though the fever afflicting Alexander was constant and gradually increased in intensity over the initial few days after the onset of symptoms. The characteristic sweats and chills of malaria are not mentioned in this account, suggesting typhoid as the likely cause. Later in his disease, it is quite possible that Alexander entered a "typhoid state" manifested by his apathetic appearance. Indeed, the only element of typhoid fever that seems to be lacking from this description is the characteristic intestinal symptoms. As such, it is highly likely that the chronicle of Alexander's final days is actually one of the few specific descriptions of the course of typhoid fever in the Classical world.

The impact of Alexander's death from typhoid fever cannot be understated. For those who believe, as the ancients did, that great individuals shape history, the death of Alexander from an unknown fever demonstrates than an infectious disease shaped the history of humankind. Although it is impossible to predict what might have happened had Alexander lived past 33 years, it is certain that his death, at the height of his power, allowed the collapse of one of the greatest, unifying empires the world has ever seen. It is for this reason that the prolonged fevers of antiquity have incredible significance and enduring interest.

## Summary

It can be said that infectious diseases have shaped the way the world has developed. Particularly in the Classical world, infection has influenced the creation of empires and wars, and has contributed to the fall of some of the greatest dynasties in human history. As many texts of the period reveal, the prolonged fevers, particularly those caused by malaria and typhoid fever, had a particularly powerful impact on the course of history. These diseases proved to be a constant, powerful force against which the Mesopotamians, Egyptians, Greeks, Romans, and others were forced to struggle with to thrive as cultures. The impact of malaria on the Peloponnesian War and the development of Rome, along with the death of Alexander the Great to typhoid fever, illustrate the importance of examining these ancient fevers of unknown origin.

## References

[1] Cunha CB, Cunha BA. The great plagues of the past: remaining questions. In: Drancourt M, Raoult D, editors. Paleomicrobiology: past human infections. New York: Elsevier; 2007.
[2] Cunha CB. Anthrax: ancient plague, persistent problem. Infect Dis Pract 1999;23(4):35–9.
[3] Cunha CB, Cunha BA. Impact of plague on human history. Infect Dis Clin North Am 2006; 20:253–72.
[4] Warrell DA, Gilles HM. Essential malariology. 4th edition. New York: Arnold Publishing; 2002.
[5] Retief F, Cilliers L. Malaria in Graeco-Roman times. Acta Cl 2004;XLVII:127–9.
[6] Scurlock J, Anderson BR. Diagnoses in Assyrian and Babylonian medicine. Chicago: University of Illinois Press; 2005. p. 38.
[7] Hippocrates, epidemics, book I, XXVI Loeb Classical Library. Harvard University Press; 1995.
[8] Aicher PJ. Guide to the aqueducts of ancient Rome. Wauconda (IL): Bolchazy-Charducci Publishers, Inc; 1995.
[9] Sallares R. Malaria and Rome. New York: Oxford University Press; 2002. p. 200–4.
[10] Celsus, De Medicina, Liber III. Loeb Classical Library. Harvard University Press; 1997.
[11] Martial, Epigrams. Loeb Classical Library. Harvard University Press; 1997.
[12] Christie AB. Infectious diseases: epidemiology and clinical practice. Edinburgh (Scotland): Churchill Livingsone; 1987. p. 100–6.
[13] Cunha BA. The death of Alexander the Great: malaria or typhoid fever? Infect Dis Clin North Am 2004;18:53–63.

ELSEVIER
SAUNDERS

INFECTIOUS
DISEASE CLINICS
OF NORTH AMERICA

Infect Dis Clin N Am 21 (2007) 867–915

# Fever of Unknown Origin: Clinical Overview of Classic and Current Concepts

## Burke A. Cunha, MD, MACP[a,b,*]

[a]Infectious Disease Division, Winthrop-University Hospital, 259 First Street, Mineola,
Long Island, NY 11501, USA
[b]State University of New York School of Medicine, Stony Brook, NY, USA

One of the problems most frequently encountered in medical practice is the diagnosis of prolonged fever, with or without local signs of disease. This problem perplexes both the physician and the patient, and it has not become less important.

Chester S. Keefer, MD

Relatively few infectious diseases have the potential to cause prolonged fevers; nevertheless, prolonged and perplexing fevers have been a diagnostic challenge from antiquity. Infectious diseases that are acute, are easily diagnosed, or have localizing signs rarely remain undiagnosed over time. Typhoid fever and malaria are examples of infections that have few localizing signs and have been diagnostic difficulties through the ages [1,2]. Because malaria and typhoid fever have some features in common, some physicians in the past used "typhomalaria" as a diagnosis, which testified to their diagnostic confusion. Osler clearly differentiated malaria from typhoid fever primarily based on their different fever patterns, which remain an important differential diagnostic point to this day [1].

Keefer was the first clinician to systematically describe the diagnostic features of disorders associated with undiagnosed prolonged fevers in his classic 1955 text [2]. In 1961, Petersdorf and Beeson [3] defined fever of unknown origin (FUO) as fever lasting 3 or more weeks with temperatures at or above 101°F (38.3°C) that remained undiagnosed after a week of intensive hospital testing. Their landmark publication described the

* Infectious Disease Division, Winthrop-University Hospital, 259 First Street, Mineola, Long Island, NY 11501.

0891-5520/07/$ - see front matter © 2007 Elsevier Inc. All rights reserved.
doi:10.1016/j.idc.2007.09.002
*id.theclinics.com*

four etiologic categories of FUO: infectious, rheumatic/inflammatory, neoplastic, and miscellaneous disorders. At the time of their 1961 publication
[3], the single most frequent cause of FUOs was infectious diseases.
Decades later, Petersdorf again reviewed FUOs and found that the relative distribution among each of the four etiologic FUO categories had
changed. By the 1980s, infectious and rheumatic diseases had decreased
and neoplastic causes of FUO had increased [4]. Petersdorf described
the criteria for classic FUOs in his initial description and subsequent review [3,4].

Over the past years, the diagnostic criteria for FUO have been modified
somewhat, reflecting the changes in diagnostic modalities available. Currently, many infectious disease physicians define an FUO as fever at or
above 101°F (38.3°C) for 3 weeks or more that remains undiagnosed after
3 days of in-hospital testing or during two or more outpatient visits.
Recently, it has been suggested that an FUO should be defined according
to time-based criteria as well as diagnostic testing intensity.

Although FUOs remain one of the most common and difficult diagnostic
problems faced daily by clinicians, only three books have been devoted
entirely to FUOs: *Prolonged and perplexing fevers* [2], *Fever of unknown
origin* [5], and, most recently, *Fever of unknown origin* [6].

## Classic concepts

Fever is an important aspect of the host response to a wide variety of
infectious, rheumatic/inflammatory, neoplastic, and miscellaneous disorders. Diagnostically, the etiologies of fevers may be approached in terms
of their height, fever patterns, and duration. The potential for prolonged
fevers is limited to relatively few disorders in each of the four categories.
The potential for any disorder to elicit a prolonged febrile response is not
known. Prolonged febrile disorders have been variously termed "prolonged and perplexing fevers," "pyrexia of unknown origin," and, most
recently, "fever of unknown origin." Disorders that do not become
FUOs are those that are, in general, acute or rapidly fatal and those
with localizing signs (ie, characteristic physical or laboratory findings
that lead to an early diagnosis and fail to meet FUO timed-based diagnostic criteria) [7–18].

Often, the diagnostic significance of nonspecific laboratory abnormalities when considered together is not appreciated. Similarly, relevant historical or physical findings commonly result in failure to consider the
correct diagnosis or FUO results in a "shotgun approach" to the FUO
workup. In general, the longer an FUO remains undiagnosed, the more
likely it is to have a noninfectious basis. Other disorders likely to present
as FUOs are those with unusual clinical findings that are not recognized
by the physician. Infections readily appreciated in endemic areas may not

be recognized when they present as FUOs in nonendemic areas (Table 1) [2,5,8,11,18].

## Clinical categories

For diagnostic purposes, FUOs may be conveniently grouped into four separate categories: infectious, rheumatic/inflammatory, neoplastic, and miscellaneous disorders. The clinical presentation should suggest whether the disorder is infectious, rheumatic/inflammatory, or neoplastic. Disorders that do not fit into these three categories should be considered miscellaneous FUO disorders [2,5,15].

FUOs, by definition, are disorders with prolonged undiagnosed fevers. This term should not be applied loosely to acute undiagnosed fevers [19]. With FUOs, the dominant clinical presentation should suggest the diagnostic category. For example, fatigue may be a feature of infection, rheumatic/inflammatory, or neoplastic disorders and, taken alone, is unhelpful. However, if fatigue is combined with weight loss, an infectious or neoplastic etiology is more likely. A neoplastic FUO etiology is favored if the weight loss is accompanied by a dramatic, sustained loss of appetite. A rheumatic/inflammatory etiology of FUO is likely if the clinical presentation is dominated by prominent arthralgias/myalgias in addition to fever and fatigue.

Details from the history, physical examination, and initial nonspecific laboratory tests narrow diagnostic possibilities. FUO-relevant findings in the history, physical examination, and initial nonspecific laboratory tests should direct the diagnostic process. From the initial history, physical examination, and nonspecific laboratory tests, it is usually possible to eliminate many disorders from further diagnostic considerations. The shotgun approach to diagnostic testing should be avoided. It is no substitute for a focused FUO laboratory test battery directed by the predominant signs/symptoms of the clinical presentation [2,5,6]. The FUO diagnostic workup should be relevant and focused rather than irrelevant.

Table 1
Disorders with prolonged and perplexing fevers

| Disorders not usually presenting as FUOs | Potential to present as FUOs |
| --- | --- |
| Acute or self-limiting disorders | Any disorder with prolonged fevers |
| Fulminant or rapidly fatal disorders | not easily diagnosed |
| Disorders with localizing signs that | Travel-related/tropical infections with |
| suggest the diagnosis | prolonged fevers presenting |
| Readily recognizable, easily diagnosable | in nonendemic areas |
| disorders | Any relapsing or recurrent disorder with |
| | prolonged fevers |
| | Any disorder with prolonged fevers |
| | presenting with unusual clinical findings |

**Infectious diseases**

*Common causes of infectious diseases*

FUOs may be approached diagnostically on a frequency distribution basis—that is, by considering the frequency of etiologies in each category. If there are aspects of the initial FUO history, physical examination, or non-specific laboratory tests to suggest the most common diagnoses, further tests should be pursued along these lines before less common etiologies are considered.

*Endocarditis*

Subacute bacterial endocarditis (SBE) is still a common cause of FUOs, mostly because practitioners have failed to consider the diagnosis or not appreciated associated clinical findings. The diagnosis of SBE should be considered historically in a patient with a history of a heart murmur, an invasive diagnostic or surgical procedure, or dental work or periodontal disease. Patients presenting with acute bacterial endocarditis present with high fevers (ie, ≥ 102°F) and a fulminant course with a new or rapidly changing heart murmur, often with peripheral manifestations. In contrast, SBE has a more indolent course, with temperatures at or less than 102°F and a slowly changing cardiac murmur with or without accompanying peripheral manifestations, depending on the duration of SBE before diagnostic evaluation.

Heart murmur alone, of course, may be due to a variety of reasons, from anemia to calcific aortic stenosis. However, if SBE is being considered as a possible diagnosis, the essential diagnostic criteria are a heart murmur plus a continuous/prolonged bacteremia (with a high degree of blood culture positivity, ie, 3/4–4/4) owing to a known endocarditis pathogen. The likelihood of peripheral manifestations depends on the duration of SBE before clinical presentation [20–22].

SBE should not be considered in the diagnosis of an FUO if the patient does not have a heart murmur or high-grade/continuous bacteremia. "Culture-negative" SBE refers to patients who have a heart murmur and negative blood cultures but with peripheral manifestations of SBE. Transthoracic echocardiography (TTE) or transesophageal echocardiography (TEE) should be obtained only on those with a heart murmur plus a high-grade/continuous bacteremia (due to a known endocarditis pathogens) or in those with negative blood cultures with peripheral manifestations of endocarditis, true culture-negative SBE [23].

Patients with systemic lupus erythematous (SLE) may have cardiac vegetations (Libman-Sacks vegetations, eg, marantic endocarditis) that may present with a heart murmur. Alternatively, patients with a noncardiac primary neoplasm may have neoplastic cardiac vegetations (eg, atrial myxoma). Both of these entities are varieties of marantic, or nonbacterial endocarditis. Patients with a heart murmur and peripheral manifestations of SBE with negative blood cultures should have a TTE/TEE to rule out atrial myxomas [23–25].

## Intra-abdominal/pelvic abscesses

Other infectious disease etiologies that are common causes of classical FUOs include intra-abdominal/pelvic abscesses. Usually, these patients have a history of an antecedent intra-abdominal/pelvic disorder or surgical procedure, which should point to an intra-abdominal/pelvic etiology for the patient's prolonged fevers [2,5,8,11,18].

## Tuberculosis

Antecedent history or exposure to tuberculosis (TB) provides the basis for considering the possibility of miliary, renal, or TB meningitis as dictated by the clinical presentation. Miliary TB is a difficult diagnosis early when clinical signs are sparse; the course may be deceptively mild and prolonged. Extrapulmonary TB should be suspected in FUO patients with a history of a positive purified protein derivative (PPD) or TB on steroids/immunosuppressive medications [26–29].

## Typhoid fever

Typhoid fever is often missed and remains a common cause of FUOs because of its lack of localizing signs early in the clinical presentation. Patients need a travel history or a history of exposure or ingestion of contaminated food/water to have typhoid fever be considered as a potential cause of an FUO. In patients with FUO due to typhoid fever, the absence of rose spots or relative bradycardia early in the clinical presentation can make for a difficult diagnosis. Morning temperature spikes are an important clue. Later in the clinical course, relative bradycardia and splenomegaly with a normal lactate dehydrogenase (LDH) and platelet count increase the probability that the patient may have typhoid fever. Leukopenia and eosinophilia are typical of typhoid fever [1,2,5,11,18].

## Epstein-Barr virus.

In the category of common infectious causes of FUOs, unusual manifestations of Epstein-Barr virus (EBV) as well as cytomegalovirus (CMV) infectious mononucleosis need to be considered in the proper clinical context. In the elderly, EBV infectious mononucleosis may be an elusive diagnosis for several reasons. First, EBV infectious mononucleosis is thought of as a disease of young adults. When it occurs in the elderly, many physicians fail to consider this as a diagnostic possibility. Also, unlike in young adults, in the elderly, EBV infectious mononucleosis presents without prominent sore throat or cervical adenopathy. In the elderly, right upper-quadrant discomfort and slightly elevated serum transaminases are the usual clinical presentation of EBV infectious mononucleosis. Such patients are also often fatigued, so that the presentation mimics a neoplastic rather than an infectious etiology, but dramatic/profound continued loss of appetite and weight should suggest a neoplasm rather than EBV infectious mononucleosis. However, nonspecific tests may indicate a non-neoplastic etiology (ie, elevated ferritin levels are not a feature of EBV infectious mononucleosis) [30,31].

### Cytomegalovirus

CMV infectious mononucleosis may affect any age group. Often, it is not considered as a cause of FUO because most physicians consider CMV to be an opportunistic pathogen in compromised hosts rather than in normal hosts. Ferritin to consider in the diagnosis of CMV in normal and immunocompetent hosts is the most frequent presentation of CMV presenting as an FUO. As with other viruses, there are clues present from nonspecific laboratory tests that should prompt the clinician to order specific CMV serology. CMV may be suggested by the combination of leukopenia/thrombocytopenia and atypical lymphocytes. Mildly but persistently elevated serum transaminases may be the only clue to CMV normal hosts with an EBV infectious mononucleosis-like illness and negative EBV viral capsule antigen IgM titers [32,33].

### Cat scratch disease

Cat scratch disease (CSD) is being recognized more frequently than it once was and is a common cause of infectious FUOs. CSD is often in the differential diagnosis of neoplastic FUOs because regional adenopathy is prominent in the clinical presentation of CSD. Antecedent history of kitten/cat licking or scratches should alert the clinician to the possibility of regional adenopathy being due to CSD. Without an appropriate history of cat contact, toxoplasmosis or lymphoma disorders should be considered in the differential diagnosis [34,35].

### Visceral leishmaniasis (kala-azar)

Visceral leishmaniasis (kala-azar) is being seen more frequently in nonendemic areas because of international travel. Visceral leishmaniasis is an infrequent cause of FUO in endemic areas, but may be a perplexing diagnosis to clinicians unfamiliar with the clinical aspects of visceral leishmaniasis in nonendemic areas. Double quotidian fever with hepatosplenomegaly in FUO patients are key clinical findings [36,37].

### Other causes of infectious diseases

Brucellosis, Q fever, toxoplasmosis, and trichinosis are among the uncommon infectious causes of FUOs. Fungal and zoonotic infections are well represented. Brucellosis and Q fever may be particularly difficult diagnoses and should be considered when other more frequent/readily diagnosable disorders have been eliminated from consideration [2,5,6].

*Toxoplasmosis*

Toxoplasmosis presenting either as monospot negative (EBV) infectious mononucleosis or as isolated/regional adenopathy mimicking CSD or lymphoma in normal hosts are the typical toxoplasmosis FUO clinical presentations. Clinicians often fail to consider toxoplasmosis in the differential diagnosis of FUO [38,39]. Atypical lymphocytes, if present, are a clue to toxoplasmosis versus CSD or lymphoma. Toxoplasmosis is an uncommon but an important cause of FUOs in immunocompetent hosts [38,39].

*Brucellosis*

Brucellosis should be considered in a patient with an appropriate history of ingesting nonpasteurized milk or goat cheese. Because localizing findings are not present in brucellosis, the diagnosis is easily made if it is considered in view of the patient's history. Mental status changes/unusual affect may be the only clues to the diagnosis. Brucellosis should be suspected in FUOs with central nervous system (CNS) and bone involvement [40,41].

*Trichinosis*

Trichinosis presenting as an FUO may or may not be associated with eosinophilia in the peripheral smear. Trichinosis requires a previous history of exposure to or ingestion of meat containing *Trichinella* species. The initial manifestations of trichinosis (ie, conjunctival suffusion, muscle tenderness, and eosinophilia) may be absent in a patient who presents with an FUO. A near-zero erythrocyte sedimentation rate (ESR) is an important diagnostic clue to trichinosis in an FUO with myositis when other findings are lacking. Trichinosis is the only infectious FUO with an ESR approaching 0 mm/h [18,42,43].

*Q fever*

Q fever requires a history of close contact with parturient cats or sheep. Without exposure to livestock, Q fever should not be considered as a diagnostic possibility. If the zoonotic connection is not made, leptospirosis may be a difficult diagnosis; Q fever may be ruled in or out by specific Q fever serology. The clue to leptospirosis is the combination of liver and renal involvement in a patient exposed to rodent urine. Leptospirosis is a biphasic illness beginning with a leptospiremic phase followed by an immune leptospiruric phase [44–46].

*Histoplasmosis*

Histoplasmosis or coccidiomycosis, particularly from endemic areas, should be considered in the differential diagnosis of FUO. Histoplasmosis resembles TB, and disseminated histoplasmosis resembles miliary TB. In FUOs, if the differential diagnosis is between histoplasmosis and TB, eosinophilia points to histoplasmosis. Usually the CNS and kidneys are spared in histoplasmosis, but liver, spleen, and bone marrow involvement are common to both disseminated TB and histoplasmosis [47,48].

### Lymphogranuloma venererum

An antecedent history of sexually transmitted diseases should raise the possibility of lymphogranuloma venereum (LGV) as a diagnostic possibility. LGV is the only sexually transmitted disease with the potential to present as an FUO. If the diagnosis is considered in FUO patients with localized/generalized adenopathy, diagnosis is easily made serologically [49,50].

### Whipple's disease

Because of its myriad clinical manifestations, Whipple's disease is difficult to diagnose. In patients with FUO, the clinical constellation of arthritis, malabsorption, and encephalopathy should suggest the possibility of Whipple's disease. Whipple's disease is a biphasic disease with fevers for weeks or months before abdominal findings [51,52].

## Rheumatic/inflammatory disorders

### Common rheumatic/inflammatory causes

Relatively few rheumatic/inflammatory disorders present as FUOs [53–55]. In the elderly, the most common rheumatic/inflammatory cause of FUOs is temporal arteritis [54]. Temporal arteritis may not be accompanied by temporal artery tenderness; prolonged fever may be the only presenting sign. Clues include otherwise unexplained dry cough, headache, jaw pain/claudication, or tongue tenderness/ulcer and night sweats with high hectic/septic fevers that may mimic an infectious FUO [56,57].

Adult Still's disease (adult juvenile rheumatoid arthritis) remains an important cause of adult FUOs [53a,54a,58]. In an FUO patient, a double quotidian fever may be a clue to adult Still's disease. Fever often precedes arthritis by weeks or months in half of cases. Adult Still's is the only rheumatic/infectious cause of FUO associated with marked leukocytosis ($>20,000/mm^3$) in the absence of infection. In elderly patients, late onset rheumatoid arthritis may present as an FUO [59].

SLE [62] may present with fever owing to flare or infection. Single, daily fever spikes are typical of SLE (without infection). Neither liver involvement nor eosinophilia is a feature of SLE. Leukopenia is the rule in SLE, but marked leukocytosis/left shift suggests superimposed infection [60].

Periarteritis nodosa (PAN) [61–64] spares the CNS but commonly involves the middle-sized vessels of the liver, mesentery, kidney, and coronary arteries. Glomerulonephritis with otherwise unexplained hypertension is a clue to the diagnosis of PAN. PAN is the only rheumatic/inflammatory infectious cause of FUOs with eosinophilia [61–64].

*Uncommon rheumatic/inflammatory causes*

Uncommon causes of rheumatic/inflammatory FUOs include Takayasu's arteritis [65–67], Kikuchi's disease [68], and familial Mediterranean fever (FMF) [69].

FMF is suggested by a recurrent serositis/episcleritis with hypophyon in FUO patients with a positive family history of FMF [69]. Takayasu's arteritis and Kikuchi's disease should be considered when symptoms are present in an FUO patient, referable to aortic arch involvement or cervical adenopathy, respectively [65–68]. The only clue to Takayasu's arteritis may be pain when lifting the arms over the head [65–67]. Both pseudogout and polyarticular gout are uncommon causes of FUO [53].

Sarcoidosis is usually an afebrile disorder. Sarcoidosis with fever is associated with uveoparotid fever (Heerfordt's syndrome), erythema nodosum, massive hepatic granulomas, or basilar meningitis [70,71]. Sarcoidosis may be accompanied by fever if complicated by infection (eg, TB). Patients with sarcoidosis presenting as FUOs usually have extensive multiorgan involvement or may have a superimposed lymphoma (ie, "sarcoidosis-lymphoma" syndrome) [72].

Among the categories of FUOs, the rheumatic/inflammatory disorders are the most likely to cause relapse or present with fevers lasting for 1 year or longer [73]. As with other categories of FUOs, the pattern of organ involvement as suggested by history, physical examination, and nonspecific laboratory abnormalities limits the differential diagnosis possibilities in most cases. Tissue biopsy is necessary to make a definitive diagnosis as Kikuchi's disease (cervical lymph node), PAN (sural nerve), or temporal arteritis (temporal artery/bone marrow) [53–55,65–68,70,71].

## Neoplastic disorders

*Lymphomas*

Among neoplastic FUOs, lymphomas—both Hodgkin's lymphoma and non-Hodgkin's lymphoma—as well as hypernephromas are the most common causes [74–78]. Hodgkin's lymphoma often presents as regional adenopathy and spreads by contiguous lymph node involvement, whereas non-Hodgkin's lymphoma is discontinuous and multifocal. Otherwise unexplained leukopenia in an elderly FUO patient should suggest lymphoma if accompanied by an elevated alkaline phosphatase level. A minority of lymphoma FUO patients may present with high-spiking fevers. Lymphoma fevers may be indolent and/or prolonged. Elevated serum ferritin levels and an increase in $\alpha_1/\alpha_2$ globulins (SPEP) may be the only clues to a lymphoma if eosinophilia and/or basophilia is not present.

### Hypernephromas

Hypernephromas (ie, renal cell carcinomas) remain an important cause of FUOs. Hypernephromas or renal cell carcinomas have been known as the "internist tumor" because of the diverse clinical manifestations of this malignancy, which may make diagnosis difficult. Most patients with hypernephromas do not present with flank masses or hematuria. Hypernephroma is one of the few malignancies that may present with high fever. A new left hydrocele in an FUO patient should suggest the diagnosis. The only clues to a hypernephroma may be an elevated gamma glutamyl transferase (GGT) or alkaline phosphatase level [79–81].

### Leukemias

Myeloproliferative disorders, particularly chronic myelogenous leukemia with blast transformation and chronic lymphatic leukemia with Richter's lymphoma transformation, are variants of these myeloproliferative disorders likely to present as FUOs [82,83]. Multiple myelomas are a recognized but uncommon cause of FUOs [84,85]. Preleukemias due to acute myelogenous leukemia not infrequently present as FUOs, with fever and sternal tenderness being the sole clinical manifestations. Preleukemia is likely if these findings are accompanied by a highly elevated serum ferritin level and/or immature red blood cells in the peripheral smear indicative of a myelophthisic process in the bone marrow [86].

### Carcinomas

Colon carcinoma, missed by most imaging techniques, is becoming more frequently recognized as a cause of FUOs, particularly in those without gastrointestinal symptoms [87]. Recently, pancreatic carcinomas have become increasingly frequent but remain an uncommon cause of FUOs. Small pancreatic carcinomas present with nonspecific symptoms (eg, mental status changes, abdominal bloating), which do not suggest a specific diagnosis. If imaging studies such as abdominal CT or MRI scans or total body gallium/indium scans are not part of the FUO workup, pancreatic carcinomas are missed [88].

### Central nervous system malignancies

Because the thermoregulatory center is located in the anterior hypothalamus, expectedly primary metastatic CNS tumors are uncommon causes of FUOs because the usual diagnostic workup does not include CT or MRI scanning of the head. These diagnostic possibilities are overlooked if no signs are present (eg, cranial nerve palsy) to suggest a CNS explanation for the patient's FUO [2,5,6,77,78].

**Miscellaneous disorders**

*Common miscellaneous disorders*

*Alcoholic cirrhosis*

It is often forgotten that the alcoholic cirrhosis is commonly accompanied by fever ($\leq 102°F$) for extended periods of time [89]. If the relationship
of low-grade fevers ($\leq 102°F$) to alcoholic cirrhosis is not appreciated, unnecessary diagnostic tests are conducted [90]. If there are signs suggesting
a hepatoma (eg, highly elevated alkaline phosphatase in a patient with
cirrhosis), the workup should be directed accordingly [89–91].

*Drug fevers*

Drug fevers are a frequently overlooked cause of FUOs. Drug fevers
should be suspected when patients are on potentially sensitizing medications, particularly sulfa-containing diuretics or stool softeners, anti-arry-
hythmics, sleep medications, pain medications, tranquilizers, antiseizure
medications, or narcotics. Antibiotics commonly associated with drug
fever include the beta-lactams (but not monobactams or carbapenems)
and the sulfa component of antimicrobials (eg, the SMX component
of TMP-SMX) [92]. It is a common misconception that the "longer
the patient is on a medication, the less likely the medication is to cause
the patient's drug fever." Instead, the opposite is true [75,93]. Some
patients develop drug fevers or drug rashes early during the course of
therapy. However, most patients who develop hypersensitive reactions
to medications have been on them for long periods of time (ie, for
months or years). The longer patients are on potentially sensitizing medications, the more likely the medication is responsible for the patient's
drug fever [75,92,93].

Patients with drug fevers have negative blood cultures, excluding contam-
inants, and look "relatively well" for their degree of fever. The cause of fever
in patients with a drug rash is readily diagnosable and does not meet the
time criteria for undiagnosed prolonged fevers. Drug fever may be a difficult
diagnosis because it does not have localizing signs, and for this reason may
present as an FUO. Patients with drug fevers may have temperatures from
100°F to 107°F, but in the FUO setting, temperature is usually at or less
than 102°F. An important clinical clue to drug fever is the presence of
relative bradycardia, which is invariably present. Clinicians must be wary
not to use relative bradycardia as a diagnostic sign in FUO patients who
are on beta blockers, diltiazem, or verapimil, or have cardiac arrhythmias
or pacemaker-induced rhythms. In such patients, pulse-temperature deficits
have no diagnostic significance.

Patients with relative bradycardia frequently have eosinophils and atypical lymphocytes in their peripheral smears. Eosinophilia is less common
than atypical lymphocytes in the peripheral smear. Atypical lymphocytes
in patients with drug fevers are present in low concentration—that is,

usually less than 5%. An elevated ESR accompanies drug fever, as do mildly/transiently elevated serum transaminase levels.

Drug fever is a diagnosis of exclusion. FUO patients with an elevated ESR, relative bradycardia, and eosinophils and/or atypical lymphocytes in the peripheral smear with mildly elevated serum transaminase levels are likely to have drug fever. The diagnosis of drug fever is confirmed by discontinuing the sensitizing medication. In the absence of rash, the temperature with drug fever will normalize or return to normal within 72 hours. There is no need to rechallenge patients with the sensitizing medication to establish the diagnosis of drug fever. Rechallenge should be avoided as it may be harmful to patients with some medications. For example, α-methyldopa may be hepatoxic, and TMP-SMX may result in Stevens-Johnson syndrome (Table 2) [75,92,93].

### Crohn's disease

Unlike ulcerative colitis, regional ileitis is a transaminal process that may present as an FUO. Crohn's disease without intestinal manifestations presenting with prolonged unexplained fever is an easily missed diagnosis. In patients with intestinal complaints, extra-interstitial findings may provide the only clues to the diagnosis (eg, episcleritis) [94].

### Subacute thyroiditis

If an antecedent history of thyroid disease/autoimmune disorders is not sought, the subtle presenting symptoms of acute thyroiditis may be missed.

Table 2
Recently described and emerging causes of fevers of unknown origin

| Patient population | Infectious causes | Noninfectious causes |
| --- | --- | --- |
| Children/young adults | Scrub typhus[a]<br>Murine typhus[a]<br>Picornavirus[b] | Antiphospholipid antibody syndrome[a] |
| Adults | Bartonella[a]<br>HIV[a]<br>Visceral leishmaniasis (kala-azar)[a]<br>Babesiosis[a]<br>Ehrlichiosis[a]<br>Melioidosis[a]<br>Chicungunya fever[b] | Pancreatic carcinoma[b]<br>Cervical carcinoma[b]<br>Antiphospholipid antibody syndrome[b] |
| Elderly | EBV<br>CMV<br>Aortitis[b] | CML (with AML blast transformation)[b]<br>CLL (with Richter's transformation)[a]<br>Rectal carcinoma[b]<br>Colon carcinoma[b] |

*Abbreviations:* AML, acute myelogenous leukemia; CLL, chronic lymphatic leukemia; CML, chronic myelogenous leukemia; CMV, cytomegalovirus; EBV, Epstein-Barr virus.
[a] Emerging cause of FUO.
[b] Recently described cause of FUO.

Subacute thyroiditis is suggested by otherwise unexplained neck/jaw angle pain in patients with a history of thyroid/autoimmune disorders [95–97].

## Uncommon miscellaneous causes

### Cyclic neutropenia

In the category of uncommon miscellaneous disorders, cyclic neutropenia is an enigmatic entity. Fevers recur with cyclic neutropenia in multiples of 7 days (usually at intervals of 21 days) and are accompanied by neutropenia (often with eosinophilia). The patient is "well" in between febrile episodes and is not neutropenic. Unless the periodicity of the fever is appreciated— that is, occurring in cycles (multiples of 7 days)—the diagnosis of cyclic neutropenia is easily missed [98].

### Pseudolymphomas

Pseudolymphomas are drug induced and usually due to diphenyl hydantoin. In the FUO setting, pseudolymphomas present in the differential diagnosis of adenopathy. The history of medications associated with pseudolymphomas is critical in suspecting the diagnosis. Obviously, lymphomas need to be ruled out before pseudolymphoma is considered as the cause of the patient's adenopathy [2,5,99].

### Factitious fevers

Factitious fevers do not occur in children or in the elderly; they occur most often in young adults. Patients presenting with factitious fever are not infrequently medical personnel. Factitious fever should be suspected in FUO patients who otherwise "look well" with relative bradycardia and have no other explanation for their fever. Usually temperature is the clue to factitious fever. Induced fevers from intravenous injections of organisms is another form of factitious fever [5,100–102].

### Rare miscellaneous causes

Schnitzler's syndrome and hyper-IgD syndrome are rare disorders that may present as FUOs. These entities should be suspected in patients on the basis of SPEP with obscure FUOs. An elevated IgM spike on SPEP is a clue to suspect Schnitzler's syndrome [103,104]. An FUO patient with an IgD spike should suggest hyper-IgD syndrome, particularly if decreased IgA is also present (Table 3) [105].

## Current concepts

### Clinical perspective

In approaching the patient with an FUO, the classic causes should first be considered. The classic infectious, rheumatic/inflammatory, and neoplastic

Table 3
Classic causes of fevers of unknown origin

| Category | Very common | Common | Uncommon |
|---|---|---|---|
| Infectious diseases | Subacute bacterial endocarditis<br>Intra-abdominal abscesses<br>Pelvic abscesses<br>Renal/perinephric abscesses<br>Typhoid/enteric fevers<br>Miliary TB<br>Renal TB<br>TB meningitis | Epstein-Barr virus mononucleosis (elderly)<br>Cytomegalovirus<br>Cat scratch disease | Toxoplasmosis<br>Brucellosis<br>Q fever<br>Leptospirosis<br>Histoplasmosis<br>Coccidioidomycosis<br>Trichinosis<br>Relapsing fever<br>Rat bite fever<br>Lymphogranuloma venereum<br>Chronic sinusitis<br>Relapsing mastoiditis<br>Subacute vertebral osteomyelitis<br>Whipple's disease |
| Rheumatic/ inflammatory disorders | Adult Still's disease (adult juvenile rheumatoid arthritis)<br>Polymyalgia rheumatica/ temporal arteritis | Late onset rheumatoid arthritis<br>Systemic lupus erythematosus<br>Periarteritis nodosa/ microscopic polyangiitis | Takayasu's arteritis<br>Kikuchi's disease<br>Polyarticular gout<br>Pseudogout<br>Familial Mediterranean fever<br>Sarcoidosis |
| Neoplastic disorders | Lymphomas (HL/NHL)<br>Hypernephromas | Hepatomas/liver metastases<br>Myeloproliferative disorders (CML/CLL)<br>Preleukemias (AML)<br>Colon carcinomas | Atrial myxomas<br>Primary/metastatic CNS tumors |
| Miscellaneous disorders | Drug fever<br>Alcoholic cirrhosis | Crohn's disease (regional enteritis)<br>Subacute thyroiditis | DVTs/pulmonary emboli (small multiple/recurrent)<br>Hypothalamic dysfunction<br>Pseudolymphomas<br>Schnitzler's syndrome<br>Hyper-IgD syndrome<br>Factitious fever |

*Abbreviations:* AML, acute myelogenous leukemia; CLL, chronic lymphatic leukemia; CML, chronic myelogenous leukemia; CNS, central nervous system; DVTs, deep vein thrombosis; HL, Hodgkin's lymphoma; NHL, non-Hodgkin's lymphoma; TB, tuberculosis.

disorders are the most common and constitute the majority of disorders responsible for FUOs.

In addition to classic causes, current causes of FUO include underappreciated or newly described entities associated with prolonged and perplexing fevers [13,106,107]. Newly emerging causes of FUOs consist of either known entities that uncommonly present as FUOs or newly described FUO disorders such as picornavirus infection in children [108]. Alternatively, disorders occurring in other than the usual peak age group for the disorder (eg, EBV infections, mononucleosis in the elderly) may present as FUOs. Virtually any emerging infectious disease, when accompanied by prolonged fevers, can present as scrub/murine typhus in children [109]. Newly described infectious diseases associated with prolonged courses of fever may present as an FUO—chikungunya fever, for example [110,111]. Because of increased international travel, entities commonly recognized and diagnosed in the endemic areas are not recognized by physicians unfamiliar with their clinical presentation in nonendemic areas (eg, meliodosis) [1,112]. Clinicians should be familiar with the emerging and newly described entities that may present as FUOs (see Table 2).

*Prolonged fevers in select populations*

*Children*

Among infectious causes of FUOs in children, viral infections such as EBV predominate. As in adults, CSD is an important cause of FUO in children because many children are in close proximity to cats. Children accompanying parents as returning travelers may present with FUOs due to malaria, typhoid fever, or TB. Common among the noninfectious causes of FUOs in children are neoplastic disorders. Age-related neoplastic disorders include Wilms' tumor, neuroblastoma, and lymphoma. Juvenile rheumatoid arthritis is the most frequently encountered rheumatic/inflammatory cause of FUO in the pediatric age group. Lastly, inflammatory bowel diseases (particularly Crohn's disease), which may be difficult to diagnose at an early stage, are not uncommon as the cause of FUOs in children [113,114].

*Organ transplants*

With organ transplants, the organ transplant pathogens should be considered in patients with fevers of prolonged duration. In transplant recipients, the severity of the associated host defense defect determines the sequence of opportunistic pathogens presenting clinically with prolonged fevers. Among the noninfectious causes of prolonged fevers in transplant recipients, neoplastic disorders secondary to immunosuppression, pulmonary emboli, and drug fevers (secondary to immunosuppressive medications) are prime considerations [115].

*HIV*

In HIV patients with prolonged fevers, infectious causes are related to the $CD_4$ count. The sequential appearance of opportunistic pathogens in HIV patients is well known. For example, an HIV patient with a microbacterial infection is more likely to be infected with *Mycobacterium tuberculosis* if he or she has a mild-to-moderately decreased count, whereas a very low count predisposes the patient to *M avium-intracellulare* late in course of HIV [116,117]. Prolonged fevers in HIV patients may be due to HIV itself or to opportunistic pathogens such as histoplasmosis, toxoplasmosis, or CMV, and in endemic areas, visceral leishmaniasis. Among HIV patients, noninfectious disorders associated with prolonged fevers include neoplasms and drug fevers secondary [116–124].

### Returning travelers

Prolonged fevers in returning travelers reflect the epidemiology of the recently visited area [125,126]. Among infectious diseases with the appropriate epidemiologic history, typhoid fever, malaria, and visceral leishmaniasis are the most common causes of prolonged unexplained fevers in returning travelers [1,5,127–129]. Among noninfectious disorders are deep venous thrombosis and/or pulmonary emboli caused by venous stasis from inactivity during long aircraft flights [130,131].

### Hospitalized patients

Hospitalized patients with prolonged fevers, if they have an explanation for their fever, are most likely to have device- or procedure-related endocarditis, central intravenous line infections, or *Clostridium difficile* colitis. Noninfectious causes of prolonged fevers in hospitalized patients include deep venous thrombosis, pulmonary emboli, and drug fevers (often due to sulfa-containing medications such as Colace) [131–134].

### Febrile neutropenia

In febrile neutropenia presenting with prolonged fevers, the physician should consider causes related to febrile neutropenia—that is, semipermanent central venous line infections (eg, Broviac or Hickman catheters). If a patient with febrile neutropenia remains febrile and has prolonged fevers after a week of antimicrobial therapy, the physician should consider, in addition to central line infections, invasive fungal infection due to either *Candida* spp. or *Aspergillus* spp. The patient with febrile neutropenia who has prolonged fevers and febrile neutropenia for over a week and develops right upper-quadrant pain with an otherwise unexplained increase in alkaline phosphate should be considered as having hepatosplenic candidiasis, a subset of disseminated/invasive candidiasis [135].

Alternatively, patients with febrile neutropenia may develop multiple small pulmonary emboli as an obscure cause of fever. Pulmonary emboli secondary to a hypercoagulable state and secondary to their underlying disorder may present with multiple small pulmonary emboli being clinically manifested as prolonged fevers [130,131].

*Elderly*

In addition to the diagnostic categories, the causes of FUO have an age distribution. For example, SBE is primarily a disease of middle-aged and elderly adults but is rare in children. To be an FUO, the disorder must be accompanied by prolonged fevers that elude diagnosis for at least 3 weeks. Implied in the clinical definition of FUO is that the cause of the FUO is not readily diagnosable from localizing signs or laboratory tests or has not been considered as a diagnostic possibility. Any disorder associated with prolonged fevers may present as an FUO if not considered in the differential diagnosis. Because of newly described entities, changes in available FUO diagnostic modalities, and international travel, a variety of infectious and noninfectious disorders are included as causes of FUOs [136–140].

## Diagnostic approach

*Clinical perspective*

Because FUOs are caused by such a wide variety of disorders, the diagnostic approach to the FUO patient is often extensive but is not focused or directed by the most likely diagnostic possibilities. A routine history and physical examination are inadequate in evaluating the FUO patient [141]. The diagnostic approach to FUO should consist of three phases. The initial FUO evaluation should include a relevant FUO history as well as a physical examination that looks particularly for diagnostic findings relevant to FUO. Initial nonspecific laboratory tests also provide clues pointing toward a particular diagnosis while simultaneously eliminating other diagnoses from further consideration. The initial evaluation should narrow diagnostic possibilities and determine the direction of the subsequent diagnostic workup. The second phase of FUO evaluation consists of a focused history, physical examination, and additional relevant nonspecific laboratory tests in patients who remain undiagnosed after the initial FUO evaluation [141,142].

Most of the FUO literature stresses the importance of a "complete history" and "comprehensive physical examination." Only rarely are physicians told what to look for or its diagnostic significance.

The focused FUO phase of diagnostic evaluation is based on a more detailed history that has FUO relevance. The FUO physical exam similarly concentrates on areas that have high diagnostic yield in FUO patients. Clinicians should be aware of the diagnostic significance of physical findings relevant to both infectious and noninfectious FUO disorders. Focused FUO laboratory testing is not specific, but is directed by the focused history and physical examination and leads to further diagnostic refinement. Lastly, the third phase of the FUO workup is the definitive diagnostic testing, which incorporates specific laboratory testing or biopsy to confirm the diagnosis [143,144].

A common error in the diagnostic approach to the FUO involves laboratory testing. All too often, undue relevance is placed on use of laboratory testing to arrive at a diagnosis. Not enough attention is paid to FUO historical details and physical examination. In FUO patients, the history and physical examination should be limited and relevant [141]. A comprehensive neurological evaluation is unhelpful in FUO patients presenting with an intra-abdominal abscess. It is a common misconception that extensive laboratory testing constitutes a thorough workup that will lead to the correct diagnosis in patients with FUO [142].

The diagnostic significance of nonspecific laboratory test abnormalities in the FUO workup is often missed if results are not considered together. Nonspecific laboratory abnormalities and clinical syndromic presentation, when taken together, may limit or eliminate various diagnoses from further diagnostic consideration and should be interpreted in the context of the FUO [143,144].

Even though subacute thyroiditis is listed as a cause of FUO in various series, it makes little sense to order tests for thyroid antibodies if a patient has no history of thyroid or autoimmune disorders or no symptoms referable to thyroiditis by history and physical examination. Such tests are needless, have no diagnostic relevance, and are a waste of health care resources. Testing should be focused and directed by the differential diagnosis suggested by the focused FUO history and physical and nonspecific laboratory tests [141–144].

Because endocarditis is a common cause of FUOs, many patients are subjected to TTE/TEE to rule out endocarditis. The diagnosis of SBE as a cause of FUO should be entertained only in patients that have a heart murmur. Blood cultures for SBE also have utility for other infections and are reasonable to obtain on most patients. The likelihood of SBE is greatest in patients with a heart murmur and in those with a high- grade/continuous bacteremia (due to a known endocarditis pathogen) with or without peripheral manifestations of SBE. All too often, TTE/TEE is ordered in patients who have a heart murmur with negative blood cultures to rule out the possibility of culture-negative endocarditis. Culture-negative endocarditis is rare to begin with and is an uncommon cause of SBE. The diagnosis of culture-negative endocarditis should be entertained in patients who have a heart murmur, negative blood cultures, *and* peripheral manifestations of SBE. TTE/TEE also may be helpful in elucidating the etiology of marantic endocarditis. Marantic endocarditis presents with a heart murmur and negative blood cultures with or without peripheral manifestations of SBE. Marantic endocarditis may be due to the vegetations associated with SBE (Liebman-Sachs vegetations) or sterile valvular vegetations secondary to a distant neoplasm [5,6,23–25].

*Initial diagnostic approach*

The physical examination relevant to potential infectious disease etiology should pay particular attention to the fundi, adenopathy, hepatic/splenic enlargement, heart murmur, and intra-abdominal or other masses [141–145]. The initial FUO history relevant to rheumatic disorders should include the patient's medical history and family medical history of rheumatic disorders, history of rheumatic/inflammatory disorders, headache/mental confusion, eye symptoms, neck or throat pain, mouth ulcers, intermittent/recurrent abdominal pain, heart murmur, myalgias and arthralgias, joint swelling, and effusion.

*Nonspecific laboratory tests*

The diagnostic significance of nonspecific tests is increased when test results are combined with clinical findings. Diagnostic specificity of non-specific laboratory abnormalities is further enhanced when considered as a group and when evaluated in the appropriate clinical context. The constellation of nonspecific laboratory testing abnormalities should prompt specific diagnostic testing to limit differential diagnostic possibilities and/or prompt testing for specific infectious diseases. Arguably, the three most underused and underappreciated tests for FUOs are the SPEP, serum alkaline phosphatase, and serum ferritin levels (Table 4) [60,146–150].

*Imaging studies*

Imaging tests have been very helpful in localizing the pathology, which in itself may suggest the diagnosis. Since infectious and noninfectious disorders have a characteristic pattern of organ involvement, positive imaging tests with CT/MRI scanning and/or gallium or indium scanning may localize the process to a single organ or may indicate multi-organ involvement and be of value in further directing the diagnostic workup. PET scans may reveal obscure abnormalities missed by other imaging techniques, such as aortitis [120,121,151–154].

**Diagnostic significance of fever patterns**

Relatively few disease entities causing FUOs have distinctive fever patterns with diagnostic significance. Nevertheless, fever patterns are especially helpful in situations in which the diagnosis is elusive and the history and physical examination are noncontributory or elusive (Table 5). In difficult cases, fever patterns may provide an important clue to the diagnosis. Fever patterns are most helpful with the most difficult diagnostic problems and should prompt the clinician to go back and re-evaluate the patient with a history, physical examination, and additional laboratory tests that are suggested by the differential diagnosis associated with a particular pattern. Fevers have a diurnal rhythm that is related to the diurnal output. When patients have a fever due to a noninfectious or infectious disorder, the temperature elevation exacerbates the normal afternoon/early evening temperature rise seen in normal individuals. Therefore, virtually all disorders

Table 4
Fevers of unknown origin: diagnostic clues from nonspecific laboratory tests

| Laboratory tests[a] | FUO: infectious causes | FUO: noninfectious causes |
|---|---|---|
| CBC | | |
| Leukopenia | Typhoid fever | SLE |
| | HIV | |
| | EBV | |
| | CMV | |
| | TB | |
| Lymphocytosis | TB | Lymphomas |
| | Toxoplasmosis | CLL |
| | EBV | |
| | CMV | |
| Atypical lymphocytes | CMV | Drug fever |
| | EBV | |
| | Malaria | |
| | Ehrlichiosis/anaplasmosis | |
| | Toxoplasmosis | |
| | Brucellosis | |
| Abnormal lymphocytes | | CLL[b] |
| Lymphopenia (relative) | Malaria | Temporal arteritis |
| | Ehrlichiosis/anaplasmosis | Sarcoidosis |
| | TB | SLE |
| | HIV | Lymphomas |
| | EBV | |
| | CMV | |
| | Whipple's disease | |
| Monocytosis | SBE | Crohn's disease |
| | TB | Sarcoidosis |
| | Histoplasmosis | LORA |
| | Visceral leishmaniasis | Neoplasms |
| | (kala-azar) | MPDs |
| | Brucellosis | SLE |
| | | Temporal arteritis |
| Eosinophilia | Trichinosis | PAN |
| | | Sarcoidosis |
| | | MPDs |
| | | Lymphoma |
| | | Drug fever |
| Basophilia | None | Neoplastic disorders |
| | | MPDs |
| Thrombocytopenia | Malaria | Neoplastic disorders |
| | Ehrlichiosis/anaplasmosis | |
| | Leptospirosis | |
| | Relapsing fever | |
| | TB | |
| | Histoplasmosis | |
| | EBV | |
| | CMV | |
| | HIV | |

(*continued on next page*)

Table 4 (*continued*)

| Laboratory tests[a] | FUO: infectious causes | FUO: noninfectious causes |
| --- | --- | --- |
| Thrombocytosis | TB | Lymphomas |
| | Osteomyelitis | Carcinomas |
| | Abscess | MPDs |
| | SBE | Temporal arteritis |
| Erythrocyte sedimentation rate | | |
| Highly elevated (> 100 mm/h) | Abscesses | Neoplastic disorders |
| | SBE | Rheumatic/inflammatory |
| | Osteomyelitis | disorders |
| | | Drug fever |
| Very low (~0 mm/h) | Trichinosis | None |
| Liver function tests | | |
| ↑ SGOT/SGPT | EBV | Drug fever |
| | CMV | Adult Still's disease |
| | Q fever | Alcoholic cirrhosis |
| | Brucellosis | |
| | Leptospirosis | |
| | Relapsing fever | |
| | Malaria | |
| | E/A | |
| | Babesiosis | |
| ↑ Alkaline phosphatase | TB | Lymphoma |
| | Histoplasmosis | Hypernephroma |
| | Liver abscess | PAN |
| | Charcot's fever | Temporal arteritis |
| | | Hepatoma |
| | | Liver metastases |
| | | Subacute thyroiditis |
| | | Adult Still's disease |
| ↑ GGT | None | Alcoholic cirrhosis |
| | | Hypernephroma |
| Serum ferritin | | |
| Highly elevated (> 2 × normal) | None | Neoplastic disorders |
| | | SLE |
| | | Adult Still's disease |
| | | Temporal arteritis |
| | | Lymphomas |
| | | CLL |
| | | CML |
| | | MPDs |
| + Cryoglobulins | SBE | SLE |
| | | LORA |
| | | CLL |
| | | Lymphomas |
| | | Crohn's disease |
| Cold agglutinins | | |
| Mild/moderately elevated titers | CMV | CLL |
| | EBV | CML |
| | Malaria | |

(*continued on next page*)

Table 4 (*continued*)

| Laboratory tests[a] | FUO: infectious causes | FUO: noninfectious causes |
|---|---|---|
| Rheumatoid factors | | |
| ↑ Rheumatoid factors | SBE | SLE |
| | | LORA |
| | | Sarcoidosis |
| | | Alcoholic cirrhosis |
| | | MPDs |
| SPEP | | |
| ↑ $\alpha_1/\alpha_2$ globulins | None | Lymphomas |
| | | SLE |
| | | MPDs |
| Monoclonal spike | None | Multiple myeloma |
| | | Hyper IgD syndrome |
| | | Schnitzler's syndrome |
| | | (IgM) |
| Polyclonal gammopathy | HIV | Sarcoidosis |
| | Malaria | Alcoholic cirrhosis |
| | LGV | MPDs |
| | | Atrial myxomas |
| LDH | | |
| ↑ LDH | Malaria | Lymphomas |
| | Babesiosis | Leukemias |
| | | MPDs |

*Abbreviations:* CBC, complete blood count; CLL, chronic lymphocytic leukemia; CML, chronic myologenous leukemia; CMV, cytomegalovirus; E/A, ehrlichiosis/anaplasmosis; EBV, Epstein-Barr virus; GGT, gamma glutamyl transferase; LDH, lactate dehydrogenase; LGV, lymphogranuloma venereum; LORA, late onset rheumatoid arthritis; MPDs, myeloproliferative disorders; PAN, periarteris nodosa; SBE, subacute bacterial endocaridits; SGOT, serum glutamic-oxaloacetic transaminase; SGPT, serum glutamic pyruvic transaminase; SLE, systemic lupus erythematosus; SPEP, serum protein electrophoresis; TB, tuberculosis.

[a] When presenting as FUOs.

[b] Abnormal nonreactive lymphocytes.

that are associated with fevers have a fever spike in the late afternoon or early evening [122,123].

## Focused diagnostic approach

### Clinical syndromic approach

Focused FUO laboratory tests add further refinement to the initial laboratory tests in limiting diagnostic possibilities. With FUO syndromic diagnosis, the pattern of organ involvement should be apparent from aspects of the history, physical examination, and laboratory tests. The pattern of organ involvement based on the focused FUO evaluation determines diagnostic possibilities for prompt and definitive diagnostic testing. The focused FUO workup should be detailed but directed as the most likely diagnosis, based on each disorder's pattern of organ involvement as determined by the focused FUO history, physical examination, and selected nonspecific laboratory tests (Table 6) [2,5,8,11,141–145].

Table 5
Diagnostic significance of fever patterns

| Fever pattern | Infectious causes | Noninfectious causes |
| --- | --- | --- |
| Morning temperature spikes | TB<br>Typhoid fever | PAN<br>Intermittent antipyretic therapy |
| Relative bradycardia | Malaria<br>Typhoid fever<br>Leptospirosis | Drug fever<br>Lymphomas<br>CNS disorders<br>β-blockers/verapamil/ diltiazem<br>Factitious fever |
| Double quotidian fevers | Miliary TB<br>Visceral leishmaniasis (kala-azar)<br>Mixed malarial infection | Intermittent antipyretic therapy<br>Adult Still's disease |
| Camel back (dromedary) fevers | Leptospirosis<br>Brucellosis<br>E/A | Intermittent antipyretic therapy |
| Relapsing fevers | Typhoid fever<br>Malaria<br>Rat bite fever (*Streptobacillus moniliformis*)<br>Relapsing fever (*Borrelia recurrentis*)<br>Whipple's disease<br>Brucellosis<br>Babesiosis<br>Bartonella<br>E/A<br>Leptospirosis<br>Q fever<br>TB<br>Histoplasmosis<br>Coccidioidomycosis<br>Visceral leishmaniasis (kala-azar)<br>Inappropriately treated infections<br>Partially treated infections | Cyclic neutropenia<br>Hyper IgD syndrome<br>Schnitzer's syndrome<br>FMF<br>SLE<br>Vasculitis<br>FAPA<br>APA |

*Abbreviations:* APA, antiphospholipid syndrome; CNS, central nervous system; E/A, ehrlichiosis/anaplasmosis; FAPA, fever, adenitis, pharyngitis, and aphthous ulcers; FMF, familial Mediterranean fever; PAN, periarteritis nodosa; SLE, systemic lupus erythematosus; TB, tuberculosis.

*Fevers of unknown origin due to infectious diseases*

After the initial and focused FUO evaluation of infectious disease causes, there are relatively few infections whose diagnosis remains elusive. These infections are not rare or difficult to diagnose, but are missed in the initial and focused FUO evaluation (eg, relapsing mastoiditis, chronic sinusitis, subacute bacterial osteomyelitis, periapical dental abscesses). These entities are readily diagnosed with appropriate imaging studies (Table 7) [10,124,142,155].

Table 6
Fevers of unknown origin: initial diagnostic approach

| FUO history | FUO physical exam | Initial laboratory tests | Focused FUO workup |
|---|---|---|---|
| History suggesting an infectious disorder: | | | |
| PMH/FMH of infections | Fever pattern | **Blood tests** | *If initial history/physical* |
| Similar illness exposure | Heart murmur | CBC | *examination and laboratory* |
| Surgical/invasive procedures | Adenopathy | LFTs | *tests suggest an infectious* |
| Recent travel (Asia, Africa, Latin America) | Splenomegaly | ESR | *disorder, proceed with* |
| Chills or night sweats | | SPEP | *a focused infectious disease* |
| Weight loss | | Blood cultures | *workup (see Table 7)* |
| Insect/rodent exposure | | **Radiology tests** | |
| Zoonotic exposure | | Chest x-ray[a] | |
| | | Abdominal CT/MRI[b] | |
| History suggesting a rheumatic disorder: | | | |
| PMH/FMH of rheumatic disorders | Fever pattern | **Blood tests** | *If initial history/physical* |
| Arthralgias/arthritis | Eye signs | CBC | *examination and laboratory* |
| Serositis | Adenopathy | LFTs | *tests suggest a rheumatic* |
| Eye symptoms | Splenomegaly | ESR | *disorder, proceed with* |
| Splenomegaly | Heart murmur | ANA | *a focused rheumatic/* |
| | Arthritis/joint effusion | RF | *inflammatory disorder* |
| | | SPEP | *workup (see Table 8)* |
| | | Ferritin levels | |
| | | **Radiology tests** | |
| | | Chest x-ray[a] | |
| | | Abdominal CT/MRI[b] | |

| History | Physical examination | Blood tests | Radiology tests | |
|---|---|---|---|---|
| History suggesting a neoplastic disorder: | | **Blood tests** | | If initial history/physical examination and laboratory tests suggest a neoplastic disorder, proceed with a focused neoplastic disorder workup (see Table 9) |
| PMH/FMH malignancy | Fever pattern | CBC | | |
| Weight loss (with ↓ appetite) | Sternal/bone tenderness | LFTs | | |
| Fatigue | Heart murmur | ESR | | |
| Night sweats | Adenopathy | SPEP | | |
| Abdominal discomfort/pain | Splenomegaly | Ferritin levels | | |
| | | | **Radiology tests** | |
| | | | Chest x-ray[a] | |
| | | | Abdominal CT/MRI[b] | |
| History suggesting a miscellaneous disorder: | | **Blood tests** | | If initial history/physical examination and laboratory tests suggest a miscellaneous disorder, proceed with a focused miscellaneous disorder workup (see Table 10) |
| Negative HPI/PMH for infectious, rheumatic, and neoplastic disorders (see above) | Fever pattern | CBC | | |
| Drugs/medications | Signs of alcoholic cirrhosis | LFTs | | |
| Alcoholism | | ESR | | |
| IBD | | SPEP | | |
| Thyroid/autoimmune disorders | | | **Radiology tests** | |
| Medical personnel | | | Abdominal CT/MRI[b] | |

*Abbreviations:* ANA, antinuclear antibody; CBC, complete blood count; ESR, erythrocyte sedimentation rate; IBD, inflammatory bowel disease; LFTs, liver function tests (SGOT, SGPT, alkaline phosphatase); RF, rheumatoid factor; SPEP, serum protein electrophoresis.

[a] If signs/symptoms referable to the chest.
[b] If signs/symptoms referable to the abdomen/pelvis.

Table 7
Focused infectious disease history and physical examination

| Focused history | Differential diagnosis | Focused physical examination | Differential diagnosis |
|---|---|---|---|
| **HPI** | | **Vital signs** | |
| Headache/mental status changes | Malaria, babesiosis, typhoid fever, Q fever, CNS, TB, HIV, brucellosis, E/A, CSD, Whipple's disease, leptospirosis | Relative bradycardia | Babesiosis, malaria, typhoid, Q fever, E/A, leptospirosis |
| Tongue pain | Relapsing fever, histoplasmosis | **HEENT** | |
| | | Premature graying/ temporal muscle wasting | HIV |
| Sore throat | Leptospirosis | Conjunctival suffusion | Relapsing fever, leptospirosis, trichinosis, E/A |
| Neck pain | Relapsing mastoiditis, subacute vertebral osteomyelitis | Roth spots | SBE |
| Prominent myalgias/ back pain | Brucellosis, SBE | Choroid tubercules | TB |
| Persistent joint pain | Whipple's disease, rat bite fever, brucellosis, LGV | Chorioretinitis | TB, toxoplasmosis, histoplasmosis |
| Thigh pain | Brucellosis | Abducens (CN VI) palsy | TB |
| Early satiety | Brucellosis, Q fever, EBV, CMV, SBE | Palatal petechiae | CMV, toxoplasmosis, EBV |
| Malabsorption symptoms | Whipple's disease | Tongue: leukoplakia, ulcer | HIV, histoplasmosis |
| **PMH** | | **Cardiovascular** | |
| Dental work/heart murmur | SBE | Heart murmur | SBE |
| Surgical/invasive procedures | SBE, abscess | **Back spine** | |
| | | Spinal tenderness | Brucellosis, subacute vertebral osteomyelitis, SBE, typhoid fever, TB |
| Infections (pulmonary, GI, GU, etc) | TB, HIV, histoplasmosis, Q fever, abscess | Trapezius tenderness | Abdominal abscess |
| Blood transfusions | HIV, CMV | Splenomegaly | SBE, TB, EBV, CMV, typhoid fever, brucellosis, relapsing fever |
| | | Hepatomegaly | Q fever, typhoid fever, brucellosis, liver abscess |

(*continued on next page*)

Table 7 (*continued*)

| Focused history | Differential diagnosis | Focused physical examination | Differential diagnosis |
|---|---|---|---|
| **Contact history** | | | |
| TB | TB, HIV, relapsing fever | Localized and/ or generalized | HIV, EBV, CMV, CDS, LGV, |
| HIV | HIV, TB, CMV | cervical/ supraclavicular, epitrochlear, axillary, inguinal adenopathy | Whipple's disease |
| Contaminated water/food | Leptospirosis, typhoid fever | **Genitourinary** Epididymo-orchitis/ epididymal nodule | EBV, TB, brucellosis, |
| IVDAs | HIV, CMV, SBE | | leptospirosis |
| **Zoonotic history** | | | |
| Insect (ticks, mites, fleas, flies, toxoplasmosis, mosquitoes, etc), exposure/bites | Visceral leishmaniasis, ehrlichiosis/ anaplasmosis, RF, malaria | | |
| Cats, dogs, birds, rodents, and the like | Bartonella, leptospirosis, Q fever | | |
| Cattle, sheep, goats, horses, and the like | RF, RBF, Q fever, brucellosis | | |
| Contaminated/ nonpasteurized milk/cheese | Q fever, brucellosis, TB | | |
| **Travel history** | | | |
| Africa, Asia, Latin America | Malaria, typhoid fever, bartonella, visceral leishmaniasis (kala-azar), TB, leptospirosis, brucellosis, Q fever | | |

*Abbreviations:* CMV, cytomegalovirus; CNS, central nervous system; CSD, cat scratch disease; E/A, ehrlichiosis/anaplasmosis; EBV, Epstein Barr virus; LGV, lymphogranuloma venereum; RF, relapsing fever; SBE, culture positive and negative causes; TB, tuberculosis.

*Fevers of unknown origin due to rheumatic/inflammatory disorders*

Physical findings relevant to rheumatic/inflammatory disorders require careful attention to the eyes, the fundi, neck, and the throat. Careful evaluation of adenopathy/splenomegaly and heart murmur is important. Clearly, joint swelling or effusion or arthritis is of paramount importance in this group (Table 8).

Table 8
Focused rheumatic/inflammatory disorder history, physical examination, and laboratory tests*

| Focused history | Differential diagnosis | Focused physical examination | Differential diagnosis | Presumptive rheumatic/inflammatory diagnosis | Focused laboratory tests |
|---|---|---|---|---|---|
| Profound depression | TA | Morning temperature spike | PAN | SLE | Relative leukopenia, lymphocytopenia, monocytosis, ↑ ferritin, DsDNA, anti-SM, ↓ $C_3$, APA, + cryoglobulins, SPEP: polyclonal gammopathy, TTE/TEE[b] |
| Headache | TA, sarcoidosis[a] | Double quotidian fever | Adult Still's disease | | |
| Transient facial edema | Takayasu's arteritis | Hectic/septic fevers | TA | | |
| Amaurosis fugax | TA, Takayasu's arteritis, SLE | Night sweats | TA | | |
| Dry eyes | Sarcoidosis | Hypertension | PAN, Takayasu's arteritis | | |
| Wet eyes | PAN | Lacrimal gland enlargement | SLE, LORA, sarcoidosis | | |
| Eye pain/symptoms | SLE, adult Still's disease, Takayasu's arteritis, TA, sarcoidosis | Conjunctivitis | Adult Still's disease, SLE, PAN, sarcoidosis | PAN | Eosinophilia, SPEP: polyclonal-gammopathy, sural nerve biopsy |
| | | | | LORA | ↑ RF, ↑ copper, ↑ CCP |
| | | | | Adult Still's disease | ↑ Ferritin |
| | | | | TA | TA biopsy |
| | | | | Takayasu's arteritis | PET scan (aorta) |
| | | | | Kikuchi's disease | Cervical node biopsy |

| Clinical clue | Diagnostic considerations | Diagnostic tests |
|---|---|---|
| Nasal stuffiness | Sarcoidosis | |
| Sore throat | SLE, adult Still's disease | |
| Jaw claudication pain | TA, Takayasu's arteritis | |
| Neck pain | Kikuchi's disease | |
| Tongue tenderness/pain | TA | |
| Dry cough | Sarcoidosis, TA | |
| Abdominal pain | SLE, adult Still's disease, PAN, FMF | |
| Conjunctival nodules | Sarcoidosis | |
| Dry eyes | Sarcoidosis | |
| Wet eyes | PAN | |
| Argyll-Robertson or Adies' pupils | Sarcoidosis | |
| Band keratopathy | Adult Still's disease, sarcoidosis | |
| Episcleritis | TA, LORA, PAN | |
| Scleritis | SLE | |
| Iritis | Adult Still's disease, SLE, sarcoidosis | |
| Uveitis | Adult Still's disease, SLE, LORA, sarcoidosis | |
| Fundi: optic neuritis with "macular star" | PAN | |
| Fundi: cytoid bodies (cotton wool spots) | SLE, TA, PAN | |
| Fundi: "candlewax drippings" | Sarcoidosis | |
| Fundi: Roth spots | SLE, PAN | |
| Fundi: central/branch retinal artery occlusion | SLE, TA, Takayasu's arteritis | |
| Fundi: central retinal vein occlusion | SLE, sarcoidosis | |
| | FMF | Colchicine trial, MEFV gene studies |
| | Sarcoidosis | Relative lymphocytopenia, eosinophilia, ↑ ACE, polyclonal, SPEP: gammopathy, ↑ urinary calcium, PFTs, ↓ $D_{L}CO$, gallium/indium scan: (Panda sign) |

(continued on next page)

Table 8 (*continued*)

| Focused history | Differential diagnosis | Focused physical examination | Differential diagnosis | Presumptive rheumatic/inflammatory diagnosis | Focused laboratory tests |
|---|---|---|---|---|---|
| | | Cranial nerve palsies (CNs III, IV, or VI) | PAN, SLE, sarcoidosis | | |
| | | Tongue ulcers | TA | | |
| | | Parotid enlargement (bilateral) | Sarcoidosis | | |
| | | Adenopathy (generalized) | SLE, LORA | | |
| | | Splenomegaly | Adult Still's disease, SLE | | |
| | | Heart murmur | SLE[b] | | |
| | | Epididymoorchitis/epididymal nodule | SLE, PAN, sarcoidosis | | |
| | | Tender fingertips | SLE | | |
| | | Arthritis/joint effusion | Adult Still's disease, SLE, LORA, FMF, sarcoidosis | | |

*Abbreviations:* ACE, angiotensin converting enzyme; anti-SM, anti-Smith antibody; APA, antiphospholipid antibody; CCP, cyclic citrillated peptide; $D_LCO$, carbon monoxide diffusing capacity; DsDNA, double-stranded DNA; FMF, familial Mediterranean fever; LORA, late onset rheumatoid arthritis; PAN, periarteritis nodosa; PFTs, pulmonary function tests; PMR, polymyalgia rheumatica; RF, rheumatoid factor; SLE, systemic lupus erythematous; SPEP, serum protein electrophoresis; TA, temporal arteritis; TTE/TEE, transthoracic echocardiography/transesophageal echocardiography.

* When presenting as an FUO.
[a] If CNS sarcoidosis.
[b] If Libman-Sacks vegetations.

*Fevers of unknown origin due to neoplastic disorders*

Important aspects of the focused FUO history for neoplastic disorders include the careful evaluation of the PMH/FMH of malignancies. Particular attention should be paid to the presence or absence of night sweats, pruritis after a hot bath or shower, and weight loss, particularly when accompanied by a dramatic decrease in appetite.

Important aspects of the physical examination include abnormalities of the cranial nerves, the eyes (including the fundi), the throat, heart murmur, adenopathy, hepatosplenomegaly, sternal tenderness, and bone tenderness (Table 9).

*Fevers of unknown origin due to miscellaneous disorders*

Miscellaneous disorders should be considered if the predominant clinical presentation does not point to an infectious, rheumatic/inflammatory, or neoplastic etiology. A relevant history for miscellaneous disorders includes medications or exposure to fumes. History of alcoholism should be included as well as thyroid/autoimmune disorders. Inquiries should be made regarding inflammatory bowel disease, particularly for extra intestinal complaints.

In patients with a history of alcoholism/cirrhosis, physical examination for miscellaneous causes should focus on the myriad manifestations. Physical examination in patients with drug fevers is notable for the absence of physical findings. An exception is pseudolymphoma due to drugs (eg, diphenylhidantoin). On physical examination, the findings related to subacute thyroiditis are related to the phase of the disease (ie, the patient is most likely to be euthyroid or slightly hypothyroid when subacute thyroiditis presents as an FUO) (Table 10).

## Sequential evaluation

*Other diagnostic tests*

A sequential (initial, focused, definitive) diagnostic approach to FUOs sequentially diagnoses or rules out causes of FUO. This three-tiered diagnostic approach leaves few FUOs undiagnosed [7,10,141–145,155–157]. The FUOs that remain undiagnosed are obscure and require special diagnostic testing (Table 11).

*Diagnostic usefulness of the Naprosyn test*

The Naprosyn (naproxen) test, which was first developed by Chang, uses Naprosyn, a nonsteroidal anti-inflammatory drug (NSAID), to differentiate neoplastic from infectious causes of fever. This test is useful to further define the diagnostic workup so that diagnostic efforts may be focused on determining a neoplastic or infectious etiology [158–160]. Naprosyn, 375 mg, is given orally every 12 hours for 3 days. Patients with infectious disorders

Table 9
Focused neoplastic disorder history, physical examination, and laboratory tests*

| Focused history | Differential diagnosis | Focused physical examination | Differential diagnosis | Presumptive neoplastic diagnosis | Focused laboratory tests |
| --- | --- | --- | --- | --- | --- |
| Headache/mental status changes | Lymphoma, CNS neoplasms, pre-leukemias (AML), CLL, CML, atrial myxomas | Relative bradycardia | Lymphomas, CNS neoplasms | Lymphomas | ↑ ferritin, ↑ calcium, ↑ copper, ↑ LDH, + Coombs test, ↑ cold agglutinins, ↑ LAP, ↑ haptoglobin, ↑ uric acid, ↑ $\alpha_1$-antitrypsin, ↓ $B_{12}$[a], ↓ folate |
| | | Cranial nerve palsies | CNS lymphomas, CNS neoplasms | | |
| | | Fundi: Roth spots | Lymphomas, atrial myxomas | | |
| Early satiety | Lymphomas, CML, CLL | Fundi: Cytoid bodies (cotton wool spots) | Atrial myxomas | | |
| Pruritus (post-hot shower/bath) | Lymphomas, CML, CLL | Fundi: retinal hemorrhages | Leukemias | Hypernephromas | ↑ GGT |
| Abdominal fullness/pain | Hepatoma, CML | Sternal tenderness | Leukemias, MPDs | Hepatomas/liver metastases | ↑ $\alpha$-fetoprotein, ↓ FBS, +HBV serology, + HCV serology, ↑ calcium, ↓ folate levels |
| | | | | CNS neoplasms | CSF: ↑ protein/+ RBCs |
| | | | | Preleukemia (AML) | ↑ LDH, ↑ ferritin, basophilia[b] |
| | | | | CML (with AML blast transformation) | ↓ LAP, ↓ LDH, ↑ uric acid, ↑$B_{12}$, + Coombs test, SPEP: ↑$\alpha$1/$\alpha$2 globulins, + Philadelphia chromosome |

| | | | |
|---|---|---|---|
| Heart murmur (marantic endocarditis) | Atrial myxomas, neoplastic vegetation (due to distant primary neoplasm) | CLL (with Richter's transformation) | ↑ LAP, + Coombs test, + cryoglobulins, ↑ $B_{12}$ level, SPEP: hypo-gammaglobulinemia, + urine immunoglobulins |
| Adenopathy | Lymphomas, CML, CLL | | SPEP: polyclonal gammopathy, TTE/TEE |
| Splenomegaly | Lymphomas, CML, CLL | Atrial myxomas | |
| Abdominal (hepatic) bruit | Hepatoma | | |
| Epididymo-orchitis/ epididymal nodule | Lymphoma | | |
| Splinter hemorrhages | Atrial myxomas | | |

*Abbreviations:* AML, acute myelogenous leukemia; CLL, chronic lymphatic leukemia; CML, chronic myelogenous leukemia; CNS, central nervous system; FBS, fasting blood sugar; FMF, familial Mediterranean fever; GGT, $\gamma$-gamma glutamyl transferase; HBV, hepatitis B virus; HCV, hepatitis C virus; LAP, leukocyte alkaline phosphatase; LDH, lactate dehydrogenase; SPEP, serum protein electrophoresis; TTE/TEE, Transthoracic echocardiography/transesophageal echocardiography.

\* When presenting as an FUO.

[a] $B_{12}$ is normal in HL, but may be decreased in NHL.

[b] May be the first sign of blast transformation in CML.

Table 10
Focused miscellaneous disorder history, physical examination, and laboratory tests*

| Focused history | Differential diagnosis | Focused physical examination | Differential diagnosis | Presumptive miscellaneous disorder diagnosis | Focused laboratory tests |
|---|---|---|---|---|---|
| On sensitizing medication | Drug fever | Relative bradycardia | Drug fever, factitious fever | Alcoholic cirrhosis | ↑ GGT, ↑ LAP, ↓ folate, SPEP: polyclonal gammopathy |
| Hypercoagulable state | DVTs/PE | Episcleritis | Crohn's disease | Crohn's disease | ↑ Ileal uptake on gallium, indium, or PET scans |
| Arthralgias/joint pain | Cyclic neutropenia, hyper-IgD syndrome, Schnitzler's syndrome | Oral ulcers ↑ | Hyper-IgD syndrome | Drug fever | D/C responsible drug |
| | | Neck/jaw angle tenderness | Subacute thyroiditis | Subacute thyroiditis | ↑ TPO, ↑ ATG |
| | | Adenopathy | Hyper-IgD syndrome | Cyclic neutropenia | Serial CBCs, (↓ WBC counts/eosinophilia during fever/attacks) |
| Sore throat | Subacute thyroiditis, hyper-IgD syndrome | Splenomegaly | Alcoholic cirrhosis, hyper-IgD syndrome | DVTs | ↑ FSPs, + LE dopplers |
| Thyroid/autoimmune disorders | Subacute thyroiditis | | | Hyper-IgD syndrome | SPEP: ↑ IgD/↓ IgA |
| Chronic alcoholism | Alcoholic cirrhosis | | | Schnitzler's syndrome | SPEP: ↑ IgM, ↑ urinary mevaconic acid/neopterin levels |
| Intermittent urticaria | Schnitzler's syndrome, hyper-IgD syndrome | | | | |
| Abdominal pain | Crohn's disease, hyper-IgD syndrome | | | Factitious fever | Urine temperature < body temperature |

*Abbreviations:* ATG, anti-thyroid globulins; DVTs, ↑ FSPs, + LE dopplers; DVTs/PE, deep vein thrombosis/pulmonary emboli; FSPs, fibrin split products; GGT, gamma glutyl transminase; LAP, leukocyte alkaline phosphatase; SPEP, serum protein electrophoresis.
* When presenting as an FUO.

Table 11
Selected causes of fevers of unknown origin appropriate for empiric therapy

| Infectious causes | Noninfectious causes |
|---|---|
| Miliary tuberculosis | Polymyalgia rheumatica/ |
| Culture-negative subacute | temporal arteritis |
| bacterial endocarditis[a] | Familial Mediterranean |
| Whipple's disease | fever |
| Febrile neutropenia | |

[a] HACEK-negative causes.

have little or no decrease in temperature during the test period, whereas those with neoplasms have a prompt and dramatic decrease in temperature for all or most of the 3-day test period. The Naprosyn test works with neoplasms that generate fevers from the malignancy itself (not an associated complication of malignancy). Although there is less experience with other NSAIDs, it appears that other NSAIDs have no effect on infectious fevers while having inhibitory effect on neoplastic fevers. As with other tests, the Naprosyn test should not be applied in situations where its use has not been defined [158,159].

The Naprosyn test does not differentiate neoplastic causes of fever from rheumatic or miscellaneous causes.

*Exploratory laparotomy*

Exploratory laparotomy was an important diagnostic modality in the past when signs and symptoms of an FUO pointed to an intra-abdominal process. With the widespread use of imaging techniques such as CT and MRI as well as gallium/indium scanning, the need for exploratory laparotomy has all but been eliminated. Currently, exploratory laparotomy should be viewed as a test of last resort when the patient has findings suggesting intra-abdominal pathology and no other tests are able to confirm the diagnosis. If exploratory laparotomy is necessary for diagnosis in a patient with FUO, laparoscopic laparotomy, which is less invasive, is preferable to an open procedure (Table 12) [161].

**Recurrent fevers of unknown origin**

*Fevers of unknown origin that remained undiagnosed*

A focused and phased FUO workup should diagnose all but the most rare and obscure causes of an FUO. FUOs that remain undiagnosed over long periods of time are unlikely to be due to an infectious or neoplastic etiology. FUOs that persist intermittently for months or years are difficult to diagnose but at least are benign in nature. Undiagnosed FUOs may be

Table 12
Fevers of unknown origin: focused diagnostic approach

| Initial FUO tests | Focused FUO tests | Definitive diagnostic tests | Remain undiagnosed after FUO workup |
|---|---|---|---|
| CBC | CBC (manual differential) | Serology for visceral leishmaniasis, brucellosis, Q fever, E/A, leptospirosis, trichinosis, coccidioidomycosis, histoplasmosis serology (if likely by history and physical findings) | Special testing needed for diagnosis |
| ESR | ANA | | |
| SGOT/SGPT | RF | | |
| SPEP | Cold agglutinins | | |
| Creatinine | Ferritin | | |
| Blood cultures | Blood smears for malaria, E/A, babesia, RBF (*S. minus*), RF (*B. recurrentis*) if likely by history and physical findings | | |
| CT/MRI chest, abdomen, and pelvis (if likely by history and physical findings) | Blood cultures ($\uparrow$ CO$_2$/6 weeks) | | |
| | TTE/TEE (if heart murmur present) | | |
| | EBV, CMV, toxoplasmosis, LGV1-3 Bartonella, salmonella IgM/IgG titers (if likely by history and physical findings) | | |
| | CSF for AFB smear/culture, cytology, ANA (if likely by history and physical findings) | | |

| | Likely to be diagnosed after *initial* FUO history, physical examination, and nonspecific tests | Likely to be diagnosed after *focused* FUO history, physical examination, and nonspecific tests | Likely to be diagnosed after *definitive* FUO history, physical examination, and nonspecific tests | Remain undiagnosed after FUO workup |
|---|---|---|---|---|
| **Infectious diseases** | SBE | CMV | Miliary TB | Relapsing mastoiditis |
| | Intra-abdominal/pelvic abscess | EBV | Visceral leishmaniasis | Chronic sinusitis |
| | Renal/perinephric abscess | Toxoplasmosis | Brucellosis | Subacute vertebral osteomyelitis |
| | | Typhoid fever | Q fever | Periapical dental abscess |
| | | CSD | Trichinosis | Aortitis |
| | | Renal TB | Coccidioidomycosis | |
| | | TB meningitis | Histoplasmosis | |
| | | | Whipple's disease | |
| **Rheumatoid/inflammatory disorders** | None | SLE | See Table 8 | See Table 8 |
| | | Adult Still's disease | FMF | Polyarticular gout, pseudogout |
| | | PAN | Takayasu's arteritis | APA |
| | | PMR/TA | Kikuchi's disease | FAPA |
| | | LORA | Antiphospholipid syndrome | |
| | | Sarcoidosis | | |
| **Neoplastic disorders** | Hypernephroma | Atrial myxomas | See Table 9 | See Table 9 |
| | Hepatoma | | MPDs (CML/CLL) | Colon carcinoma |
| | Pancreatic carcinoma | | Preleukemia (AML) | Cervical carcinoma |
| | | | | CNS malignancies |
| **Miscellaneous disorders** | Cirrhosis | Subacute thyroiditis | See Table 10 | See Table 10 |
| | Drug fever | Crohn's disease | Pseudolymphoma | Fume fever |
| | | Hyper-IgD syndrome | Cyclic neutropenia | Hypothalamic dysfunction |
| | | Schnitzler's syndrome | DVTs/PE | Factitious fever |

*Abbreviations*: ANA, antinuclear antibody; APA, antiphospholipid syndrome; CBC, complete blood count; ESR, erythrocyte sedimentation rate; E/A, ehrlichiosis/anaplasmosis; **RBF**, rat bite fever; RF, relapsing fever; SGOT/SGPT, serum glutamic oxaloacetic transaminase/serum glutamic pyruvic transaminase; UA/UC, urinalysis/urine culture.

recurrent or persistent. After a focused FUO workup, an undiagnosed FUO of prolonged duration is usually due to a miscellaneous cause, including periodic fever syndromes. Rare causes of recurrent or persistent FUOs are shown in Box 1 [73].

Clinicians should pursue these diagnoses only after all other diagnostic possibilities have been exhausted.

The underlying cause of an FUO determines its potential for recurrence. Infectious diseases causing FUOs are self-limiting from either therapeutic/surgical intervention or natural resolution. Some infectious diseases responsible for FUOs may present as relapsing fevers, others may present as recurrent FUOs. Relapsing fevers remit, and patients have little or no fever between episodes. The periodicity and fever pattern of relapsing fevers may be clues to their infectious etiology. Certain infectious diseases—for example, relapsing fever (*Borrelia recurrentis*). In general, intracellular pathogens (eg, viruses) that may cause FUOs have the potential to be recurrent, depending on the efficacy of host defense-suppressive mechanisms.

Similarly, benign neoplastic disorders may recur periodically and present as recurrent FUOs if the initial etiology of the fever is not initially determined. Malignant neoplasms are self-limiting naturally or with therapeutic interventions. Rheumatic inflammatory causes are, by nature, disorders that tend to periodicity with episodic exacerbations and remissions. Among all the categories of FUOs, rheumatic inflammatory diseases are the most likely to manifest as recurrent FUOs.

Other miscellaneous causes of recurrent fever include cyclic neutropenia. Other FUOs prone to relapse include relapsing polychondritis, periapical dental abscesses, Crohn's disease, and alcoholic cirrhosis.

---

**Box 1. Rare causes of recurrent or persistent fevers of unknown origin**

- Aortic enteric fistulas
- Castleman's disease
- Gaucher's disease
- Fabry's disease
- FAPA (fever, adenitis, pharyngitis, and aphthous ulcers) syndrome
- Systemic mastocytosis
- Rosai-Dorfman syndrome
- TNF receptor I-associated periodic syndrome (familial Hibernian fever)
- Erdheim-Chester disease
- Muckle-Well's disease
- Habitual hypothermia

The clinician approaching a patient with recurrent FUO should reevaluate the patient with additional focused history, physical examinations, and laboratory tests as needed in an attempt to diagnose the cause. Often, over time, clinical features that were not present initially are manifested, and these are important in establishing a definitive diagnosis. Although unlikely, the possibility also exists that the patient has a separate disorder presenting as an FUO after the initial one, giving the appearance of a recurrent FUO. For these reasons, a focused reevaluation with each episode of recurrent FUO is appropriate. If a definitive diagnosis is established as to the cause of the recurrent FUOs, the clinician and patient should be reassured when there is recurrence that the underlying cause (usually rheumatic/inflammatory) is a disorder prone to febrile recurrences (eg, SLE, FMF). If during the recurrent episodes of FUO the clinical presentation remains unchanged, an additional workup is not needed [2,5,13,18,73].

## Empiric therapy

The disorders responsible for FUOs are numerous and their manifestations protean; therefore, emphasis is properly on the diagnostic approach to determining the cause of the FUO. With many FUOs, patients and physicians frequently attempt to lower the patient's fever. Fever is a cardinal sign that serves as the impetus to determine a diagnosis in both acute fevers and FUOs. Suppression of fever serves no physiologic or clinical purpose. Antipyretics should be avoided because they obscure the febrile response and alter fever patterns that may be important diagnostically. Altering the febrile manifestation of the FUO eliminates important diagnostic information, often resulting in a more difficult or delayed diagnosis. Not only should fever not be suppressed, but patients should be encouraged to plot their fevers along with simultaneous pulse rates, which often demonstrate characteristic fever patterns and may be helpful diagnostically [2,5].

In some situations, empiric therapy in patients with FUOs is reasonable and necessary. The empiric treatment of true culture-negative endocarditis is reasonable if the patient meets the previously discussed criteria for culture-negative endocarditis. Empiric therapy for SBE should not be started in patients who have fever, heart murmur, and negative blood cultures without peripheral manifestations of endocarditis. Empiric therapy for temporal arteritis is vital and may prevent permanent blindness. Vasculitic doses of corticosteroids should be used in the treatment of such patients. If miliary TB is suspected and the patient is deteriorating clinically, empiric anti-TB therapy is reasonable and may be life-saving. Miliary TB is a difficult diagnosis to confirm and requires biopsy of liver or bone marrow. Biopsy results take time, and patients deteriorating with potential miliary TB should be given empiric trial of anti-tuberculous therapy at least until biopsy results

Table 13
Fevers of unknown origin: diagnostic pearls and pitfalls

| Pearls | Examples |
|--------|----------|
| The clinical significance of subtle or nonspecific diagnostic findings taken together often suggest a particular diagnosis | Lymphoma (with ↑ $\alpha_1/\alpha_2$ globulins and ↑ alkaline phosphatase) Lymphomas with ↑ LDH and ↑ alkaline phosphatase |
| Subtle or initial signs/symptoms are easily missed findings | SLE (with cytoid bodies) Adult Still's disease (with ↑ ferritin levels) |
| With FUOs, repeat history, physical examination, and laboratory tests until diagnostic clues become apparent | SBE (with new appearing/appreciated Roth spots) Miliary TB (with choroid tubercules) CLL (with Richter's transformation) |
| Serial laboratory tests often reveal abnormalities not initially present. Such findings should prompt further testing to rule out or confirm the presumptive diagnosis | CML (with blast transformation) |
| With FUOs, clinical manifestations often change over time | SLE (with cerebritis, then pneumonitis, and then abdominal pain) Whipple's disease (with mental confusion, then abdominal symptoms, and then arthritis) |
| The longer an FUO remains undiagnosed, the less likely it is due to infection. Exceptions are Charcot's fever due to intermittent biliary tract obstruction and miliary TB. | Hyper-IgD syndrome (with recurrences >1 year) Cyclic neutropenia (with recurrences >1 year) |
| Relapsing/recurrent FUOs are usually due to rheumatic/inflammatory disorders | SLE (with recurrent fevers) FMF (with recurrent fevers) |
| In FUO cases in which the diagnosis remains elusive, fever patterns may be the only clue to the correct diagnosis | Ehrlichiosis (with camel back fever curve) Drug fever (with relative bradycardia) Adult Still's disease (with double quotidian fever) PAN (with morning temperature spikes) |
| Rheumatic/inflammatory disorders (uninfected) are not associated with leukocytosis and typically have leukopenia/normal WBC count | Adult Still's disease (with WBC count ≥20 K/mm$^3$) |
| FUOs with fatigue, weight loss, anorexia, and hepatomegaly are most likely due to malignancy rather than infection | Lymphoma (with hepatomegaly) |
| With FUOs, highly elevated serum ferritin levels are important in eliminating infectious diseases from further diagnostic consideration | Highly elevated ferritin levels (limit diagnostic possibilities to neoplastic and rheumatic/infectious disorders) |

| Pitfalls | Examples |
|----------|----------|
| Failure to consider the diagnosis because classic findings are not present | Crohn's disease (without abdominal complaints) EBV infectious mononucleosis (in the elderly without sore throat or cervical adenopathy) |

(*continued on next page*)

Table 13 (*continued*)

| Pitfalls | Examples |
|---|---|
| Diagnosis not considered because late-appearing clinical/laboratory findings not recognized as part of the usual clinical presentation | Typhoid fever (with fingertip/spinal tenderness) Q fever (with SBE) |
| Extensive "shotgun testing" should be avoided; it only misdirects the relevant FUO workup | Subacute thyroiditis (no need for thyroiditis tests in patients without PMH of thyroid disease/autoimmune disorders or symptoms/signs of subacute thyroiditis) |
| Doing a "complete and comprehensive" but irrelevant and nonfocused history and physical examination in FUO patients is diagnostically unhelpful | Regional enteritis (with episcleritis without abdominal complaints as the initial manifestation of Crohn's disease) |
| FUOs are usually due to a rheumatic/inflammatory disorder, but a mild/protracted course does not rule out infection or malignancy | Deceptive mild/prolonged course miliary TB, SBE, or lymphomas |
| In FUO patients, a complete and comprehensive history and physical examination are futile if the physician does not know what findings to look for and their diagnostic significance | PAN (with hearing loss as the initial presenting sign) |
| With few exceptions (TA, miliary TB), empiric treatment of FUOs should be avoided as antimicrobial therapy may delay or obscure the diagnosis | Doxycycline (will partially treat some zoonoses) Quinolones (will partially treat tuberculosis) |
| In FUO patients, the Naprosyn test should be used only to differentiate neoplastic from infectious fevers | Naprosyn test (initial does not differentiate neoplastic from non-neoplastic fevers) |
| The diagnostic significance of an elevated alkaline phosphatase level is often overlooked in FUOs | Increased alkaline phosphatase may be an important clue (with lymphoma, temporal arteritis, or subacute thyroiditis) |
| In FUOs, atypical lymphocytes in the peripheral smear may be an important clue to nonviral disorders | Atypical lymphocytes in the peripheral smear (manual CBC with a differential count) not necessarily in the peripheral smear. Initial atypical lymphocytosis should suggest drug fever, malaria, ehrlichiosis/anaplasmosis, or toxoplasmosis |
| SPEP is an underused test that often provides important clues to a variety of FUOs | SPEP is useful to identify monoclonal spikes, (multiple myeloma); polyclonal gammopathy may be a clue to sarcoidosis, LVG, atrial myxoma, or malaria; $\uparrow \alpha_1/\alpha_2$ globulins may point to lymphomas, SLE |
| Elevated serum ferritin levels in FUOs should not be dismissed as being nonspecific and an "acute phase reactant" | A highly elevated ferritin level in an FUO is chronically an often important diagnostic clue (with rheumatic and neoplastic disorders) |

are available to rule out or confirm the diagnosis of miliary TB. Most other infectious diseases presenting as FUOs (eg, Q fever, SBE) are usually not rapidly progressive, and appropriate therapy can be initiated after the diagnosis is confirmed serologically or by PCR [162].

With these few exceptions, empiric treatment of FUOs should be avoided, and efforts should be directed at arriving at a definitive diagnosis.

## Lessons learned

Prolonged unexplained fevers have perplexed clinicians from antiquity to the present. FUOs remain a challenging exercise in differential diagnosis. The diagnostic workup should be directed by features of the clinical presentations, which almost always suggest an infectious, rheumatic/inflammatory, neoplastic, or miscellaneous disorder. Using the approach outlined in this article, clinicians can diagnose all but the most obscure causes of FUOs. Most undiagnosed FUOs are due to a failure to consider a diagnosis or a comprehensive but misguided workup. The most common errors in FUO diagnostics are defects in diagnostic reasoning (eg, either the significance of abnormal clinical/laboratory findings were not appreciated or key tests were not included during the FUO workup).

A comprehensive and careful history and physical examination and exhaustive laboratory testing are no substitute for a focused FUO diagnostic evaluation.

Clinicians faced with FUOs should be familiar with the clinical and laboratory findings associated with each disorder included in the differential diagnosis. Clinicians should also be aware of time relationships in the appearance and disappearance of clinical and laboratory findings. Often, early or late clinical or laboratory findings are overlooked because physicians often recognize only the most common clinical findings.

Experience over the years has led to a distillation of diagnostic FUO principles (ie, FUO pearls). Pearls are aphorisms summarizing the lessons learned from experience over the years with FUOs. Pitfalls are aphorismically expressed potential diagnostic problems to avoid in the diagnostic approach to FUOs (Table 13) [2,5,6,8,141].

## References

[1] Cunha BA. Osler on typhoid fever: differentiation of typhoid from typhus and malaria. Infect Dis Clin North Am 2004;18:111–26.

[2] Keefer CS, Leard SE. Prolonged and perplexing fevers. Boston: Little Brown; 1955.

[3] Petersdorf RG, Beeson PB. Fever of unexplained origin: report on 100 cases. Medicine (Baltimore) 1961;40:1–30.

[4] Larson EB, Featherstone HJ, Petersdorf RG. Fever of undetermined origin: diagnosis and follow-up of 105 cases, 1970–80. Medicine 1982;61:269–92.

[5] Murray HW, editor. Fever of undetermined origin. Mount Kisco (NY): Informa Healthcare; 1983.

[6] Cunha BA, editor. Fever of unknown origin. New York: Informa Healthcare; 2007.

[7] Molavi A, Weinstein L. Persistent perplexing pyrexia. Some comments on etiology and diagnosis. Med Clin North Am 1970;54:379–96.

[8] Louria DB. Fever of unknown etiology. Del Med J 1971;43:343–8.

[9] Jacoby GA, Swartz MN. Fever of undetermined origin. N Engl J Med 1973;289:1407–10.

[10] Wolf SM, Fauci AS, Dale DC. Unusual etiologies of fever and their evaluation. Annu Rev Med 1975;26:277–81.

[11] Brusch JL, Weinstein L. Fever of unknown origin. Med Clin North Am 1988;72:1247–61.

[12] Kazanjian PH. Fever of unknown origin. Review of 86 patients treated in community hospital. Clin Infect Dis 1992;15:968–73.

[13] Knockaert DC, Vanneste LJ, Vannester SB, et al. Fever of unknown origin in the 1980s: an update of the diagnostic spectrum. Arch Intern Med 1992;152:51–5.

[14] Lortholary O, Bletry LG, Godeau P. Fever of unknown origin: a retrospective multicentre study of 103 cases, 1980–88. Eur J Med 1992;3:109–20.

[15] Cunha BA. Fever of unknown origin. Infect Dis Clin North Am 1996;10:111–28.

[16] Bryan CS. Fever of unknown origin. Arch Intern Med 2003;163:1003–4.

[17] Amin K, Kauffman C. Fever of unknown origin. Postgrad Med 2003;114:69–76.

[18] Cunha BA. Fever of unknown origin. In: Gorbach SL, Bartlett JG, Blacklow NE, editors. Infectious diseases. 3rd edition. Philadelphia: Lippincott Williams & Wilkins; 2005. p. 1568–77.

[19] Nubile MJ. Acute fevers of unknown origin. A plea for restraint. Arch Intern Med 1993; 153:2525–6.

[20] Brusch JL. Diagnosis of infective endocarditis I. Infective endocarditis management in the era of intravascular devices. New York: Informa Healthcare; 2006. p. 241–54.

[21] Cunha BA, Gill MV, Lazar J. Acute infective endocarditis. Infect Dis Clin North Am 1996; 10:811–34.

[22] Cunha BA. MSSA/MRSA acute bacterial endocarditis (ABE): clinical pathway for diagnosis and treatment. Antibiotics for Clinicians 2006;10:29–34.

[23] Brusch JL. Culture negative infective endocarditis. Infectious Disease Practice 2006;30: 545–8.

[24] Brusch JL. HACEK endocarditis. Infectious Disease Practice 2007;31:616–7.

[25] Cunha BA. The mimics of endocarditis. In: Brusch JL, editor. Infective endocarditis management in the era of intravascular devices. New York: Informa Healthcare; 2006. p. 345–54.

[26] Mert A, Bilir M, Tabak F. Miliary tuberculosis: clinical manifestations, diagnosis and outcome in 38 adults. Respiration 2001;6:217–24.

[27] Collazos J, Guerra E, Mayo J, et al. Tuberculosis as a cause of recurrent fever of unknown origin. J Infect 2000;41:269–72.

[28] Wang JY, Hsueh PR, Wang SK, et al. Disseminated tuberculosis: a 10-year experience in a medical center. Medicine 2007;86:39–46.

[29] Fitzgerald DW. Miliary tuberculosis. In: Schlossberg D, editor. Tuberculosis & nontuberculosis mycobacterial infections. New York: McGraw-Hill; 2006. p. 332–44.

[30] Axelrod P, Finestone AJ. Infectious mononucleosis in older adults. Am Fam Physician 1990;42:1599–606.

[31] Cunha BA. CMV infectious mononucleosis presenting as fever of unknown origin. Emerg Med 2001;33:73–5.

[32] Manfredi R, Calza L, Chiodo F. Primary cytomegalovirus infection in otherwise healthy adults with fever of unknown origin: a 3-year prospective survey. Infection 2006;34: 87–90.

[33] Mickail N, Navsheen S, Cunha BA. Fever of unknown origin: cytomegalovirus (CMV) in an immuno-competent host. Infectious Disease Practice 2007;21:629–30.

[34] Jacobs RF, Schutze GE. *Bartonella henselae* as a cause of prolonged fever and fever of unknown origin in children. Clin Infect Dis 1998;26:80–4.

[35] Tsujino K, Tsukahara M, Tsuneoka H, et al. Clinical implication of prolonged fever in children with cat scratch disease. J Infect Chemother 2004;10:227–33.

[36] Manson-Bahr PH. Leishmaniasis. In: Manson's tropical diseases. 16th edition. London: Balliere, Tindall and Cassell; 1966. p. 107–43.

[37] Pearson RD, Sousa AQ. Clinical spectrum of leishmaniasis. Clin Infect Dis 1996;22:1–13.

[38] Shanley FM. Toxoplasmosis and prolonged FUO. Hosp Pract 1986;21:18.

[39] Farid Z, Ibrahim FH, Safwat Y. Toxoplasma lymphadenitis presenting as prolonged fever. J Egypt Public Health Assoc 1990;65:236–41.

[40] Young EJ, Corbel MJ, editors. Brucellosis: clinical and laboratory aspects. Boca Raton (FL): CRC Press; 1989.

[41] Madkour MM. Madkour's Brucellosis. 2nd edition. Berlin: Springer; 2001.

[42] Tinoco-Velazques I, Gomez-Priego A, Menoza R, et al. Searching for antibodies against *Trichinella spiralis* in the sera of patients with fever of unknown cause. Ann Trop Med Parasitol 2002;96:391–5.

[43] Nausheen S, Cunha BA. Trichinosis: current concepts. Infectious Disease Practice 2007;31: 613–5.

[44] Tissot-Dupont H, Raoult D, Brouqui P, et al. Epidemiologic features and clinical presentation of acute Q fever in hospitalized patients: 323 French cases. Am J Med 1992;93: 427–534.

[45] Fergusson RJ, Shaw TR, Kitchin AH, et al. Subclinical chronic Q fever. Q J Med 1985;57: 669–76.

[46] Brouqui P, Tissot-Dupont H, Drancourt M, et al. Chronic Q fever: ninety-two cases from France including 27 cases without endocarditis. Arch Intern Med 1993;153: 642–8.

[47] Al-Agha OM, Mooty M, Salarieh A. A 43-year-old woman with acquired immunodeficiency syndrome and fever of unknown origin. Disseminated histoplasmosis. Arch Pathol Lab Med 2006;130:120–3.

[48] Saluja S, Sunita, Bhasin S, et al. Disseminated histoplasmosis with reactive haemophagocytosis presenting as PUO on immunocompetent host. J Assoc Physicians India 2005;53: 906–97.

[49] Schachter J, Osaba AO. Lymphogranuloma venereum. Br Med Bull 1983;39:151–4.

[50] Bernstein DI, Hubbard T, Wenman WM, et al. Mediastinal and supraclavicular lymphadenitis and pneumonitis due to Chlamydia trachomatis serovars L1 and L2. N Engl J Med 1984;311:1543–6.

[51] Varvolgyi C, Buban T, Szakall S, et al. Fever of unknown origin with seronegative spondyloarthropathy: an atypical manifestation of Whipple's disease. Ann Rheum Dis 2002;61: 377–8.

[52] Garcia A, Batlle C, Losada E, et al. Whipple disease as a cause of fever of unknown origin. Med Clin North Am 2005;125:635.

[53] Carsons SE. Fever in rheumatic and autoimmune disease. Infect Dis Clin North Am 1996; 10:67–84.

[53a] Mert A, Ozaras R, Tabak F, et al. Fever of unknown origin: a review of 20 patients with adult-onset Still's disease. Clin Rheumatol 2003;22:89–93.

[54] Cunha BA. Fever of unknown origin in rheumatic diseases. In: Cunha BA, editor. Fever of unknown origin. New York: Informa Healthcare; 2007. p. 59–64.

[54a] Crispin JC, Martinez-Banos D, Alcocer-Varela J. Adult-onset still disease as the cause of fever of unknown origin. Medicine 2005;84:331–7.

[55] Harmouche H, Maamar M, Sahnoune I, et al. Fever revealing Behçet's disease. Two new cases. Eur J Intern Med 2007;18:146–7.

[56] Ghosh MK, Shensa S, Lerner PI. Arteritis of the aged (giant cell arteritis) and fever of unexplained origin. Am J Med 1976;60:429–36.

[57] Calamia KT, Hunder GG. Giant cell arteritis (temporal arteritis) presenting as fever of undetermined origin. Arthritis Rheum 1981;24:1414–8.

[58] Cunha BA. Fever of unknown origin due to adult onset juvenile rheumatoid arthritis (adult onset still's disease): the diagnostic significance of a double quotidian fever and elevated serum ferritin levels. Heart Lung 2004;33:417–21.

[59] Cunha BA, Syed U, Hamid N. Fever of unknown origin (FUO) due to late onset of rheumatoid arthritis (LORA). Heart Lung 2006;35:70–3.

[60] Beyan E, Uzuner A, Beyan C. An uncommon cause of fever in the elderly: late-onset systemic lupus erythematosus. Clin Rheumatol 2003;22:481–3.

[61] Stollerman GH. Fever of unknown origin with polyarteritis nodosa. J Tenn Med Assoc 1975;68:709–14.

[62] Henderson J, Cohen J, Jackson J, et al. Polyarteritis nodosa presenting as pyrexia of unknown origin. Postgrad Med J 2002;78:685–6.

[63] Kamimura T, Hatakeyama M, Torigoe K, et al. Muscular polyarteritis nodosa as a cause of fever of undetermined origin: a case report and review of the literature. Rheumatol Int 2005; 25:394–7.

[64] Zenone T, Knefati Y, Sabatier JC. Polyarteritis nodosa presenting with jaw claudication and headache. Joint Bone Spine 2007;74:301–2.

[65] Wu YJJ, Martin BR, Ong K, et al. Takayasu's arteritis presenting as a cause of fever of unknown origin. Am J Med 1989;87:476–7.

[66] Erten N, Saka B, Karan MA, et al. Takayasu's arteritis presenting with fever of unknown origin: two case reports. J Clin Rheumatol 2004;10:16–20.

[67] Tato F, Weiss M, Hoffman U. Takayasu's arteritis without manifest arterial stenoses as cause of fever of unknown origin. Dtsch Med Wochenschr 2006;131:1727–30.

[68] Bailey EM, Klein N, Cunha BA. Kikuchi's disease with liver function presenting as fever of unknown origin. Lancet 1989;2:986.

[69] Ben-Chetrit E, Levy M. Familial Mediterranean fever. Lancet 1998;351:659–64.

[70] Baughman RP, editor. Sarcoidosis. New York: Informa Healthcare; 2006.

[71] Miller AC, Chacko T, Rashid RM, et al. Fever of unknown origin and isolated noncaseating granuloma of the marrow: could this be sarcoidosis? Allergy Asthma Proc 2007;28:230–5.

[72] DeLeon DG, Shifteh S, Cunha BA. Fever of unknown origin due to Sarcoidosis-Lymphoma Syndrome. Heart Lung 2004;33:124–9.

[73] Knockaert DC. Recurrent fever of unknown origin. In: Cunha BA, editor. Fever of unknown origin. New York: Informa Healthcare; 2007. p. 133–50.

[74] Luft FC, Risssing JP, White A, et al. Infections or neoplasm as causes of prolonged fever in cancer patients. Am J Med Sci 1969;272:67–72.

[75] Cunha BA. Fever of unknown origin in malignant disorders. Infectious Disease Practice 2004;26:335–6.

[76] Cunha BA. Fever of unknown origin in malignancies. In: Cunha BA, editor. Fever of unknown origin. New York: Informa Healthcare; 2007. p. 27–34.

[77] Hazani A, Isaac B. Unexplained fever in hematologic disorders: section I benign hematologic discorders. In: Isaac B, Kernbaum S, Burke M, editors. Unexplained fever. Boca Raton: CRC Press; 1991. p. 189–208.

[78] Kuviliev E, Glamour T, Shekar R, et al. Angiotropic large cell lymphoma presenting as fever of unknown origin. Am J Med Sci 1999;317:266–8.

[79] Berger L, Sinkoff MW. Systemic manifestations of hypernephroma: a review of 273 cases. Am J Med 1957;22:791–76.

[80] Cronin RS, Keahny WD, Miller PD, et al. Renal cell carcinoma: unusual systemic manifestations. Medicine 1976;55:291–318.

[81] Weinstein EC, Geraci JE, Green LF. Hypernephroma presenting as fever of unknown origin. Proc Mayo Clin 1961;36:12–9.

[82] Cunha BA. Fevers of unknown origin (FUO): Chronic myelogenous leukemia (CML) with blast transformation. Infectious Disease Practice 2007;31:606–8.

[83] Cunha BA, Mohan S, Parchuri S. Fever of unknown origin: CLL vs lymphoma (Richter's transformation). Heart Lung 2005;34:437–41.

[84] Mueller PS, Terrel CL, Gertz MA. Fever of unknown origin caused by multiple myeloma: report of 9 cases. Arch Intern Med 2002;162:1305–9.

[85] Lambotte O, Royer B, Genet P, et al. Multiple myeloma presenting as fever of unknown origin. Eur J Intern Med 2003;14:94–7.

[86] Cunha BA, Goldstein O. Fever of unknown origin (FUO): pre-leukemia due to acute myelogenous leukemia (AML). Infectious Disease Practice 2006;30:540–1.

[87] Agmon-Levin N, Ziv-Sokolovsky N, Shull P, et al. Carcinoma of colon presenting as fever of unknown origin. Am J Med Sci 2005;329:322–6.

[88] Strollo S, Eisenstein L, Cunha BA. Fever of unknown origin (FUO): pancreatic carcinoma. Infectious Disease Practice 2006;30:497–8.

[89] Tisdale WA, Klatskin G. The fever of Laennec's cirrhosis. Yale J Biol Med 1960;33:94–106.

[90] Signh N, Yu VL, Wagener MM, et al. Cirrhotic fever in the 1990s: a prospective study with clinical implications. Clin Infect Dis 1997;24:1135–8.

[91] Admani A, Smith LG. Fever of unknown origin in Cirrhosis. In: Cunha BA, editor. Fever of unknown origin. New York: Informa Healthcare; 2007. p. 21–6.

[92] Cluff LE, Johnson JE. Drug fever. Prog Allergy 1969;168:41–51.

[93] Johnson DH, Cunha BA. Drug fever. Infect Dis Clin North Am 1996;10:85–92.

[94] Dominguez A, Pena JM, Barbado FJ, et al. Prolonged course fever as presentation form of Crohn's disease. An Med Interna 1990;7:39–41.

[95] Daloviso JR, Blonde L, Cortez M, et al. Subacute thyroiditis with increased serum alkaline phosphatase. Ann Intern Med 1978;88:505–7.

[96] Brendan MW, Matthew JH, Dennis PM. Subacute thyroiditis manifesting as fever of unknown origin. South Med J 2000;93:926–9.

[97] Cunha BA, Thermidor M, Mohan S, et al. Fever of unknown origin: subacute thyroiditis versus typhoid fever. Heart Lung 2005;34:147–51.

[98] Dale DC, Bolyard AA, Aprikyan A. Cyclic neutropenia. Semin Hematol 2002;39:89–94.

[99] Knockaert DC, Scheurmans A, Vlayen J, et al. Fever of unknown origin due to inflammatory pseudotumor of lymph nodes. Acta Clin Belg 1998;53:367–70.

[100] Murray HW, Tuazon CU, Guerrero IC, et al. A clue to early diagnosis of factitious fever. N Engl J Med 1977;296:23–4.

[101] Murray HW. Factitious fever updated. Arch Intern Med 1979;139:739–40.

[102] Aduan RP, Fauci AS, Dale DC, et al. Factitious fever and self-induced infection. A report of 32 cases and review of the literature. Ann Intern Med 1979;90:230–42.

[103] Lipsker D, Veran Y, Grunenberger F, et al. The Schnitzler syndrome. Four new cases and review of the literature. Medicine 2001;80:37–44.

[104] de Koning HD, Bodar EJ, van der Meer JW, et al. Schnitzler syndrome: beyond the case reports: review and follow-up of 94 patients with an emphasis on prognosis and treatment. Semin Arthritis Rheumatol 37:in press.

[105] Simon A, Cuisset L, Vincent MF, et al. Molecular analysis of the mevalonate kinase gene in a cohort of patients with the hyper-IgD and periodic fever syndrome: its application as a diagnostic tool. Ann Intern Med 2001;135:338–43.

[106] Zenone T. Fever of unknown origin in adults: evaluation of 144 cases in a non-university hospital. Scand J Infect Dis 2006;38:625–31.

[107] Diaz MM, Barbado Hernandez FJ, Gomez Cerezo J, et al. Fever of unknown origin: differences in two different clinical series in a university hospital. Rev Clin Esp 2007;207: 13–5.

[108] Jones MS, Lukashov VV, Ganac RD, et al. Discovery of a novel human picornavirus from a pediatric patient presenting with fever of unknown origin. J Clin Microbiol 2007;45: 2144–50.

[109] Silpapojakul K, Chupuppakarn S, Yuthasompob S, et al. Scrub and murine typhus in children with obscure fever in the tropics. Pediatr Infect Dis J 1991;10:200–3.

[110] Bodenmann P, Genton B. Chikungunya: an epidemic in real time. Lancet 2006;368:186–7.
[111] Nausheen S, Cunha BA. Chikungunya fever: current concepts. Infectious Disease Practice 2006;31:548–50.
[112] Handa R, Bhatia S, Wali JP. Melioidosis: a rare but not forgotten cause of fever of unknown origin. Br J Clin Pathol 1996;50:116–7.
[113] Majeed HA. Differential diagnosis of fever of unknown origin in children. Curr Opin Rheumatol 2000;12:439–44.
[114] Krilov LR. Fever of unknown origin in children. In: Cunha BA, editor. Fever of unknown origin. New York: Informa Healthcare; 2007. p. 17–20.
[115] Bouza E, Loeches B, Muno P. Fever of unknown origin in solid organ transplant recipients. In: Cunha BA, editor. Fever of unknown origin. New York: Informa Healthcare; 2007. p. 79–100.
[116] Cunha BA. Fever of unknown origin in HIV/AIDS patients. Drugs Today 1999;35: 429–34.
[117] Armstrong WS, Katz JT, Kazanjian PH. Human immunodeficiency virus-associated fever of unknown origin a study of 70 patients in the United States and review. Clin Infect Dis 1999;28:341–5.
[118] Lozano F, Torre-Cisneros J, Pena JM, et al. Impact of a highly active antiretroviral therapy of fever of unknown origin in HIV-infected patients. Eur J Clin Microbiol Infect Dis 2002; 21:132–9.
[119] Armstrong WS, Kazanjian P. Fever of unknown origin in HIV patients. In: Cunha BA, editor. Fever of unknown origin. New York: Informa Healthcare; 2007. p. 65–78.
[120] Blockmans D, Knockaert D, Maes A, et al. Clinical values of (18) F fluorodeoxyglucose position emission tomography or patients with fevers of unknown origin. Clin Infect Dis 2001;32:191–6.
[121] Rijinders AJ, Bleeker-Rovers CP, Vos FJ, et al. A prospective multicenter study of the value of FDG-PET as part of a structured diagnostic protocol in patients with fever of unknown origin. Eur J Nucl Med Mod Imaging 2007;34:694–703.
[122] Woodward TE. The fever pattern as a clinical diagnostic aid. In: Mackowiak PA, editor. Fever basic mechanisms and management. 2nd edition. Philadelphia: Lippincott-Raven; 1997. p. 215–36.
[123] Cunha BA. The diagnostic significance of fever curves. Infect Dis Clin North Am 1996;10: 33–44.
[124] Cunha BA. Diagnostic significance of relative Bradycardia. Clin Microbiol Infect 2000;6:633–4.
[125] Maegraith B. Unde venis? Lancet 1963;1:401–3.
[126] Saxe SE, Gardner P. The returning traveler with fever. Infect Dis Clin North Am 1992;6: 427–39.
[127] Cunha BA. Malaria or typhoid fever: a diagnostic dilemma? Am J Med 2005;118:1442–3.
[128] Sharma BK, Kumari S, Varma SC, et al. Prolonged undiagnosed fever in Northern India. Trop Geogr Med 1992;44:32–6.
[129] Chin C, Chen YS, Lee SS, et al. Fever of unknown origin in Taiwan. Infection 2006;34: 75–80.
[130] AbuRahma AF, Saiedy S, Robinson PA, et al. Role of venous duplex imaging of the lower extremities in patients with fever of unknown origin. Surgery 1997;121:366–71.
[131] Murray HW, Ellis CG, Blumenthal DS, et al. Fever and pulmonary thromboembolism. Am J Med 1979;67:232–5.
[132] Jagneaux T, Lopez FA, Sanders CV. Postoperative fever of unknown origin. In: Cunha BA, editor. Fever of unknown origin. New York: Informa Healthcare; 2007. p. 115–33.
[133] Cunha BA. Fever in the critical care unit. In: Cunha BA, editor. Infectious disease in critical care medicine. 2nd edition. New York: Informa Healthcare; 2007. p. 41–72.
[134] Cunha BA. Nosocomial fever of unknown origin. In: Cunha BA, editor. Fever of unknown origin. New York: Informa Healthcare; 2007. p. 101–8.

[135] Antoniadou A, Giamarellou H. Fever of unkown origin in Febrile Leukopenia. In: Cunha BA, editor. Fever of unknown origin. New York: Informa Healthcare; 2007. p. 35–8.

[136] Esposito AL, Gleckman RA. Fever of unknown origin in the elderly. J Am Geriatr Soc 1978;26:498–505.

[137] Kauffman CA, Jones PG. Diagnosing fever of unknown origin in older patients. Geriatrics 1984;39:46–51.

[138] Knockaert DC, Vanneste LJ, Bobbears HJ. Fever of unknown origin in elderly patients. J Am Geriatr Soc 1993;41:1187–92.

[139] Cunha BA. Fever of unknown origin in the elderly. Infectious Disease Practice 1993;2: 380–3.

[140] Norman DC, Wong MB. Fever of unknown origin in older persons. In: Cunha BA, editor. Fever of unknown origin. New York: Informa Healthcare; 2007. p. 109–14.

[141] Tumulty PA. The history and physical examination. In: Murray HW, editor. FUO of undetermined origin. Mount Kisco (NY): Futura Publishing Company; 1983. p. 125–40.

[142] Esposito AL, Gleckman RA. A diagnostic approach to the adult with fever of unknown origin. Arch Intern Med 1979;139:575–8.

[143] Esposito AL. Planning and proceeding with the diagnostic evaluation. In: Murray HW, editor. Fever of undetermined origin. Mount Kisco (NY): Futura Publishing; 1983. p. 141–55.

[144] Cunha BA. Fever of unknown origin: a focused diagnostic approach. In: Cunha BA, editor. Fever of unknown origin. New York: Informa Healthcare; 2007. p. 9–16.

[145] Bleeker-Rovers CP, Vos FJ, de Kleijn EM, et al. A prospective multicenter study on fever of unknown origin: the yield of a structured diagnostic protocol. Medicine 2007;86: 26–38.

[146] Cunha BA. Nonspecific tests in the diagnosis of fever of unknown origin. In: Cunha BA, editor. Fever of unknown origin. New York: Informa Healthcare; 2007. p. 151–8.

[147] Cunha BA. Polyclonal gammopathy on SPEP. Infectious Disease Practice 1996;20: 39–40.

[148] Brensilver HL, Kaplan MM. Significance of elevated liver alkaline phosphatase in serum. Gastroenterology 1975;58:1556–9.

[149] Hamid N, Krol V, Eisenstein L. Fever of unknown origin (FUO) due to preleukemia/myelodysplastic syndrome: diagnostic importance of monocytosis and elevated serum ferritin levels. Heart Lung 2006;35:277–82.

[150] Cunha BA, Parchuri S, Mohan S. Fever of unknown origin: temporal arteritis presenting with persistent cough and elevated serum ferritin levels. Heart Lung 2006;35:112–6.

[151] Cunha BA. Fever of unknown origin (FUO): diagnostic importance of serum ferritin levels. Scand J Infect Dis 2007;39:651–2.

[152] Knockaert DC, Mortelmans LA, DeRoo MC, et al. Clinical value of gallium-67 scintography in evaluation of fever of unknown origin. Clin Infect Dis 1994;18:601–5.

[153] Kjaer A, Lebeh A-M. Diagnostic value of in-granulocyte scintigraphy in patients with fever of unknown origin. J Nucl Med 2002;43:140–4.

[154] Trivedi Y, Yung E, Katz DS. Imaging in fever of unknown origin. In: Cunha BA, editor. Fever of unknown origin. New York: Informa Healthcare; 2007. p. 209–28.

[155] Purnendu S, Louria DB. Non-invasive and invasive diagnostic procedures and laboratory methods. In: Murray WH, editor. FUO of undetermined origin. Mount Kisco (NY): Futura Publishing; 1983. p. 159–90.

[156] Kosmin AR, Lorber B. Specific tests in the diagnosis of fever of unknown origin. In: Cunha BA, editor. Fever of unknown origin. New York: Informa Healthcare; 2007. p. 159–208.

[157] Buckley RM. Miscellaneous and unusual cases of fever of unknown origin. In: Murray HW, editor. FUO of undetermined origin. Mount Kisco (NY): Futura Publishing; 1983. p. 109–24.

[158] Chang JC. How to differentiate neoplastic fever from infectious fever in patients with cancer: usefulness of the Naproxen test. Heart Lung 1987;16:122–7.

[159] Reme P, Cunha BA. NSAIDs and the Naprosyn test in fever of unknown origins. Infectious Disease Practice 2000;24:32.

[160] Cunha BA, Boyaren M, Hamid N. Multiple myeloma presenting as a fever of unknown origin: the diagnostic importance of the Naprosyn test. Heart Lung 2006;15:358–62.

[161] Ozaras R, Celik AD, Zengin K, et al. Is laparotomy necessary in the diagnosis of fever of unknown origin? Acta Chir Belg 2005;105:89–92.

[162] Elko LM, Bryan CS. Empiric therapy in fever of unknown origin: a cautionary note. In: Cunha BA, editor. Fever of unknown origin. New York: Informa Healthcare; 2007. p. 229–36.

INFECTIOUS
DISEASE CLINICS
OF NORTH AMERICA

Infect Dis Clin N Am 21 (2007) 917–936

ELSEVIER
SAUNDERS

# Fever of Unknown Origin: Historical and Physical Clues to Making the Diagnosis

Jill Tolia, MD[a,b,*], Leon G. Smith, MD[a]

[a]Department of Infectious Diseases, St. Michael's Medical Center,
111 Central Avenue, Newark, NJ 07104, USA
[b]Staten Island University Hospital, Staten Island, NY, USA

*"Humanity has but three great enemies: fever, famine and war; of these by far the greatest, by far the most terrible is fever"*
—Sir William Osler, MD, 1896 [1]

Fever of unknown origin (FUO), defined in 1961 by Petersdorf and Beeson [2] as an illness of more than 3 weeks' duration with a temperature greater than 101°F on several occasions with a diagnosis uncertain after 1 week of study in the hospital, remains as elusive today as it did then nearly 50 years ago [3]. There are no published guidelines on the approach to the diagnosis of FUO [4,5], which is not surprising considering some published studies report as many as 200 different causes of FUO [5]. Numerous retrospective case series and prospective studies report that a diagnosis is never established in up to 30% of cases of FUO [6–8]. In addition, the definition of FUO has changed over time, most notably in the revised definition of Durack and Street [9] with emphasis on four different types of FUO (Table 1). Specifically, the work-up of classical FUO has shifted from 1 week of study in the hospital to 3 days or three outpatient visits. Notably, the advent of HIV-AIDS and highly active antiretroviral therapy adds a new dimension to the approach to FUO with infections and drug fever representing a higher proportion of cases and previously uncommon infections occurring frequently [10].

Historically, the "big three" causes of FUO have fallen into three categories: (1) infection, (2) neoplasm, and (3) collagen vascular disease [2].

---

\* Corresponding author. Department of Infectious Diseases, St. Michael's Medical Center, 111 Central Avenue, Newark, NJ 07104.

*E-mail address:* sachitatolia@hotmail.com (J. Tolia).

0891-5520/07/$ - see front matter © 2007 Elsevier Inc. All rights reserved.
doi:10.1016/j.idc.2007.08.011

*id.theclinics.com*

Table 1
New definitions for fever of unknown origin

| | Classic FUO | Nosocomial FUO | Immune-Deficient FUO | HIV-Related FUO |
|---|---|---|---|---|
| Definition | > 38°C, > 3 wk, > 2 visits or 3 d in hospital | > 38°C, 3 d, not present or including on admission | > 38°C, > 3 d, negative cultures after 48 h | > 38°C, > 3 wk for outpatients, > 3 d for inpatients, HIV infection confirmed |
| Patient location | Community, clinic, or hospital | Acute care hospital | Hospital or clinic | Community, clinic, or hospital |
| Leading causes | Cancer, infections, inflammatory conditions, undiagnosed, habitual hyperthermia | Nosocomial infections, postoperative complications, drug fever | Most caused by infections, but cause documented in only 40%–60% | HIV (primary infection), typical and atypical mycobacteria, CMV, lymphomas, toxoplasmosis, cryptococcosis |
| History emphasis | Travel, contacts, animal and insect exposure, medications, immunizations, family history, cardiac valve disorder | Operations and procedures, devices, anatomic considerations, drug treatment | Stage of chemotherapy, drugs administered, underlying immunosuppressive disorder | Drugs, exposures, risk factors, travel, contacts, stage of HIV infection |
| Examination emphasis | Fundi, oropharynx, temporal artery, abdomen, lymph nodes, spleen, joints, skin, nails, genitalia, rectum or prostate, lower limb deep veins | Wounds, drains, devices, sinuses, urine | Skin folds, IV sites, lungs, perianal area | Mouth, sinuses, skin, lymph nodes, eyes, lungs, perianal area |

| | | | | |
|---|---|---|---|---|
| Investigation emphasis | Imaging, biopsies, sedimentation rate, skin tests | Imaging, bacterial cultures | CXR, bacterial cultures | Blood and lymphocyte count; serologic tests; CXR; stool examination; biopsies of lung, bone marrow, and liver for cultures and cytologic tests; brain imaging |
| Management | Observation, outpatient temperature chart, investigations, avoidance of empirical drug treatments | Depends on situation | Antimicrobial treatment protocols | Antiviral and antimicrobial protocols, vaccines, revision of treatment regiments, good nutrition |
| Time course of disease | Months | Weeks | Days | Weeks to months |
| Tempo of investigation | Weeks | Weeks | Hours | Days to weeks |

*Abbreviations:* CMV, cytomegalovirus; CXR, chest radiograph; HIV, human immunodeficiency virus; IV, intravenous.
*From* Mackowiak P, Durack D. Fever of unknown origin. In: Mandell, Douglas and Bennett's principles and practice of infectious diseases. 6th edition. Elsevier; 2005. p. 718–29; with permission.

The percentage of cases of FUO in each of these three categories has shifted over time, reflecting a change in diagnostic capabilities and disease prevalence [6,11]. For example, many case series of FUO report a decrease in the incidence of FUO caused by neoplasm, likely caused in part by earlier diagnosis before the disease meets the criteria for FUO [6]. Other diseases that previously remained undiagnosed, such as Lyme disease, are now routinely diagnosed because of the use of a previously unavailable diagnostic test [12]. A comprehensive history and physical is the key to establishing a diagnosis in a patient with FUO. This article provides a systematic approach to the diagnosis of FUO by delineating the most important elements of a comprehensive history and physical. In addition, shared anecdotes are equally valuable (Dr. Donald Louria, MD, personal communication, 2007) and the body of this article and Box 1 contain numerous examples of causes of FUO encountered in practice, which in addition to providing an interesting example of a case of FUO serve further to exemplify the approach to diagnosis of FUO.

The history of presenting illness is of critical importance in the patient with FUO and is often difficult to obtain because many symptoms relevant to the diagnosis are vague, intermittent, or seemingly insignificant [13]. At times, the patient with FUO may have forgotten early events and recalls them only if specifically prodded. In some cases, it may be necessary on repeat history and physical examination literally to start with the hair and systematically move down the body to the toes (Dr. Donald Louria, MD, personal communication, 2007). In certain patient populations, notably elderly patients, no symptoms related to the underlying illness are elicited in the history of presenting illness. In the study by Esposito and Gleckman [14] of 111 patients greater than age 65 with FUO, intra-abdominal abscess was the most common infectious etiology of FUO; however, in 13 of 41 patients with this diagnosis no symptoms related to the abdomen were present [15]. In all patients, specific questions about constitutional symptoms including weight change, chills, and night sweats should be elicited. Questions should be asked about the true onset of symptoms, regardless of how mild or insidious. For example, in a patient with inflammatory bowel disease, bowel symptoms may be intermittent or be of such long standing as to be accepted as normal [16]. No symptom should be regarded as irrelevant, keeping in mind that it is well regarded that most patients with FUO exhibit atypical manifestations of common illnesses [2].

In addition to a comprehensive list of all previously documented medical conditions, the past medical history should include information about previously treated chronic infections, such as tuberculosis (TB), endocarditis, and rheumatic fever. Any prior diagnosis of cancer, no matter how remote, with specific information about timing and type of therapy should be listed. Prior surgery with specific information about type of surgery performed, postoperative complications, and any indwelling foreign materials should also be included. Questions about prosthetic devices should include

**Box 1. Clinical pearls for the diagnosis of fever
of unknown origin**

1. Alkaline phosphatase is the most important single laboratory test; may be elevated in temporal arteritis, hypernephroma, thyroiditis, tuberculosis.
2. Thrombocytosis >600,000 mm$^3$ suggests cancer or bone marrow disease and less often tuberculosis or infections with yeasts or fungi.
3. Nucleated red cells in the periphery in the absence of hemolysis suggests marrow invasion.
4. Free blood anywhere (pericardium, chest, abdomen, brain) can produce FUO and this may last for weeks, sometimes with rigors.
5. Rectus sheath hematoma can produce FUO or shock.
6. Trapezius soreness suggests subdiaphragmatic abscess.
7. Up to 20% of FUO cases may be caused by cytomegalovirus infection.
8. Fever, leukopenia, and palpable spleen in middle-aged men suggest either tuberculosis or lymphoma.
9. With granulomatous hepatitis, liver function studies may be normal; a liver biopsy or steroid trial may be needed.
10. Tumors may produce fever for many months or even up to 7 or more years.
11. Alcoholic hepatitis and hepatic cirrhosis can both be associated with low-grade or substantial fever (up to 104°F).
12. Juvenile rheumatoid arthritis should always be considered in adults, especially if arthralgias or myalgias are present. The erythrocyte sedimentation rate should be increased and there may be a transient rash. There may also be hepatosplenomegaly.
13. One or more liver abscesses can be present even with normal liver function tests. If they are small enough, sonograms and CT scans can be negative.
14. Pulmonary emboli with or without a positive chest radiograph is an important cause of FUO; even angiograms can be initially negative.
15. Bowel disease is an important cause of FUO; regional ileitis, colitis, and Whipple's disease all can present as an FUO.
16. Sinusitis must be considered as a cause of FUO; the history may be surprisingly negative.
17. In older patients with FUO, intra-abdominal infection should always be considered carefully; a bowel leak, subacute appendicitis, and cholecystitis may be very hard to diagnose.

18. Sarcoidosis can produce FUO if there is extensive central nervous system or lung involvement.
19. Tender cartilage on the nose, ear, or sternum with episcleritis and Raynaud's syndrome is polychondritis.
20. Pain on raising the arms over the head suggests Takayasu's disease.
21. Recurrent fever with erythema multiforme suggests herpes simplex.
22. Blindness, deafness, and central nervous system stupor suggests Whipple's disease.
23. Low-grade fever with anemia and abnormal liver function tests suggests Wilson's disease.
24. Recurrent fever with joint pain and petechial rash suggests chronic meningococcemia.
25. Recurrent shock and fever with abdominal trauma or sex suggests anaphylaxis caused by leaking echinococcus.
26. Postprostate resection with fever and progressive dementia suggests cryptococcus or tuberculosis.
27. Hectic fever, right upper quadrant tenderness, and elevated alkaline phosphatase suggest Charcot's fever.

prosthetic valves, indwelling venous catheters, pacemakers and implantable defibrillators, prosthetic joints, and cosmetic implants. Any history of psychiatric illness should be sought, because psychogenic or factitious fever is an important differential diagnosis. Prior history of intra-abdominal inflammatory conditions even without surgical intervention, such as cholecystitis or diverticulitis, should be sought. Information about recent inpatient or outpatient hospital stay is important for diagnosing nosocomial and iatrogenic causes of FUO.

A comprehensive list of all medications including over-the-counter and herbal remedies should be included. Drug fever is a well-documented cause of FUO and has been noted to occur with greater frequency in older patients and patients with HIV. Certain medications highly associated with drug fever are listed in Box 2. Drug fever can occur at any time during the course of drug therapy [17]. An absence of other signs of inflammation and relative bradycardia are seen with drug fever; however, relative bradycardia is a nonspecific finding in drug fever, and has been described in association with a selected number of specific infections as shown in Box 3. Typically, the fever resolves within 2 days of discontinuation of the drug and persistence of fever beyond 72 hours after the drug is removed allows one to conclude that the drug is not the offending agent in producing the fever [5]. It should be kept in mind, however, that the disappearance of fever is related to the rate of secretion of metabolites of drug from the body and with certain slowly

**Box 2. Commonly used medications that can cause fever of unknown origin**

*Antimicrobial agents*
Carbapenems
Cephalosporins
Minocycline HCl
Nitrofurantoin
Penicillins
Rifampin
Sulfonamides

*Anticonvulsants*
Barbiturates
Carbamazepine
Phenytoin

*Antihistamines*

*Cardiovascular drugs*
Hydralazine HCl
Procainamide HCl
Quinidine

*Histamine$_2$ blockers*
Cimetidine
Ranitidine HCl

*Iodides*

*Herbal remedies*

*Nonsteroidal anti-inflammatory drugs*
Ibuprofen
Sulindac
*Phenothiazines*
*Salicylates*

---

*From* Amin K, Kauffman C. Fever of unknown origin: a strategic approach to this diagnostic dilemma. Postgrad Med 2003;114:69–75; with permission.

metabolized agents may take up to 1 week to be completely eliminated [18]. Response of fever to naproxen has been shown in some case reports to be significant; specifically, fevers caused by solid tumors subside promptly, whereas fevers caused by other entities may persist [11].

A history of previous allergic reactions to medications may again point to a diagnosis of drug fever when a related agent is used. Multiple drug and

## Box 3. Physical clues to diagnosing fever of unknown origin

*Arthritis or joint pain*
Familial Mediterranean fever
Pseudogout
Rat-bite fever
Rheumatoid arthritis
Systemic lupus erythematosus
Lyme disease
Lymphogranuloma venereum
Whipple's disease
Brucellosis
Hyperimmunoglobulinemia D syndrome

*Band keratopathy*
Adult Still's disease
Adult juvenile rheumatoid arthritis
Sarcoidosis

*Bruit over spine*
Tumor
Arteriovenous fistula

*Calf tenderness*
Rocky Mountain spotted fever
Polymyositis
Pneumococcal bacteremia

*Conjunctivitis*
Tuberculosis
Cat-scratch disease
Systemic lupus erythematosus
*Chlamydia* infection
Histoplasmosis

*Conjunctival suffusion*
Leptospirosis
Relapsing fever
Rocky Mountain spotted fever

*Costo-vertebral angle tenderness*
Perinephric abscess
Chronic pyelonephritis

*Dry eyes*
Rheumatoid arthritis
Systemic lupus erythematosus

Periarteritis nodosa
Sjögren's syndrome

*Epididymo-orchitis*
Tuberculosis
Lymphoma
Brucellosis
Leptospirosis
Periarteritis nodosa
Infectious mononucleosis
Blastomycosis
Carcinoma

*Epistaxis*
Relapsing fever
Psittacosis
Rheumatic fever

*Heart murmur*
Subacute bacterial endocarditis
Atrial myxoma (changes with position)

*Hepatomegaly*
Lymphoma
Metastatic carcinoma
Alcoholic liver disease
Hepatoma
Relapsing fever
Granulomatous hepatitis
Q fever
Typhoid fever

*Lymphadenopathy*
Lymphoma
Cat-scratch fever
Tuberculosis
Lymphomogranuloma venereum
Epstein-Barr virus mononucleosis
Cytomegalovirus infection
Toxoplasmosis
HIV infection
Adult Still's disease
Brucellosis
Whipple's disease
Pseudolymphoma
Kikuchi's disease

*Orbital involvement*
Lymphoma
Metastatic carcinoma

*Relative bradycardia*
Typhoid fever
Malaria
Leptospirosis
Psittacosis
Central fever
Drug fever

*Rose spots*
Typhoid
Psittacosis

*Subconjunctival hemorrhage*
Endocarditis
Trichinosis

*Skin hyperpigmentation*
Whipple's disease
Hypersensitivity vasculitis
Hemochromatosis
Addison's disease

*Splenic abscess*
Subacute bacterial endocarditis
Brucellosis
Enteric fever

*Splenomegaly*
Leukemia
Lymphoma
Tuberculosis
Brucellosis
Subacute bacterial endocarditis
Cytomegalovirus infection
Epstein-Barr virus mononucleosis
Rheumatoid arthritis
Sarcoidosis
Psittacosis
Relapsing fever
Alcoholic liver disease
Typhoid fever

Rocky Mountain spotted fever
Kikuchi's disease

*Spinal tenderness*
Subacute vertebral osteomyelitis
Subacute bacterial endocarditis
Brucellosis
Typhoid fever

*Sternal tenderness*
Myeloproliferative diseases
Metastatic carcinoma (marrow invasion)
Brucellosis
Leukemia
Osteomyelitis

*Tender cartilage*
Raynaud's syndrome
Polychondritis
Cytomegalovirus infection

*Thigh tenderness*
Brucellosis
Polymyositis

*Thrombophlebitis*
Psittacosis

*Tongue tenderness*
Relapsing fever
Giant cell arteritis
Amyloidosis

*Trapezius tenderness*
Subdiaphragmatic abscess

*Uveal tract involvement*
Tuberculosis
Adult juvenile rheumatoid arthritis
Toxoplasmosis
Sarcoidosis
Systemic lupus erythematosus

*Uveitis*
Tuberculosis
Adult Still's disease
Sarcoidosis

Systemic lupus erythematosus
Behçet's syndrome

*Watery eyes*
Periarteritis nodosa

---

*Data from* References [13,19–21].

environmental allergies may identify an atopic individual in whom certain inflammatory diseases may be more likely. Finally, an allergy history in a patient with a seemingly unrelated and incongruous list of allergies may be the means to identify an underlying psychiatric disorder contributing to either factitious or psychogenic fever.

The portion of the history defined as the social history includes many important aspects of a patient's lifestyle that prove important in the diagnosis of FUO. Country of origin, prior countries of residence, and travel history provide important information about exposure to endemic diseases, such as malaria and histoplasmosis (Figs. 1 and 2). Specific questions should be asked about travel, with details about activities during travel and prophylactic medications and vaccinations; vaccination status; occupation and volunteer positions including history of contact with hospitalized patients, nursing home residents, or young children; recreational drug use; recreational

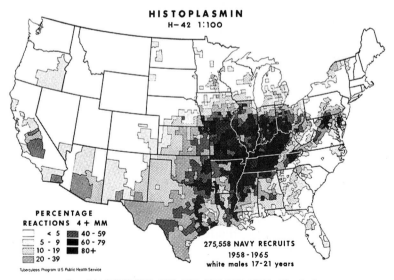

Fig. 1. Epidemiology of histoplasmosis. (*From* Mackowiak P, Durack D. Fever of unknown origin. In: Mandell, Douglas and Bennett's principles and practice of infectious diseases. 6th edition. Elsevier; 2005. p. 718–29; with permission.)

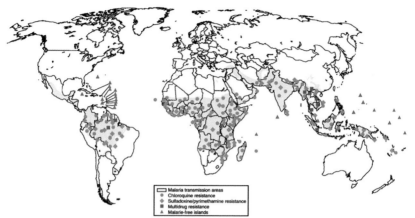

Fig. 2. Distribution of drug-resistant malaria. (*From* Mackowiak P, Durack D. Fever of unknown origin. In: Mandell, Douglas and Bennett's principles and practice of infectious diseases. 6th edition. Elsevier; 2005. p. 718–29; with permission.)

activities, such as gardening, swimming in lakes, or exploring caves; living conditions and prior episodes of homelessness, unusual dietary habits, such as consumption of unpasteurized dairy products or rare meats; pets; animal and tick exposure; fresh water exposure; and sexual activity. In patients with underlying immunologic compromise, questions about specific recent travel are of limited perspective. For example, a patient with HIV can present with FUO caused by disseminated histoplasmosis, even though the last travel to an endemic histoplasma geographic area was 10 or 15 years earlier (Dr. Donald Louria, MD, personal communication, 2007). Some examples of specific diagnoses that can be elicited in the social history are shown in Box 4.

The family history is important both for prior illnesses in family members, who may have a genetic link to the patient, and recent illnesses in family members to which the patient may have been exposed. Certain rare hereditary causes of FUO are listed in Table 2. Prior family history of cancer is important in considering an occult cancer in the patient. A history of current similar symptoms in a family member may represent a shared exposure.

The importance of a good physical examination is exemplified by the study in which positive physical findings were directly related to the diagnosis in 26 (59%) of 44 patients in whom the diagnosis was made [22]. It is important to note that in most cases in this study, repeated physical examinations were required before the findings pointing to the diagnosis were noted.

Much has been written about the measurement of fever and fever patterns in the diagnosis of FUO. Prior studies reveal that there is no significant relationship between the pattern of fever and diagnosis [23]. Certain generalizations can be made based on anecdotal reports, however, which provide some guidance in the work-up of a patient with an obscure cause of fever.

**Box 4. Historical clues to diagnosing fever of unknown origin**

*Abdominal pain*
Periarteritis nodosa
Familial Mediterranean fever
Relapsing fever

*Animal contact*
Psittacosis
Leptospirosis
Brucellosis
Toxoplasmosis
Cat-scratch disease
Q fever
Rat-bite fever

*Back pain*
Brucellosis
Subacute bacterial endocarditis
Enterococcal endocarditis, myeloma (in older patients)

*Cardiovascular accident*
Subacute bacterial endocarditis
Takayasu's arteritis
Periarteritis nodosa
Rocky Mountain spotted fever

*Chronic conjunctivitis*
Tuberculosis
Systemic lupus erythematosus
Polyarteritis nodosa
Cat-scratch disease
Sarcoidosis

*Fatigue*
Carcinoma
Lymphoma
Infectious mononucleosis
Typhoid fever
Systemic lupus erythematosus
Rheumatoid arthritis
Toxoplasmosis
Anicteric hepatitis

*Foul breath*
Lung abscess
Liver failure

Esophageal diverticulum
Renal failure

*Headache*
Malaria
Brucellosis
Relapsing fever
Rat-bite fever
Chronic meningitis-encephalitis
Malaria
Brucellosis
Central nervous system neoplasm
Rocky Mountain spotted fever

*Headache and myalgias*
Psittacosis
Q fever
Streptobacillary fever
Leptospirosis

*Medication and toxic substances*
Drug fever
Fume fever

*Mental confusion*
Sarcoid meningitis
Tuberculous meningitis
Cryptococcal meningitis
Carcinomatous meningitis
Central nervous system neoplasm
Brucellosis
Typhoid fever
HIV infection

*Myalgias*
Trichinosis
Subacute bacterial endocarditis
Periarteritis nodosa
Rheumatoid arthritis
Familial Mediterranean fever
Polymyositis
Juvenile rheumatoid arthritis

*Neck pain*
Subacute thyroiditis
Adult Still's disease

Temporal arteritis
Relapsing mastoiditis
Septic jugular phlebitis

*Nonproductive cough*
Tuberculosis
Q fever
Typhoid fever
Legionnaires' disease

*Tick exposure*
Relapsing fever
Rocky Mountain spotted fever
Lyme disease

*Vision disorders or eye pain*
Temporal arteritis
Subacute bacterial endocarditis
Relapsing fever
Brain abscess
Takayasu's arteritis

---

*Data from* References [13,19–21].

Diurnal variation is absent in 50% of noninfectious conditions associated with fever [23]. Double quotidian fever defined as two peaks in 24 hours is seen in 50% of cases of gonococcal endocarditis [23]. It has also been described in cases of leishmaniasis, malaria, miliary TB, and adult Still's disease [3]. A sustained fever occurs frequently in gram-negative pneumonia or severe central nervous system damage [19]. Pel-Ebstein fever, a daily fever that occurs for days to weeks then disappears and reappears later in the same pattern (Fig. 3), has been associated with Hodgkin's disease [15]. Periodic or relapsing fever is seen in malaria, lymphoma, borrelia, cyclic neutropenia, and rat-bite fever. An early morning fever spike has been described in TB, *Nocardia*, polyarteritis nodosa, brucellosis, and salmonellosis.

Other vital signs are important in the evaluation of FUO, specifically in relation to the presence of fever. Relative bradycardia, shown in Fig. 4, has been described in prior case reports in association with the following conditions: drug fever, leishmaniasis, typhoid fever, Legionnaire's disease, psittacosis, leptospirosis, brucellosis, and Kikuchi's disease. In general, the patient's blood pressure, pulse, and respiratory rate relative to the temperature are important in differentiating an acute infectious condition from a chronic indolent infectious or inflammatory condition or a long-standing noninfectious condition.

Table 2
Features of hereditary periodic fever syndromes

| | FMF | HIDS | TRAPS | Muckle-Wells syndrome |
|---|---|---|---|---|
| Age of onset | Variable <20–30 y | Mostly <1 y | Variable; mostly infancy or childhood | Infancy or childhood |
| Mode of inheritance (autosomal) | Recessive | Recessive | Dominant | Dominant |
| Chromosomal location of genetic defect | 16 p | 12 q | 12 q | 1 q |
| Duration of attacks | 1–4 d | 3–7 d | 1–3 wk | 1–2 d |
| Abdominal symptoms | | | | |
| Pains | + | ++ | + | + |
| Diarrhea | – | + | – | – |
| Chest pain | + | – | – | – |
| Skin involvement | Rather rare erysipelas-like (only below the knee) | ++ Macules, papules | ++ Painful erythematous patches (erysipelas-like) | ++ Urticaria |
| Arthralgia or arthritis | +/+ | +/+ | +/– | +/+ |
| Lymphadenopathy | – | + Cervical, inguinal, axillar, abdominal | + Cervical, inguinal, axillar | – |
| Splenomegaly | +/– | + (childhood) | – | + |
| Risk for amyloidosis | + | Very rare | Rare | + |
| Typical features | Testicular pain (prepubertal) | | Conjunctivitis, periorbital edema, testicular pain | Conjunctivitis, deafness later in life |
| Effective treatment | Colchicine | None | Corticosteroids | None |

*Abbreviations:* FMF, Familial Mediterranean fever; HIDS, hyperimmunoglobulin D and periodic fever syndrome; TRAPS, tumor necrosis factor receptor-1–associated periodic syndrome.

*From* Knockaert DC, Vanderschueren S, Blockmans D. Fever of unknown origin in adults: 40 years on. J Intern Med 2003;253:263–75; with permission.

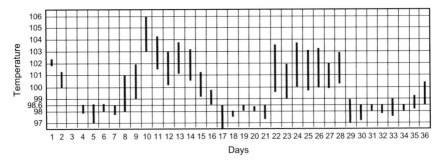

Fig. 3. Relative bradycardia (typhoid fever). (*From* Mackowiak P, Durack D. Fever of unknown origin. In: Mandell, Douglas and Bennett's principles and practice of infectious diseases. 6th edition. Elsevier; 2005. p. 718–29; with permission.)

The physical examination of a patient with FUO should be thorough and conducted in systematic manner with attention to all body systems. Many prior case series of FUO have established lists of physical examination findings and associated diagnosis of causes of FUO. A previously published comprehensive list is shown in Box 3. In general, physical findings that ultimately lead to a diagnosis of FUO can be categorized as follows: typical findings but an atypical presentation of a well-known disease, obscure physical findings that are pathognomonic for a particular disease, physical findings in areas that are not extensively examined in a routine physical examination, and common physical findings of common causes of FUO. Representative examples of each category are outlined next.

An atypical presentation of a well-known disease is commonly seen in cases of FUO: isolated lymphadenopathy as the only manifestation of disseminated TB; retroperitoneal lymphadenopathy in lymphoma that can easily be missed on physical examination; vascular findings (subconjunctival hemorrhages,

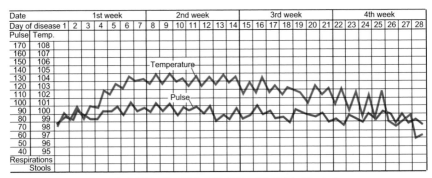

Fig. 4. Pel-Ebstein fever (Hodgkin's disease). (*From* Mackowiak P, Durack D. Fever of unknown origin. In: Mandell, Douglas and Bennett's principles and practice of infectious diseases. 6th edition. Elsevier; 2005. p. 718–29; with permission.)

Janeway lesions) in bacterial endocarditis; or bone pain or constitutional symptoms of metastatic cancer with no symptoms of the primary disorder.

Some obscure physical findings are so rare and yet so well associated with specific diseases as to be significant. Relative bradycardia as previously outlined is an important example. Some other examples include skin hyperpigmentation and Whipple's disease, a heart murmur that changes with position and atrial myxoma, choroid lesions of the eyes and TB, rose spots and salmonellosis, and Roth's spots and bacterial endocarditis.

Physical findings that can be easily missed on routine physical examination can point to a diagnosis of FUO when a careful and thorough examination is conducted [24]. Some specific areas as presented by Tumulty [25] include eye grounds, gums and oral cavity, clavicles, trapezius muscle, sternal tenderness, auscultation for bruits, rectal examination, testicular examination, and diaphragmatic mobility. Uveitis could be the only finding in autoimmune disease or cotton wool spots may be the only manifestation of cytomegalovirus disease in an immunocompromised patient. The list of eye findings and associated diseases is extensive as shown in Box 3 and Table 2. Poor oral hygiene can point to the diagnosis of infective endocarditis or lung abscess. Tongue pain can be indicative of temporal arteritis or infiltrative diseases, such as amyloid or sarcoid. Pain over the clavicles can be sign of localized painful lymph nodes caused by metastatic cancer from a remote location (gastrointestinal, ovarian). Pain over the trapezius muscle indicates an inflammatory process, which causes irritation of the diaphragm, such as a subdiaphragmatic abscess or pancreatic cancer. Sternal tenderness can be the result of anything that causes myeloproliferative changes of the bone marrow (metastatic tumor). Auscultation over the entire vascular system could elicit an occult vascular tumor or splenic infarct. Epididymitis can be seen as the only manifestation of disseminated TB. Sinus tenderness caused by chronic sinusitis can be easily overlooked if not examined specifically.

Some examples of common physical findings of well-known causes of FUO include temporal artery tenderness in temporal arteritis, diffuse lymphadenopathy in lymphoma, and heart murmur in bacterial endocarditis.

Despite changes in definition, categorization, and approach, FUO continues to exist as a diagnostic dilemma. In this condition, unlike many others, the successful diagnosis depends on a thorough history and physical examination rather than modern diagnostic procedures. Attention to detail, recognition of certain patterns, and disregarding nothing increases the chances of success. In addition, repetition of both history and physical examination is often necessary to arrive at a diagnosis in this very difficult endeavor.

## References

[1] Osler W. The study of the fevers of the south. J Am Med Assoc 1896;26(21):999–1004.
[2] Petersdorf R, Beeson P. Fever of unexplained origin: report on 100 cases. Medicine 1961;40: 1–30.

[3] Louria D. Fever of unknown etiology. Del Med J 1971;343–8.

[4] Larson E, Featherstone H, Petersdorf R. Fever of undetermined origin: diagnosis and follow-up of 105 cases, 1970-1980. Medicine 1982;61(5):269–93.

[5] Mourad O, Palda V, Detsky A. A comprehensive evidence-based approach to fever of unknown origin. Arch Intern Med 2003;163(5):545–51.

[6] Gaeta G, Fusco F, Nardiello S. Fever of unknown origin: a systematic review of the literature for 1995–2004. Nucl Med Commun 2006;27:205–11.

[7] Jitendranath L, Slim J. Work-up of fever of unknown origin in adult patients. Hosp Physician 2005;9–15.

[8] Mackowiak P, Durack D. Fever of unknown origin. In: Mandell, Douglas and Bennett's principles and practice of infectious diseases. 6th edition. Elsevier; 2005. p. 718–29.

[9] Durack D, Street A. Fever of unknown origin: reexamined and redefined. Curr Clin Top Infect Dis 1991;11:35–51.

[10] Bissuel F, Leport C, Perronne C, et al. Fever of unknown origin in HIV-infected patients: a critical analysis of a retrospective series of 57 cases. J Intern Med 1994;236(5):529–35.

[11] Arnow P. Fever of unknown origin. Lancet 1997;350:575–80.

[12] Kazanjian P. Fever of unknown origin: review of 86 patients treated in community hospitals. Clin Infect Dis 1992;15:968–73.

[13] Cunha B. Fever of unknown origin in the elderly. Geriatrics 1982;37(6):30–44.

[14] Esposito A, Gleckman R. A diagnostic approach to the adult with fever of unknown origin. Arch Intern Med 1979;139:575–9.

[15] Woolery W, Franco F. Fever of unknown origin: keys to determining the etiology in older patients. Geriatrics 2004;59(10):41–5.

[16] Jacoby G, Swartz M. Fever of undetermined origin. N Engl J Med 1973;289(26):1407–10.

[17] Amin K, Kauffman C. Fever of unknown origin: a strategic approach to this diagnostic dilemma. Postgrad Med 2003;114(3):69–75.

[18] Brusch J, Weinstein L. Fever of unknown origin. Med Clin North Am 1988;72(5):1247–59.

[19] Cunha B. Fever of unknown origin. In: Infectious diseases. 2nd edition. Philadelphia: WB Saunders; 1996. p. 1678–88.

[20] Cunha B. Fever of unknown origin. Infect Dis Clin North Am 1996;10(1):112–27.

[21] Knockaert DC, Vanderschueren S, Blockmans D. Fever of unknown origin in adults: 40 years on. J Intern Med 2003;253:263–75.

[22] Lohr J, Hendley J. Prolonged fever of unknown origin: a record of experiences with 54 childhood patients. Clin Pediatr (Phila) 1977;16(9):768–73.

[23] Musher D, Fainstein V, Young E, et al. Fever patterns: their lack of clinical significance. Arch Intern Med 1979;139:1225–8.

[24] Hirschmann J. Fever of unknown origin in adults. Clin Infect Dis 1997;24:291–302.

[25] Tumulty P. The patient with fever of undetermined origin: a diagnostic challenge. Johns Hopkins Med J 1967;120:95–106.

INFECTIOUS
DISEASE CLINICS
OF NORTH AMERICA

Infect Dis Clin N Am 21 (2007) 937–945

ELSEVIER
SAUNDERS

# Fever of Unknown Origin in Older Persons

Dean C. Norman, MD[a,b,*],
Megan Bernadette Wong, BS[b],
Thomas T. Yoshikawa, MD[a,b]

[a]*University of California, Los Angeles David Geffen School of Medicine,
Los Angeles, CA, USA*
[b]*VA Greater Los Angeles Healthcare System (11), 11301 Wilshire Boulevard,
Los Angeles, CA 90073, USA*

Infectious diseases in general in the aged are associated with higher morbidity and mortality rates. Decremental biologic changes with age affect host defenses and responses to infection, and the frequent presence of comorbidities also may adversely impact host defenses, especially in frail older persons [1]. Furthermore, the geriatric patient is more likely to be on multiple medications that in turn may diminish host defenses (eg, sedative hypnotics increase the risk of aspiration). Unfortunately, infections may present differently in older persons than in younger populations, making early diagnosis difficult. Delays in diagnosis and the initiation of appropriate therapy for this already-compromised population contribute to the observed higher morbidity and mortality rates.

Fever is the cardinal sign of infection, but this most important diagnostic clue may be blunted or absent in up to one third of infected geriatric patients. Conversely, the presence of fever has special significance for the older population. A large study of febrile adults presenting to walk-in clinics or emergency departments determined that the presence of fever in the elderly was much more likely to be associated with a serious bacterial or viral infection compared with younger febrile patients [2]. Similarly, the presence of a leukocytosis and/or bandemia in a geriatric patient is also

---

* Corresponding author. US Department of Veteran Affairs, West Los Angeles Health Care Center, 11301 Wilshire Boulevard, Los Angeles, CA 90073.

*E-mail address:* dean.norman@va.gov (D.C. Norman).

0891-5520/07/$ - see front matter © 2007 Elsevier Inc. All rights reserved.
doi:10.1016/j.idc.2007.09.003

*id.theclinics.com*

more likely to be associated with a serious infection, whether or not a fever is present [3,4].

Fever of unknown origin (FUO) in the old differs significantly from FUO in younger adults because the etiology is different. Moreover, it is important to aggressively determine the etiology of FUO in this older population because it is often treatable. Unfortunately, few FUO studies in adults distinctly separate data on patients 65 years and older. However, an extensive literature review of studies of adults with FUO estimated the overall prevalence of FUO in hospitalized patients to be 2.9% [5], and a prospective study of 167 hospitalized patients with FUO determined 28% of cases occurred in patients 65 years and older [6]. A more recent retrospective study of 165 adults hospitalized in a non-university hospital with FUO determined that 42.3% of the cases were 65 and older [7].

The traditional definition of FUO as a fever higher than 38.3°C (101°F) on several occasions over a period of at least 3 weeks and whose etiology remains undetermined after 1 week of intensive study in the hospital has been modified because of broad changes in medical practice. The move from inpatient to ambulatory care and the ready availability of a wide range of diagnostic tests and procedures available in the ambulatory-care setting allow for the effective and efficient evaluation of FUO as an outpatient. Newer definitions have removed the requirement for hospitalization and added obligatory diagnostic investigations after standardized history and physical examination fail to reveal the etiology a fever before it is identified as an FUO [8]. Even so, the traditional and newer definitions requiring a minimal temperature of 38.3°C may not be applicable to older patients. This is due to the blunted or absent febrile response to infection observed in this age group [9–11]. Numerous studies confirm that approximately 20% to 30% of infected geriatric patients will not mount a robust fever response to infection [9–13]. Examples include studies of bacteremia [14,15], endocarditis [16–18], pneumonia [19–23], tuberculosis [24], and meningitis [25], all of which demonstrate that infected older persons may present with diminished or no fever compared with younger adults. Of note, a more recent study of community-acquired bacterial meningitis did not confirm a difference in fever response between old and young adults. However, 16% of meningitis cases occurring in 267 adults over 60 years old did not present with a temperature greater than 38°C [26].

On the basis of the above studies and additional studies done by Castle and colleagues [27,28] that looked at baseline temperatures and changes in temperatures with infection in a nursing home population, the definition of fever in older persons should be changed. As baseline temperatures were found to be lower in the frail nursing home patients studied, the present authors recommend the new definition to be a persistent oral or tympanic membrane temperature of 99°F (37.2°C) or greater, or persistent rectal temperature of 99.5°F (37.5°C) or greater [9]. A fever would also be considered to be present if there is a change of temperature over baseline of 2.4°F or more (1.3°C). The clinician caring for frail elderly patients should be aware that any acute change in functional status may herald the onset of an infectious disease and, if associated with a change in temperature, increases the likelihood that an infection is present [10].

FUO in older persons differs from FUO in younger individuals both in etiology and because a diagnosis can be made in a higher percentage of cases. A precise etiologic diagnosis can be made in substantial majority of cases (over 70%) of older persons with FUO, whereas up to 51% of adults of all ages with FUO remain undiagnosed despite extensive work-up [7,8,29–31]. Table 1 summarizes these comparative data, including data from several decades, and supports the aggressive approach to investigating the etiology of FUO in older persons as many of the causative diseases are treatable.

In many cases, FUO in older persons may represent atypical, nonclassic presentations of common infectious and noninfectious diseases [32–34]. Similar to the frequency observed in young patients, infection is a common etiology of FUO in older persons and occurs in 15% to 35% of cases. There are differences in etiology of these infections between young and old, and tuberculosis is much more likely to be a cause of FUO in older persons than in the young. Tuberculosis, endocarditis, intraabdominal sepsis, and HIV infection in older patients may present particular diagnostic challenges.

As mentioned above, tuberculosis is a more common disease in the older patient with FUO than it is in younger patients with FUO, and it was

Table 1
Etiology of fever of unknown origin in older versus younger patients

| | Old[a] n (%) | Young[a] n (%) | Old n (%) | Young n (%) | All ages[b] n (%) |
|---|---|---|---|---|---|
| Total patients | 204 | 152 | 61 | 83 | 220 |
| Infections | 72 (35) | 33 (21) | 9 (15) | 24 (29) | 54 (25) |
| Viral | 1 (.05) | 8 (5) | — | — | 7 (3) |
| Tuberculosis | 20 (10) | 4 (3) | — | — | 4 (2) |
| Abscess | 25 (12) | 6 (4) | — | — | 6 (3) |
| Endocarditis | 14 (7) | 2 (1) | — | — | 5 (2) |
| Other | 12 (6) | 13 (9) | — | — | 32 (15) |
| Noninfectious inflammatory diseases | 57 (28)[c] | 27(17)[c] | 22 (36) | 16 (19) | 52 (24) |
| Neoplasms | 38 (19) | 8 (5) | 9 (15) | 5 (6) | 31 (14) |
| Miscellaneous | 17 (8) | 39 (26) | 3 (5) | 19 (23) | 17 (8) |
| No diagnosis | 18 (9) | 45 (29) | 18 (30) | 19 (23) | 66 (30) |

[a] Includes subjects from the 1970s to the 1980s.

[b] Includes cases from the late 1980s to the early 1990s.

[c] In descending order of frequency: temporal arteritis, polymyalgia rheumatica, Wegener's granulomatosis, polyarteritis nodosa, rheumatoid arthritis, and sarcoidosis.

*Data from* de Kleijn E, van der Meer J. Fever of unknown origin (FUO): report on 53 patients in a Dutch university hospital. Neth J Med 1995;47:54–60.

responsible for 50% of infections in the older age group in a recent review of FUO comparing old and young FUO patients [35]. A more recent prospective study of 94 FUO patients reported from Taiwan found that tuberculosis was the cause of FUO in 23% of cases overall and was more likely to be present in older FUO patients [36]. In another prospective comparison study of tuberculosis, elderly patients were significantly less likely to have fever, hemoptysis, cough, and a positive response to 5TU purified protein derivative skin test, but were more likely to have disseminated disease [24]. Finally, in a large prevalence study of tuberculosis in nursing homes in Hong Kong, only 3 of 15 active tuberculosis cases had any classical symptoms, confirming again that atypical presentations of infectious diseases are especially likely to occur in frail older persons [37].

Infective endocarditis in the old, as compared with younger patients, is characterized by less severe clinical symptoms (eg, blunted or absent fever) and may present with vague, nonspecific constitutional symptoms such as lethargy, malaise, anorexia, and weight loss. Early use of transesophageal echocardiography facilitates timely diagnosis and may reduce diagnostic delays [17,18]. Obviously, any heart murmur in an older FUO patient should lead to the consideration that endocarditis is present; diagnostic echocardiography should be performed. Similar to endocarditis, intra-abdominal infections may present in a nonspecific manner. Even mild symptoms and findings (minimal tenderness and distention) may indicate an intra-abdominal infection, and early imaging (ultrasound, abdominal computed tomography) should be considered in these cases [38,39]. HIV infection may occur in older persons, and it is estimated that over 10% of new cases of HIV infection occur in adults over age 50. HIV should eventually be considered if no other etiology of FUO is found, but should be considered earlier if the history of sexual activity becomes a potential diagnostic clue [40].

Noninfectious inflammatory diseases such as temporal arteritis, rheumatoid arthritis, and polymyalgia rheumatica are common causes of FUO in the old, but are seen less frequently in younger adults with FUO (see Table 1). Noninfectious inflammatory diseases are at least second to infection as a cause of FUO in several FUO studies and are responsible for 25% to 36% of FUO cases in older persons (see Table 1, [35]). Conversely, FUO will occur in approximately 10% of temporal arteritis cases. A new localized headache, temporal artery abnormality (decreased pulse, tenderness or nodules), asthenia, anorexia, or weight loss is a typical clinical feature of this disease [41]. An elevated erythrocyte sedimentation rate, especially if at or above 50 mm per hour Westergren or a high C-reactive protein, provide additional diagnostic clues that should lead to prompt confirmatory temporal artery biopsy. Polymyalgia rheumatica, typically characterized by pain involving neck and shoulder girdle, is also associated with a high erythrocyte sedimentation rate and commonly coexists with temporal arteritis [41].

Finally, malignancies, usually hematological in origin, account for a significant percentage of cases of FUO in older persons (see Table 1, [29,31]).

Although unintentional weight loss in an older patient might suggest the presence of a neoplasm, unintentional weight loss commonly occurs with a variety of afflictions affecting older patients, including depression, dementia, chronic disease, or as an adverse drug reaction.

### Diagnostic approach to the older patient with fever of unknown origin

A complete history and physical examination are still an important part of the assessment of any older patient. Potential diagnostic clues to the etiology of an FUO should be elucidated to narrow the potential diagnoses and focus on further laboratory and imaging work-up. Any recent clinical changes should be explored even if the patient considers these symptoms to be part of "getting old" (eg, new onset or change in chest pain in an immobile patient should lead to the consideration of pulmonary embolism as a cause of FUO). Historical data should be obtained from a variety of sources, even if the patient appears to be cognitively intact. Family members, caregivers, and others where appropriate should be interviewed and all medical records reviewed. Records from allied health professionals should also be read because key information on functional status, nutrition, and skin integrity may be revealed. Nonspecific findings such as weight loss, depression, or "failure-to-thrive" symptoms could indicate hyperthyroidism—an entity that has a very different presentation in the older patient compared with the younger adult and may also be a cause of FUO.

The list of drugs capable of causing FUO is extensive, and it should be assumed that any drug or drug combination is capable of causing fever in older persons. Therefore, a detailed medication history that includes alcohol and illicit drug use, dietary supplements, and over-the-counter medications should be obtained. Noncompliance with medications is common in older persons, and reconciliation between what a patient is prescribed and what he or she is actually taking, including determining the actual dosage and frequency of administration, is necessary. The patient should be queried about pet and occupational exposure and given the easy availability of drugs for treatment of erectile dysfunction; a sexual activities history is mandatory. Late infections of implanted devices may occur in older persons, and inquiries should also be made about the presence of any implants such as artificial heart valves, joint replacements, and vascular grafts.

The physical examination should include a neurological examination and an assessment of cognitive function with the Mini-Mental State Examination or an equivalent test. As mentioned above, temporal arteritis is a possible cause of FUO in the older patient, and the temporal arteries should be carefully inspected and palpated for thickening, tenderness, and nodules. Occult dental or periodontal infection may be also be a cause of FUO, and the condition of the dentition should be determined, including the gentle tapping over of teeth to elicit pain. As noted above, intra-abdominal infection may present in a subtle, nonspecific fashion [38,39], and thus the entire abdomen should be carefully palpated. Digital rectal examination should be part of the physical examination to examine the prostate for bogginess, tenderness, or nodules that could indicate inflammatory disease of the prostate as a potential etiology of FUO. Patients with limited mobility are susceptible to skin breakdown and should undergo a skin examination. The clinician caring for an older immobile FUO patient should do his or her own examination. The sacrum and heels should be examined carefully and, as small sacral ulcers may be missed in obese patients, obese patients should be turned over and the skin examined. The extremities should be observed for the presence of phlebitis, especially in hospitalized patients with intravenous catheters, and the lower extremities should be examined for the presence of deep venous thrombosis. Palpation of the muscles of the shoulder girdle for tenderness and or observation of pain on motion may indicate polymyalgia rheumatica. The physical examination should be repeated at intervals to ascertain whether new physical findings develop over time (eg, a new heart murmur) [42].

## Laboratory and imaging studies

Patients with FUO by definition have already undergone a basic diagnostic assessment that minimally would include standard laboratory testing and imaging, as used as erythrocyte sedimentation rate, C-reactive protein, repeated blood cultures, and a chest radiograph. Additional testing would depend on clues derived from the history and physical examination. Before additional costly evaluation is undertaken, consideration should be given to first eliminating nonessential drugs and, if necessary, even essential drugs should be discontinued one by one as deemed clinically appropriate. Usually the fever, if the drug is the cause, resolves within a few days of discontinuance [43].

If no diagnostic clues are elucidated, further testing would next include an abdominal ultrasound and, if negative, computed CT of the abdomen and chest. An ultrasound should be also performed directed at any prosthetic devices or implant that the FUO patient might have. Many older persons have systolic heart murmurs secondary to aortic valve sclerosis, and thus transthoracic followed by transesophageal echocardiography should be strongly considered in older FUO patients with any murmur, even if no other diagnostic clues point toward the possibility of endocarditis.

Finally, one study determined that when potential diagnostic clues are found, nuclear medicine scans may be helpful in localizing inflammation [44]. A recent FUO study found that a potential cause for the FUO could be found in 12 of 19 patients (67%) with nuclear scanning. Indium-111labeled–granulocyte scintigraphy was superior to fluorine-18-fluorodeoxyglucose (FDG) positron emission tomography (PET) because FDG-PET was associated with a much higher false-positive rate [45]. Another study demonstrated FDG-PET to be clinically helpful in 37% of FUO cases where no diagnostic clues were apparent [46]. Performing FDG-PET before abdominal and chest CT has been suggested by the authors of a recent prospective study on FUO [8].

Finally, in occasional cases when diagnostic clues include abnormal liver function tests or indicate blood cell abnormalities, liver and bone marrow biopsy, respectively, should be considered if other, less invasive tests are inconclusive.

## Therapy of fever of unknown origin

A trial of antibiotics should be discouraged in older FUO patients except where there is rapid clinical deterioration. An empiric trial of corticosteroids may be initiated even before obtaining a temporal artery biopsy when temporal arteritis is a strong consideration. Corticosteroids may be held in stable patients pending biopsy results.

A prospective study of 61 FUO patients discharged from the hospital without an etiologic diagnosis and followed for a mean of 5.8 years found that fevers resolved in most patients. The age range of these study participants was between 16 years and 75 years, and a diagnosis was eventually made in 12 patients during the follow-up period; all were successfully treated. Although 10% of the cases died during the follow-up period, it was determined that only in two cases (3%) was death thought to have resulted from the disease causing the FUO [47]. A later retrospective study found that in 78% of 37 patients with FUO and no diagnosis, fever resolved after several months (only five of these cases received a trial of antibiotics) [7]. A more recent prospective study found 41% of 51 patients with FUO and no diagnosis either spontaneously recovered or their fevers resolved with nonsteroidal anti-inflammatory agents. Only one death occurred in the 12-month median follow-up period [8].

## References

[1] Yoshikawa TT. Epidemiology and special aspects of infectious diseases in aging. In: Yoshikawa TT, Ouslander JG, editors. Infection management for geriatrics in long-term care facilities. 2nd edition. New York: Informa Healthcare; 2007. p. 15–9.
[2] Keating MJ III, Klimek JJ, Levine DS, et al. Effect of aging on the clinical significance of fever in ambulatory adult patients. J Am Geriatr Soc 1984;32:282–7.
[3] Wasserman M, Levinstein M, Keller E, et al. Utility of fever, white blood cell, and differential count in predicting bacterial infections in the elderly. J Am Geriatr Soc 1989;37:534–43.
[4] Gur H, Aviram R, Or J, et al. Unexplained fever in the ED. Analysis of 139 patients. Am J Emerg Med 2003;21:230–5.
[5] Mourad O, Palda V, Detsky AS. A comprehensive evidence-based approach to fever of unknown origin. Arch Intern Med 2003;163(5):545–51.

[6] de Kleijn E, Vandenbroucke JP, van der Meer J. Fever of unknown origin (FUO): I. A prospective multicenter study of 167 patients with FUO, using fixed epidemiologic entry criteria. Medicine (Baltimore) 1997;76(6):392–400.

[7] Zenone T. Fever of unknown origin in adults: evaluation of 144 cases in a non-university hospital. Scand J Infect Dis 2006;38:632–8.

[8] Bleeker-Rovers CP, Vos FJ, de Kleijn E, et al. A prospective multicenter study on fever of unknown origin. The yield of a structured diagnostic protocol. Medicine 2007;86(1): 26–38.

[9] Norman DC. Fever and fever of unknown origin in the elderly. Clin Infect Dis 2000;31(1): 148–51.

[10] Norman DC. Clinical manifestations of infection. In: Yoshikawa TT, Ouslander JG, editors. Infection management for geriatrics in long-term care facilities. 2nd edition. New York: Informa Helathcare; 2007. p. 105–14.

[11] Norman DC. Fever of unknown origin in older persons. In: Cunha Burke A, editor. Fever of unknown origin, editor. New York: Informa Healthcare; 2007. p. 109–14.

[12] Jones SR. Fever in the elderly. In: Machowiak P, editor. Fever: basic mechanisms and management. New York: Raven Press; 1991. p. 233–41.

[13] Norman DC, Yoshikawa TT. Fever in the elderly. In: Cunha BA, editor. Fever: infectious disease clinics of North America. Philadelphia: W.B. Saunders Company; 1996. p. 93–101.

[14] Bryant RE, Hood AF, Hood CE, et al. Factors affecting mortality of gram-negative rod bacteremia. Arch Intern Med 1971;127:120–7.

[15] Gleckman R, Hibert D. Afebrile bacteremia: a phenomenon in geriatric patients. JAMA 1981;248:1478–81.

[16] Terpenning MS, Buggy BO, Kauffman CA. Infective endocarditis: clinical features in young and elderly patients. Am J Med 1987;83:626–34.

[17] Werner GS, Schulz R, Fuchs JB, et al. Infective endocarditis in the elderly in the era of transesophageal echocardiography: clinical features and prognosis compared with younger patients. Am J Med 1996;100:90–7.

[18] Dhawan VK. Infective endocarditis in elderly patients. Clin Infect Dis 2002;34:806–12.

[19] Finklestein MS, Petkun WM, Freedman ML, et al. Pneumococcal bacteremia in adults: age-dependent differences in presentation and in outcome. J Am Geriat Soc 1983;31:19–27.

[20] Marrie TJ, Haldane EV, Faulkner RS, et al. Community-acquired pneumonia requiring hospitalization: is it different in the elderly? J Am Geriatr Soc 1985;33:671–80.

[21] Fernandez-Sabe N, Carratala J, Roson B, et al. Community-acquired pneumonia in very elderly patients: causative organisms, clinical characteristics and outcomes. Medicine (Baltimore) 2003;82(3):159–69.

[22] Metlay J, Schulz R, Li YH, et al. Influence of age on symptoms at presentation in patients with community-acquired pneumonia. Arch Intern Med 1997;157(13):1453–9.

[23] Roghmann MC, Warner J, Mackowiak PA. The relationship between age and fever magnitude. Am J Med Sci 2001;322(2):68–70.

[24] Korzeniewska-Kosela M, Krysl J, Muller N, et al. Tuberculosis in young adults and the elderly: a prospective comparison. Chest 1994;106(n1):28–33.

[25] Gorse GJ, Thrupp LD, Nudleman KL, et al. Bacterial meningitis in the elderly. Arch Intern Med 1984;144:1603–7.

[26] Weisfelt M, van de Beek D, Spaniaard L, et al. Community-acquired bacterial meningitis in older people. J Am Geriatr Soc 2006;54(10):1500–7.

[27] Castle SC, Yeh M, Toledo S, et al. Lowering the temperature criterion improves detection of infections nursing home residents. Aging Immunology and Infectious Diseases 1993;4: 67–76.

[28] Castle SC, Yeh M, Norman DC, et al. Fever response in the elderly: are the older truly colder? J Am Geriatr Soc 1991;39:853–7.

[29] Esposito AL, Gleckman RA. Fever of unknown origin in the elderly. J Am Geriatr Soc 1978; 26:498–505.

[30] Berland B, Gleckman RA. Fever of unknown origin in the elderly: a sequential approach to diagnosis. Postgrad Med 1992;92:197–210.

[31] Knockaert DC, Vanneste LJ, Bobbaers HJ. Fever of unknown origin in elderly patients. J Am Geriatr Soc 1993;41:1187–92.

[32] Smith KY, Bradley SF, Kauffman CA. Fever of unknown origin in the elderly: lymphoma presenting as vertebral compression fractures. J Am Geriatr Soc 1994;42:88–92.

[33] Agmon-Levin N, Ziv-Sokolovsky N, Shull P, et al. Carcinoma of colon presenting as fever of unknown origin. Am J Med Sci 2005;329(4):322–6.

[34] Karachaliou IG, Karachalios GN, Kanakis KV, et al. Fever of unknown origin due to dental infections: case reports and review. Am J Med Sci 2007;333(2):109–11.

[35] Tal S, Guller V, Gurevich A, et al. Fever of unknown origin in the elderly. J Intern Med 2002; 252(4):295–304.

[36] Chin C, Lee S, Chen Y, et al. Mycobacteriosis in patients with fever of unknown origin. J Microbiol Immunol Infect 2003;36:248–53.

[37] Chan-Yeung M, Chan F, Cheung A, et al. Prevalence of tuberculosis infection and active tuberculosis in old age homes in Hong Kong. J Am Geriatr Soc 2006;54:1334–40.

[38] Norman DC, Yoshikawa TT. Intra-abdominal infection: diagnosis and treatment in the elderly patient. Gerontology 1984;30:327–38.

[39] Potts FE, Vukov LF. Utility of fever and leukocytosis in acute surgical abdomens in octogenarians and beyond. J Gerontol A Biol Sci Med Sci 1999;54(2):M55–8.

[40] Zanjani F, Saboe K, Oslin D. Age difference in rates of mental health/substance abuse and behavioral care in HIV-positive adults. AIDS Patient Care STDs 2007;21(5):347–55.

[41] Gonzalez-Gay MA, Garcia-Porrua C, Miranda-Filloy JA, et al. Giant cell arteritis and polymyalgia rheumatica. Pathophysiology and management. Drugs Aging 2006;23(8):627–49.

[42] Amin K, Kauffman C. Fever of unknown origin. Postgrad Med 2003;114(3):69–76.

[43] Arnow PM, Flaherty JP. Fever of unknown origin [review article]. Lancet 1997;350:575–80.

[44] de Kleijn E, van Lier J, van der Meer J. Fever of unknown origin (FUO): II. Diagnostic procedures in a prospective multicenter study of 167 patients. Medicine (Baltimore) 1997; 76(6):401–14.

[45] Kjaer A, Lebech AM, Eigtved A, et al. Fever of unknown origin: prospective comparison of diagnostic value of [18]F-FDG PET and [111]In-granulocyte scintigraphy. Eur J Nucl Med Mol Imaging 2004;31(5):622–6.

[46] Bleeker-Rovers CP, de Kleijn E, Corstens F, et al. Clinical value of FDG PET in patients with fever of unknown origin and patients suspected of focal infection or inflammation. Eur J Nucl Med Mol Imaging 2004;31(1):29–37.

[47] Knockaert DC, Dujardin KS, Bobbars HJ. Long-term follow-up of patients with undiagnosed fever of unknown origin. Arch Intern Med 1996;156(6):618–20.

ELSEVIER
SAUNDERS

INFECTIOUS
DISEASE CLINICS
OF NORTH AMERICA

Infect Dis Clin N Am 21 (2007) 947–962

# Fever of Unknown Origin Caused by Tuberculosis

Jason J. Bofinger, MD[a],
David Schlossberg, MD, FACP[b,c,*]

[a]Section of Infectious Diseases, Temple University Hospital, Parkinson Pavilion,
Fifth Floor, 3401 North Broad Street, Philadelphia, PA 19140, USA
[b]Division of Infectious Diseases, Temple University School of Medicine, PA, USA
[c]Tuberculosis Control Program, Philadelphia Department of Public Health,
500 South Broad Street, Philadelphia, PA 19146, USA

Case report: A 75-year-old woman developed fever, night sweats, and cough. Four months before admission she began taking prednisone, 20 mg/day, because of a hypoplastic bone marrow complicated by anemia and thrombocytopenia. After 4 months she noticed fever, night sweats, and a nonproductive cough. Evaluation at that time was unremarkable, although her erythrocyte sedimentation rate was 128/min. One month later, she was still febrile and reported chills; her chest radiograph at that time showed generalized nodules. Tuberculosis (TB) was suspected, and after a bone-marrow aspirate for smear and culture, empiric anti-TB therapy was begun. One month later, the marrow sample grew *Mycobacterium tuberculosis*; 2 weeks after that, the patient died [1].

The year of this case report was 1962, and the patient was Eleanor Roosevelt. The year before her illness, the seminal article on fever of unknown origin (FUO) had been published by Petersdorf and Beeson [2], and her physicians were aware of the entity and of the importance of TB as a cause. Although Mrs. Roosevelt's death from TB was widely known, and speculation about a missed diagnosis was rampant, it is not generally known that her isolate eventually was shown to be resistant to the anti-TB medications she received (isoniozid and streptomycin) for the 6 weeks before her death. This article discusses TB as a cause of FUO. At the end of the article, the Roosevelt case is revisited to see if enough has been learned in the intervening 45 years to prevent similar outcomes.

* Corresponding author. Tuberculosis Control Program, Philadelphia Department of Public Health, 500 South Broad Street, Philadelphia, PA 19146.
*E-mail address:* dschloss@ix.netcom.com (D. Schlossberg).

0891-5520/07/$ - see front matter © 2007 Elsevier Inc. All rights reserved.
doi:10.1016/j.idc.2007.08.001 *id.theclinics.com*

The major causes of FUO have traditionally been infection, malignancy, rheumatologic disorders, and a variety of miscellaneous causes. The relative contribution of each category fluctuates with geography, patient age, and immunocompetence. In parts of the world as disparate as Taiwan, Tokyo, Jordan, and Turkey, TB remains a common cause of FUO [3–6]. Regardless of its frequency, however, TB should always be considered in the differential diagnosis of this entity because of its treatability.

The concept of FUO was first defined by Petersdorf and Beeson in 1961 [2] as fever greater than 38.3°C (101°F) on several occasions, lasting for more than 3 weeks, the cause of which is uncertain despite 1 week of in-hospital evaluation. More recently, reflecting modern medicine's emphasis on outpatient management and the higher pace of in-hospital investigation, this classic definition of FUO has been modified. The hospital is no longer a necessary setting, and the required duration of investigation is now generally accepted as either three outpatient visits or 3 days of hospitalization. Because this recent modification is the most inclusive, it is used in this article and also includes the subgroups of FUO, such as nosocomial, immune-deficient, HIV-associated, and episodic FUO, a fluctuating pattern of fever with afebrile intervals of 2 weeks or more [7–9].

## Epidemiology

The most recent incidence data from the Centers for Disease Control and Prevention [10] indicate 4.6 incident cases of TB per 100,000 population reported in the United States in 2006, which represents a 3.2% decline from 2005. The TB incidence in 2006 was the lowest recorded since 1953, when recording began, but the rate of decline has slowed since the year 2000. The average annual percentage decline in the TB incidence rate was 7.3% per year in the period 1993 to 2000, but only 3.8% per year in the period 2000 to 2006. Another trend involves the forms of TB being reported: although the total number of cases of TB in the United States is declining, extrapulmonary TB is decreasing much less rapidly and accounts for approximately 20% of all reported cases [11,12].

In certain patients with FUO, TB should be high on the differential diagnosis because of susceptibility to infection (eg, travelers, diabetics, foreign-born); likelihood of disseminated infection (eg, HIV-AIDS and other immune deficiency, young children, renal failure); and atypical manifestations of infection (eg, children, elderly, HIV-AIDS). Some of these patient groups have more than one reason to suspect TB (eg, elderly patients have both a greater prevalence of TB and are more likely to manifest atypical manifestations of disease). Additional patients in whom TB should always be considered include the homeless; residents or employees of high-risk congregate settings; and patients with malignancy, malnutrition, alcoholism, gastrectomy, and silicosis. Specific patient groups whose risk for TB is particularly high or recently appreciated, or in whom TB is often clinically atypical, are discussed later. FUO in the elderly often results from an atypical presentation of a common disease. Infection is the etiology in 25% to 35%, with TB occurring much more commonly in the elderly than in younger patients with FUO [13]. In one study [14], TB was found in 12% of elderly patients with FUO, compared with 2% of younger patients. In this study, TB accounted for 50% of all infections in the elderly. In another series of elderly patients in Turkey [15], TB was the most common cause of FUO, prompting these investigators to recommend empiric anti-TB therapy in this setting.

Elderly adults are at increased risk for reactivation TB, and they frequently present with atypical symptoms and radiographic findings; hemoptysis, night sweats, and positive purified protein derivative (PPD) are all less common than in younger patients. In the experience of Korzeniewska-Kosela and colleagues [16] the PPD was positive in 86.2% of young adults with TB, but in only 67.6% of elderly patients; this difference was attributed to age-related impairment of T-cell function. In older age groups, pleural effusion may be the sole manifestation of disease, and miliary TB is more common than in younger patients [13]. Dialysis patients are at risk for developing TB because of depressed cellular immunity. Negative PPDs have been observed in 60% to 100% of cases, and extrapulmonary disease, mainly miliary and lymphadenopathic, has been observed in 30% to 90% [8]. Fever can be episodic or recurrent. TB should be strongly considered as a cause of FUO in dialysis patients, and some investigators recommend empiric treatment for this group [17].

Diabetes is a known risk for TB. Although the overall clinical presentation resembles that of nondiabetics, diabetic patients often develop atypical radiographic patterns, particularly lower lobe disease and multilobar infiltrates [18].

Foreign-born persons in the United States are affected disproportionately by TB. In 2006, the TB rate among foreign-born persons was 9.5 times greater than that of their United States–born counterparts. More than half the cases were in persons from five countries: Mexico, the Philippines, Vietnam, India, and China. TB lymphadenitis seems to be particularly common in these groups, especially in patients from Asia [11].

As world travel increases, so does the risk of infection, especially TB. The greatest TB risk for travelers is in those visiting friends or relatives. Such nontourist travel is now a recognized TB risk factor for children and a reason to screen for latent tuberculous infection [19–22]. The mechanics of travel may also expose individuals to TB, particularly airline travel, because of the possibility of close confinement with a contagious patient. Like other airborne infections, TB has been transmitted on airplanes by the droplet nuclei, which remain airborne indefinitely; in-flight transmission risk is proportionate to the duration of the flight, in that flights less than 8 hours have not been associated with acquisition of TB infection. Because air exchange is usually efficient, especially when planes are airborne, risk is also proportionate to a traveler's proximity to an infectious patient. Overall, however, the risk to the air traveler is low, and no cases of TB disease (as opposed to infection) have been documented as a result of air travel [23].

Immunosuppressed patients are at increased risk for reactivation of TB. In patients immunosuppressed because of HIV infection, TB often presents as extrapulmonary and disseminated disease, which often obscures the diagnosis and explains its relatively frequent presentation as an FUO [24]. A related phenomenon, the immune-reconstitution inflammatory syndrome, is the development of symptomatic TB as a result of improving immune status. Such improvement may result during treatment of TB, in which case immune-reconstitution inflammatory syndrome may present as TB in previously unsuspected anatomic sites or as an exacerbation of a known site of involvement. Alternatively, immune-reconstitution inflammatory syndrome may present as the initial manifestation of TB in a patient whose immune reconstitution results from antiretroviral therapy. In this manner, the initiation of highly active antiretroviral therapy may be followed by previously unsuspected TB in a patient with no history or indication of prior tuberculous infection.

HIV-negative patients who are immunosuppressed because of underlying disease or of iatrogenic immunosuppression are also at risk for reactivation of TB. Administration of corticosteroids has traditionally been associated with TB, with the risk increasing with the dose and duration of corticosteroid therapy. From an epidemiologic standpoint, the minimal dose associated with increased risk is prednisone or its equivalent, 15 mg/day for greater than 2 weeks; this is the level at which targeted testing for latent TB is recommended. Lower doses and intermittent doses may not have the associated risk, and higher doses for prolonged duration seem to have a stronger association, but specific thresholds have not been established [25].

Recently, tumor necrosis factor-$\alpha$ inhibitors have been recognized as increasing the risk for reactivation of TB and other infections characterized by a granulomatous response. The risk for TB seems greater with infliximab than with etanercept, possibly because of different mechanisms of action: infliximab is an anti–tumor necrosis factor monoclonal antibody, whereas etanercept is a soluble, tumor necrosis factor–neutralizing tumor necrosis factor receptor fusion molecule. Infliximab and adalimumab (another monoclonal antibody) reduce TB-responsive CD4 cells and suppress antigen-induced interferon-$\gamma$ production, whereas no such effect was seen by etanercept; the infliximab risk may result from the combined effect on both tumor necrosis factor and interferon-$\gamma$. In the murine model of TB, chronic infection was controlled in mice given the receptor fusion molecule, whereas the anti–tumor necrosis factor antibody produced early mortality; the difference was attributed to less penetration into the granulomata by the receptor fusion molecule [26–28].

Multiple categories of transplant recipients are at risk for TB because of iatrogenic immunosuppression. Liver transplant recipients are well-known to be at risk, and some have advocated treatment of latent tuberculous infection in PPD-positive patients during their candidacy period [29]. Heart-lung transplants with reactivated TB frequently develop extrapulmonary disease [30]. Some observers have noted a high mortality among this patient population if TB is not identified and treated pretransplant [31]. Renal transplant patients with TB also have a predisposition for extrapulmonary reactivation; most cases appear after the first year, with a mean elapsed time of 38 months [32].

## Clinical presentations

The clinical forms of TB that most commonly present as FUO are those that feature nonspecific signs and symptoms and are difficult to diagnose. Disseminated disease without the characteristic miliary pattern on chest radiograph or extrapulmonary disease without clear localizing features are the most frequent presentations [7]. Bacteriologic confirmation of extrapulmonary disease can be difficult because the affected body sites are often relatively inaccessible to diagnostic instruments. Moreover, even though there may be extensive tissue damage, affected tissues are typically paucibacillary, reducing the sensitivity of both acid-fast bacilli (AFB) smear and culture [33].

Some patients with FUO caused by TB have fever that is described as "intermittent" or "recurrent." One group of such patients had a median duration of symptoms of 5 months, with febrile episodes ranging in duration from a few hours to 1 week. Constitutional symptoms and abdominal pain were the most commonly associated complaints [8]. Other temperature patterns that have been associated with TB (with varying degree of documentation in the literature) are temperature-pulse dissociation, or relative bradycardia, reversal of the normal diurnal variation, and double quotidian fever: two temperature spikes per day. Along with these various fever patterns, TB has traditionally been associated with night sweats, but there are many other causes of this phenomenon, including infectious and noninfectious etiologies and numerous medications.

Disseminated or miliary TB is TB that has entered the bloodstream. Its presence can be suggested by a miliary pattern on chest radiograph or inferred by documented involvement of bone marrow, liver, or two or more noncontiguous anatomic sites. The exact incidence of miliary TB is unclear. Symptoms are nonspecific and can mimic a variety of diseases, which often leads to delayed or missed diagnosis. In reported series of autopsied cases, from 33% to 80% of diagnoses had been missed antemortem. Misdiagnosis has grave implications: treatment delay of even 1 to 8 days apparently contributes to the high mortality rate [34]. This observation, plus the inherent delay in diagnosing TB, stresses the importance of empiric treatment in ill patients in whom disseminated TB is suspected but not yet confirmed.

In a retrospective review from Taiwan [34], over half of patients who fulfilled the criteria for disseminated TB had underlying comorbidities, most commonly AIDS (14%) and diabetes (14%), followed by malignancy, end-stage renal disease, cirrhosis, organ transplant, autoimmune disease, and alcoholism. The presence of comorbidities was found to be significantly associated with prognosis. The most commonly involved organs were the lung (87.2%); musculoskeletal system (19.5%); and genitourinary tract (17.1%). AIDS patients had a higher incidence of mycobacteremia and marrow involvement, whereas TB pericarditis and peritonitis were more common in non-AIDS patients with other underlying comorbidities.

Many patients with miliary TB have localization to the lungs, from which the organism gained entry into the bloodstream, or in another organ system (eg, the central nervous system). A form exists with no localization, however, called TB sepsis or sepsis tuberculosis gravissima (Landouzy's disease). This septic picture can be fulminant or subacute. In 1881, Louis Landouzy described a typhoidal form of acute TB, which he designated as "typhobacci-lose" [35]. Patients, frequently older children, developed several weeks of continuous fever and wasting, without localizing signs. Occasional patients died, and in these no miliary granulomata were found. Most patients defervesced and recovered slowly from the initial episode, however, only to develop localized, typical TB after a few weeks, months, or even years. Recent reports in the AIDS era [36] have suggested a resurgence of the acute septic form of TB, often with a rapidly fatal course. Similarity has been noted between gram-negative sepsis and TB sepsis, because *M tuberculosis* produces lipo-polysaccharide, and investigators have described coagulopathy, disseminated intravascular coagulation, and decreased levels of protein C and antithrombin III in tuberculous patients. As a result of these observations, a recent publication [36] describes the administration of recombinant human activated protein-C in a patient with TB sepsis, with apparent transient improvement attributed to the recombinant human activated protein-C.

Although the liver is commonly involved in TB, and hepatic granulomata are often demonstrable in patients with pulmonary TB with no manifestations of liver disease, there is a subset of patients with exclusive or predominant involvement of the liver or biliary tract; this has been termed variously "miliary TB of the liver," or "primary miliary TB." The clinical presentation may suggest primary or metastatic carcinoma, with fever, weight loss, and a nodular liver. Vascular studies may reveal avascular masses, which some believe distinguishes the lesions from malignancy. Also noted as part of the tuberculous process are splenomegaly, hepatic calcifications, and pain or tenderness in the right upper quadrant of the abdomen. When jaundice is present, it may be constant or intermittent and is attributed to lymph node obstruction, either of the common bile duct at the porta hepatis or the hepatoduodenal ligament. Jaundiced patients are more likely to have elevated serum alkaline phosphatase or transaminases, but these latter studies may also be normal. Although liver biopsy typically demonstrates granulomata positive AFB stains are rare. In a large study from India, TB was the most common cause of granulomatous hepatitis, accounting for 55% of cases [37].

Splenic TB is usually associated with involvement of the liver. In the pre-antibiotic era, the spleen was affected in one third of children with TB, and was the most commonly affected abdominal organ [38]. Reviews from the antibiotic era [39,40] found approximately 10% of cases of abdominal TB with splenic involvement, although a large series of 300 patients from 1997 [41] found none. Splenic enlargement is the most common manifestation of splenic involvement, with imaging studies showing single or multiple masses resembling malignancy. Occasionally, the spleen may be the only site of tuberculous infection, and splenic rupture has been reported as a rare complication.

Tuberculous lymphadenitis is especially common among foreign-born individuals in the United States. In a retrospective review from California [11], 92% of patients presenting with TB lymph node disease were foreign-born. Most of these patients had positive PPDs, and the cervical and supraclavicular nodes were most commonly involved. Seventeen percent had bilateral involvement. Chest radiograph abnormalities consistent with pulmonary TB were seen in 38%. Interestingly, fever was relatively uncommon and was documented in only 19% of cases in this series. TB may involve lymph nodes in unusual locations, resulting in protean and often misleading clinical presentations. For example, mediastinal TB adenitis may present as cardiac tamponade or dysphagia and tracheoesophageal fistula. Infection of upper abdominal lymph nodes may result in thoracic duct obstruction with resultant chylothorax, chylous ascites, or chyluria. Enlarged portal lymph nodes have produced biliary obstruction [42–44]. Patients with intercostal adenopathy may complain of localized chest pain, and involvement of posterior iliac crest lymph nodes may present with localized discomfort and swelling. The enlargement of epitrochlear lymph nodes is seen in a variety of infectious and malignant states, including disseminated TB.

Because TB can involve virtually every organ of the body, any localization of TB may present as FUO. Renal involvement may be clinically silent and suspected only because of hematuria or the classic finding of sterile pyuria; eventually, hypodense defects may be seen in the renal cortex, but these precede any radiologic distortion of the collecting system, which takes longer to develop. Peritoneal or pericardial TB may also elude diagnosis because of minimal localizing symptoms, as can focal musculoskeletal involvement. Other presentations may be misleading (eg, the ability of TB of the gastrointestinal tract to mimic Crohn's disease, also a cause of fever).

*Physical examination*

Physical findings are occasionally helpful in diagnosis of FUO. A careful examination should include an ophthalmoscopic search for the choroidal tubercles of miliary TB. Also raising the possibility of TB is an epididymal nodule; enlarged iliac crest or epitrochlear lymph nodes; splenomegaly; and a variety of skin lesions that result from hematologic spread of

TB: lupus vulgaris, producing a nodule or plaque on the face or neck; erythema induratum's tender subcutaneous nodules that frequently suppurate (AFB smear and culture are negative, but polymerase chain reaction [PCR] may be positive); and tuberculosis cutis miliaris disseminata, an acutely developing papulovesicular rash, Gram stain of which can misleadingly seem to show gram-positive rods, although a secondary acid-fast stain may demonstrate mycobacteria [45].

## Laboratory diagnosis

Diagnostic procedures used in TB include the following:

PPD
Interferon-$\gamma$ release assays
Nucleic acid amplification tests
Adenine deaminase
Biopsy
    Liver
    Spleen
    Lymph node
    Bone marrow
    Skin lesions
    Specific lesions or lining of effusions (eg, pleura, peritoneum, pericardium, synovium)
Laparotomy or laparoscopy
Chest radiograph (remember to repeat)
CT of necrotic lymph nodes or adrenal glands

Among the noninvasive diagnostic aids, one of the most frequent is the tuberculin skin test, or PPD. The PPD may be negative in up to half of cases [7], however, especially in dialysis patients and the elderly and immunocompromised. It is also frequently negative in miliary and peritoneal TB [9]. Consequently, the PPD is not useful in the individual patient, either to support or exclude the diagnosis of TB (except in children). Smears of sputum are AFB positive in only one quarter to one half of all cases with pulmonary disease. In patients with FUO caused by TB, the helpfulness of this test is minimal. In miliary TB without pulmonary parenchymal localization, the sputum is usually negative [7].

Because of their ability to detect small amounts of nucleic acids, PCR and other nucleic acid amplification tests (NAATs) are potentially useful as diagnostic alternatives to culture-based techniques, especially in extrapulmonary or disseminated TB, which are typically paucibacillary [33]. The two available in the United States are MTD (Gen-Probe, San Diego, California) and Amplicor (Roche, Nutley, New Jersey). Ritis and colleagues [33] studied a PCR assay for the IS6110 insertion element of *M tuberculosis* in 24 HIV-negative patients with FUO in whom clinical suspicion for extrapulmonary

TB was high. Both tissues suspected of being infected and samples of bone marrow proved to be of high diagnostic yield for this assay. The yield for peripheral blood was low, consistent with previous findings that the incidence of mycobacteremia in HIV-negative patients with extrapulmonary disease is lower than it is in those who are HIV-positive [46,47]. In HIV negative patients with suspected extrapulmonary TB, PCR of tissues suspected of disease may be helpful. If the affected site is either inaccessible for sampling or is unknown, then PCR of bone marrow, or of peripheral blood if the patient is HIV-positive, may provide a provisional diagnosis [48]. In general, NAATs demonstrate high specificity but low sensitivity. They are most effective in respiratory secretions, as compared with cerebrospinal fluid, pleural fluid, lymph nodes, and abscesses, but even with sputum the sensitivity suffers in paucibacillary disease (eg, smear-negative patients). The combination of high specificity with low sensitivity reduces the value of NAATs in excluding disease, but they may occasionally be helpful in suggesting or confirming disease. In general these tests have not fulfilled their promise, however, and the clinician who suspects TB on other grounds should not be deterred from empiric therapy because of a negative NAAT [49–52].

Detection of adenine deaminase in sputum and cerebrospinal, pericardial, pleural, and ascitic fluids is probably more helpful in extrapulmonary than pulmonary disease. Adenine deaminase detection has the combination of high sensitivity and low specificity; this test might be complementary with NAATs, which have high specificity.

Interferon-γ release assays are available and are used increasingly to detect tuberculous infection. The Centers for Disease Control and Prevention has recommended that the QuantiFERON-GOLD (Cellestis, Carnegie, Victoria, Australia) test may be used in instances where the PPD is now used, but there is general agreement that the response of multiple subgroups of patients has not been adequately studied; these include infants and the immunosuppressed. Although overall evaluation of sensitivity and specificity awaits further study, recent experience suggests potential use of interferon-γ release assays in certain patients with negative PPDs, particularly newborns [53], immunosuppressed patients with reactivation of TB [54], and patients with unusual presentations [55].

The chest radiograph is normal in one half of patients with extrapulmonary TB. It is important to repeat the chest radiograph periodically in patients with FUO, however, because miliary lesions not apparent at first may blossom and become more apparent on subsequent films [7,9]. Miliary lesions are more common in patients with HIV. Other patterns on chest radiographs are consolidations; fibrotic changes; and, as was the case with Mrs. Roosevelt, nodules [34]. CT demonstration of necrotic lymph nodes or enlarged, necrotic, and calcified adrenal glands is highly suggestive of a mycobacterial etiology of FUO, especially in areas of high endemicity, or in patients at high risk for TB [8].

The hematologic changes seen in TB infection are protean, affecting both plasma components and cell lines. The more common of these changes,

which can provide diagnostic clues in patients with FUO caused by TB, are
as follows [56]:

Bone marrow
    Fibrosis with myelophthisis
    Hypoplasia, aplasia, necrosis
    Granulomatosis, amyloidosis
Erythrocyte
    Anemia of chronic disease
    Less common: macrocytic, autoimmune hemolytic anemia, sideroblastic
    Polycythemia from renal TB
    Elevated ferritin (often > 1000 µg/L), C-reactive protein, and erythro-
      cyte sedimentation rate
Granulocytes
    Neutrophilia, leukemoid reaction
    Neutropenia
    Pelger-Huët anomaly
    Basophilia
    Eosinophilia
    Hemophagocytic syndrome
Lymphoid
    Lymphocytosis
    Lymphocytopenia (including decreased CD4 cells even in HIV-nega-
      tive patients)
Platelets
    Thrombocytosis
    Thrombocytopenia
Coagulation
    Disseminated intravascular coagulation, hypercoagulable state

Because TB can infect virtually every endocrine gland there are endocri-
nologic manifestations of tuberculous infection that should suggest the diagnosis in patients with FUO [18]. Although less commonly than in the
preantibiotic era, TB still causes 20% of cases of adrenal insufficiency in
the developed world. Infection of the gland results from early lymphohema-
togenous spread and is often associated with concomitant foci of infection,
most often of the lungs and genitourinary tract. In most cases there is bilateral involvement. Pathologic findings are atypical, in that granulomata are
less common than in other organs, perhaps reflecting local production of
steroids. Calcification is common but not specific and is most often seen
on CT after 2 years of infection, in the context of shrunken, atrophic glands.
Treatment at this point is unlikely to result in recovery of adrenal function.
Earlier in the course of infection, CT findings may include enlarged, noncal-
cified glands with areas of lucency representing parenchymal necrosis.

Syndrome of inappropriate antidiuretic hormone has long been associated with TB patients, in whom hyponatremia is much more common

than hypernatremia; in one series of patients with disseminated disease, it was recorded in 58.9% [34]. Recent studies have demonstrated the presence of circulating arginine vasopressin in patients with pulmonary and miliary TB who are hyponatremic, and levels decrease in response to free water challenge. Syndrome of inappropriate antidiuretic hormone is most commonly associated with pulmonary infection, but is also seen in TB meningitis, miliary TB, and TB epididymo-orchitis. In most cases, the serum sodium corrects with TB treatment.

TB is a well-described cause of hypercalcemia. In most cases, it is associated with pulmonary TB, but can also be seen with miliary and other extrapulmonary involvement. Hypercalcemia may become apparent early in the course of treatment, possible reflecting a treatment-induced rise in serum albumin. Patients usually have increased serum phosphorus and decreased parathyroid hormone levels, suggesting a vitamin D–dependent mechanism as seen in other granulomatous diseases. In most cases, hypercalcemia is mild and asymptomatic and resolves within 1 to 7 months of treatment for TB [34].

## Invasive diagnostic procedures

Laparotomy and laparoscopy are frequently used in evaluation of FUO when no diagnosis is apparent. In the experience of most, however, structures that appear normal by CT are usually confirmed to be so on laparoscopy or biopsy. Laparoscopy is most helpful when clues point to abdominal disease (eg, abdominal tenderness, hepatosplenomegaly, abnormal liver function tests, CT abnormalities, and so forth), and has had a yield of only 20% when such features are absent [7]. In a study from Mexico [57] of patients with FUO who underwent laparoscopy, 12 of 15 patients were suspected of having abdominal pathology on the basis of imaging studies. Samples obtained from surgery yielded a definitive diagnosis in 10, and in four patients laparoscopic findings and samples helped to rule out the presence of infection or neoplasm.

Liver biopsy demonstrates granulomata in 80% to 90% of cases of miliary TB. About one half of granulomata show caseation, and one half is AFB positive on smear [7]. In a study from Spain of HIV-positive patients with FUO who underwent percutaneous liver biopsy, Garcia-Ordonez and colleagues [24] demonstrated a sensitivity of percutaneous liver biopsy for the diagnosis of TB of 72.5%, and in patients who were diagnosed with TB, an elevated alkaline phosphatase and hepatomegaly had a positive predictive value of 86.4%. Spain has the highest prevalence of HIV-associated TB in the western world, so the diagnostic yield of percutaneous liver biopsy in HIV patients may not be as high in other countries. Nevertheless, the literature suggests that the diagnostic yield of percutaneous liver biopsy for TB is much higher in HIV-positive patients than it is in those who are HIV-negative, probably because of the predilection of TB (and other opportunistic infections) to disseminate in patients with HIV. Percutaneous liver biopsy can be considered in any patient with FUO who has elevated alkaline phosphatase and hepatomegaly, and may be especially helpful in the setting of HIV infection.

Bone marrow biopsy may demonstrate granulomata in one half of cases, but the yield is greater than 80% when anemia, leukopenia, and monocytosis are present [7]. Combined histopathology and culture seems to be more helpful than histopathology alone: 93% versus 44.7% [34]. Bone marrow biopsy should also be considered in patients with FUO suspected of having TB who have no localizing organ-specific findings, especially if hematologic abnormalities are also present.

Although splenic biopsy is generally regarded as a high-risk procedure because of the risk of hemorrhage, fine-needle aspiration (FNA) of the organ has been shown to have a very low rate of complications [57]. The procedure is most rewarding in patients with either splenomegaly or space-occupying lesions of the spleen. In 31 patients with FUO in India, 11 were diagnosed with TB on the basis of splenic FNA [58]. Nearly two thirds of the samples from patients diagnosed with TB were AFB positive, with the highest rate of positivity in samples with inflammatory cells and necrosis without granulomata.

Lymph nodes are often accessible by aspiration, biopsy, or excision. In patients in California with TB lymphadenitis [11], granulomata were found more frequently in lymph node biopsy specimens compared with FNA, but no significant difference was demonstrated in the rate of culture positivity between FNA and biopsy. Decreased sensitivity of FNA for granulomata was noted in patients with HIV and other immunocompromised states. It seems that FNA is a reasonable initial approach in patients with FUO who have lymph node enlargement, although one should keep in mind that if the FNA is nondiagnostic and TB is still suspected, biopsy may increase the diagnostic yield, especially in HIV and other immunocompromised patients. It is important to remember that, if TB of a body cavity is suspected, the cavity lining is more likely to provide a diagnosis by histology and culture than is evaluation of the fluid itself. Biopsy and histology of pleura, peritoneum, pericardium, and synovium are usually more helpful than assessment of the corresponding fluids.

*Diagnostic and therapeutic trials*

In patients with FUO who are suspected of having TB infection and whose clinical condition is deteriorating, empiric anti-TB therapy should be considered. In many cases, the diagnosis of TB is made solely on the basis of response to therapy alone [13]. In the experience of Onal and coworkers [15], empiric therapy established the diagnosis of 43% of their FUO cases that were caused by TB. Empiric therapy should also be considered in patients with intermittent fever (especially in areas of high prevalence), with suggestive clinical, radiographic, or laboratory findings; with predisposing factors (elderly, dialysis, immunocompromised, and so forth); and in those suspected of having disseminated disease, in whom a delay in treatment could adversely affect prognosis.

A response to empiric therapy with a rifampin-containing regimen may result from nontuberculous infection, because rifampin has activity against many classes of microorganisms. It is the most powerful anti-TB drug available, however, and most clinicians include it in an empiric regimen for a potentially fatal infection. Prior administration of other antimicrobials with anti-TB activity (eg, fluoroquinolones) should also be taken into account in managing such patients, both because resistance may have emerged to the drug administered and also because a prior response may have resulted from transient antituberculous chemotherapy.

## Summary: revisiting the Roosevelt case

The diagnosis of TB should always be considered in patients with FUO, especially in those at particular risk or with suggestive clues. In the Roosevelt case, she had the dual risks of corticosteroid administration and age; in addition, she had the early clues of hematologic abnormalities (which may have resulted from her tuberculous infection) and elevated erythrocyte sedimentation rate. Eventually, she developed night sweats and diffuse nodules on her chest radiograph. In such settings, a therapeutic-diagnostic trial is certainly appropriate, and the timing of such therapy depends on the patient's clinical status and physician judgment.

It is likely that Mrs. Roosevelt would have responded to therapy if her organism were not resistant. Empiric trials must take into account the possibility of resistance, which should be considered if empiric therapy is unsuccessful, if a patient had been treated previously for TB, has lived in an area of high prevalence of resistance, or has been exposed to patients likely to be infected with resistant organisms. In such cases, consideration should be given to supplementing a standard three- or four-drug empiric regimen with two or more second-line drugs (eg, levofloxacin, amikacin, ethionamide, para-aminosalicylate, cycloserine) or even third-line drugs (eg, linezolid, imipenem, amoxicillin-clavulanate, macrolides) if the second-line agents cannot be given.

## Summary

TB is an important cause of FUO, especially in patients at risk for TB because of a variety of factors including geography, immunocompetence, age, and comorbidities. Infection may be focal or generalized. Associated physical findings and laboratory and radiologic abnormalities may suggest the diagnosis, but the index of suspicion should remain high in view of

TB's treatability, and empiric anti-TB therapy should be considered in all patients with FUO who defy diagnosis.

## References

[1] Lerner BH. Revisiting the death of Eleanor Roosevelt: was the diagnosis of tuberculosis missed? Int J Tuberc Lung Dis 2001;5:1080–5.
[2] Petersdorf RG, Beeson P. Fever of unexplained origin: report of 100 cases. Medicine 1961; 40:1–30.
[3] Goto M, Koyama H, Takahashi O, et al. A retrospective review of 226 hospitalized patients with fever. Intern Med 2007;46:17–22.
[4] Chin C, Lee SS, Chen YS, et al. Mycobacteriosis in patients with fever of unknown origin. J Microbiol Immunol Infect 2003;36:248–53.
[5] Ammari F. Fever of unknown origin in North Jordan. Trop Doct 2006;36:251–3.
[6] Erten N, Saka B, Ozturk G, et al. Fever of unknown origin: a report of 57 cases. Int J Clin Pract 2005;59:958–60.
[7] Arnow PM, Flaherty JP. Fever of unknown origin. Lancet 1997;350:575–80.
[8] Collazos J, Guerra E, Mayo J, et al. Tuberculosis as a cause of recurrent fever of unknown origin. J Infect 2000;41(3):269–72.
[9] Knockaert DC, Vanderschueren S, Blockmans D. Fever of unknown origin in adults: 40 years on. J Intern Med 2003;253:263–75.
[10] Pratt R, Robison V, Navis T, et al. MMWR 2007;56(11):245–8.
[11] Polesky A, Grove W, Bhatia G. Peripheral tuberculous lymphadenitis: epidemiology, diagnosis, treatment, and outcome. Medicine 2005;84(6):350–62.
[12] Pratt R, Robison V, Navin T, et al. Trends in tuberculosis incidence—United States, 2006. MMWR Morb Mortal Wkly Rep 2007;56(11):245–8.
[13] Tal S, Guller V, Gurevich A, et al. Fever of unknown origin in the elderly. J Intern Med 2002; 252:295–304.
[14] Knockaert DC, Vanneste LJ, Bobbaers HJ. Fever of unknown origin in elderly patients. J Am Geriatr Soc 1993;41:1187–92.
[15] Onal IK, Cankurtaran M, Cakar M. Fever of unknown origin: what is remarkable in the elderly in a developing country? J Infect. 2006;52:399–404.
[16] Korzeniewska-Kosela M, Krysl J, Muller N, et al. Tuberculosis in young adults and the elderly. Chest 1994;106:28–32.
[17] Erkoc R, Dogan E,, Sayarlioglu H. Tuberculosis in dialysis patients, single centre experience from an endemic area. Int J Clin Pract 2004;58:1115–7.
[18] Blumberg EA, Abrutyn E. Endocrine and metabolic aspects of tuberculosis. In: Schlossberg D, editor. Tuberculosis and nontuberculous mycobacterial infection. 5th edition. New York: McGraw-Hill; 2006.
[19] Angell SY, Behrens RH. Risk assessment and disease prevention in travelers visiting friends and relatives. Infect Dis Clin North Am 2005;19:49–66.
[20] MMWR Recommendations and Reports. Controlling tuberculosis in the United States. MMWR Morb Mortal Wkly Rep 2005;54(RR-12):44–5.
[21] Arguin PM, Kozarsky PE, Navin AW. Health Information for international travel 2005–2006. US Department of Health and Human Services, CDC; 2005.
[22] Sohail MR, Fisher PR. Health risks to air travelers. Infect Dis Clin North Am 2005;19:67–84.
[23] World Health Organization. TB and air travel: guidelines for control second edition, 2006. Available at: http://whqlibdoc.who.int/hq/2006/WHO_HTM_TB_2006.363_eng.pdf. Accessed June 12, 2007.
[24] Garcia-Ordonez MA, Colmenero JD, Jiminez-Onate F, et al. Diagnostic usefulness of percutaneous liver biopsy in HIV-infected patients with fever of unknown origin. J Infect 1999; 38:94–8.

[25] MMWR Recommendations and Reports. Targeted tuberculin testing and treatment of latent TB Infection. MMWR Morb Mortal Wkly Rep 2000;49(RR-6):23–5.

[26] Saliu OY, Sofer C, Stein DS, et al. Tumor-necrosis-factor blockers: differential effects on mycobacterial immunity. J Infect Dis 2006;194:486–92.

[27] Wallis RS. Reactivation of latent tuberculosis by TNF blockade: the role of interferon gamma. J Investig Dermatol Symp Proc 2007;12:16–21.

[28] Plessner HL, Lin PL, Kohno T, et al. Neutralization of tumor necrosis factor (TNF) by antibody but not TNF receptor fusion molecule exacerbates chronic murine tuberculosis. J Infect Dis 2007;195:1643–50.

[29] Singh N, Wagener MM, Gayoski T. Safety and efficacy of isoniazid chemoprophylaxis administered during liver transplant candidacy for the prevention of posttransplant tuberculosis. Transplantation 2002;74:892–5.

[30] Chou NK, Liu LT, Hsu RB, et al. Various clinical presentations of tuberculosis in heart transplant patients. Transplant Proc 2004;36:2396–8.

[31] Morales P, Briones A, Torres JJ, et al. Pulmonary tuberculosis in lung and heart-lung transplantation: fifteen years of experience in a single center in Spain. Transplant Proc 2005;37: 4050–5.

[32] Ergun I, Ekmekci Y, Sengul S, et al. Mycobacterium tuberculosis infection in renal transplant recipients. Transplant Proc 2006;38:1344–5.

[33] Ritis K, Tzoanopoulos D, Speletas M, et al. Amplification of IS6110 sequence for the detection of *Mycobacterium tuberculosis* complex in HIV-negative patients with fever of unknown origin and evidence of extrapulmonary disease. J Intern Med 2000;248:415–24.

[34] Wang JY, Hsueh PR, Wang SK, et al. Disseminated tuberculosis: a 10-year experience in a medical center. Medicine 2007;86:39–46.

[35] Landouzy L. Note Sur La Fièvre Bacillaire Prètuberculeuse à Forme Typhoide ou Typhobacillose. In: Pour L'Étude de La Tuberculose Chez L'Homme Et Chez Les Animaux. Paris: Libraire De L'Académie De Médicine; 1892. p. 619–22 [in French].

[36] Rubin ZA, Leonard MK, Martin GS. Brief report: tuberculosis sepsis and activated protein C. Am J Med Sci 2006;332:48–50.

[37] Sabharwal BD, Malhotra N, Garg R, et al. Granulomatous hepatitis: a retrospective study. Indian J Pathol Microbiol 1995;38:413–6.

[38] Yoshijima Y, Harada Y, Kohdera U, et al. Possible splenic tuberculosis presenting as unexplained fever. Pediatr Int 2000;42:705–7.

[39] Lundstedt C, Nyman R, Brismar J, et al. Imaging of tuberculosis. II. Abdominal manifestations in 112 patients. Acta Radiol 1996;37:489–95.

[40] Denton T, Hossain J. A radiological study of abdominal tuberculosis in a Saudi population, with special reference to ultrasound and computed tomography. Clin Radiol 1993;47: 409–14.

[41] Bhansali SK. Abdominal tuberculosis: experience with 300 cases. Am J Gastroenterol 1997; 67:324–37.

[42] Akcam M, Artan R, Yilmaz A, et al. Abdominal tuberculosis in adolescents: difficulties in diagnosis. Saudi Med J 2005;26:122–6.

[43] Sharma SK, Mohan A. Extrapulmonary tuberculosis. Indian J Med Res 2004;120:316–53.

[44] Bayindir Y, Sevinc A, Serefhanoglu K, et al. Cervico-mediastinal tuberculous lymphadenitis presenting as prolonged fever of unknown origin. J Natl Med Assoc 2004;96:682–5.

[45] Stein A, Purgus R, Drancourt M, et al. Photo quiz. Clin Infect Dis 1999;29:1307–8.

[46] Richter C, Kox LFF, van Leeuwen J, et al. PCR detection of mycobacteremia in Tanzanian patients with extrapulmonary tuberculosis. Eur J Clin Microbiol Infect Dis 1996;15: 813–7.

[47] Chan CM, Yuen KY, Chan KS, et al. Single-tube nested PCR in the diagnosis of TB. J Clin Pathol 1996;49:290–4.

[48] Singh UB, Bhanu NV, Suresh VN. Utility of polymerase chain reaction in diagnosis of TB from samples of bone marrow aspirate. Am J Trop Med Hyg 2006;75:960–3.

[49] Dinnes J, Deeks J, Kunst H. A systematic review of rapid diagnostic tests for the detection of TB infection. Health Technol Assess 2007;11:1–196.

[50] Osores F, Nolasco O, Verdonck K, et al. Clinical evaluation of a 16S Ribosomal RNA polymerase chain reaction test for the diagnosis of lymph node tuberculosis. Clin Infect Dis 2006; 43:855–9.

[51] Ozkutuk A, Kirdir S, Ozden S, et al. Evaluation of cobas amplicor MTB test to detect *Mycobacterium tuberculosis* in pulmonary and extrapulmonary specimens. New Microbiol 2006; 29:269–73.

[52] Michos AG, Daikos GL, Tzanetou K. Detection of *Mycobacterium tuberculosis* DNA in respiratory and nonrespiratory specimens by the Amplicor MTB PCR. Diagn Microbiol Infect Dis 2006;54:121–6.

[53] Connell T, Bar-Zeev N, Curtis N. Early detection of perinatal tuberculosis B using a whole blood interferon-gamma release assay. Clin Infect Dis 2006;42:e82–5.

[54] Ravn P, Munk ME, Andersen AB, et al. Reactivation of TB during immunosuppressive treatment in a patient with a positive quantiferon-RD1 Test. Scand J Infect Dis 2004;36: 499–501.

[55] Arend SM, Ottenhoff THM, Anderson P, et al. Uncommon presentations of tuberculosis: the potential value of a novel diagnostic assay based on the *Mycobacterium tuberculosis*-specific antigens ESAT-6 and CFP-10. Int J Tuberc Lung Dis 2001;5:680–6.

[56] Oyer RA, Schlossberg D. Hematologic changes in tuberculosis. In: Schlossberg D, editor. Tuberculosis and nontuberculous mycobacterial infection. 5th edition. New York: McGraw-Hill; 2006.

[57] Arch-Ferrer JE, Velazquez-Fernandez D, Sierra-Madero J, et al. Laparoscopic approach to fever of unknown origin. Surg Endosc 2003;17:494–7.

[58] Rajwanshi A, Gupta D, Kapoor S, et al. Fine needle aspiration biopsy of the spleen in pyrexia of unknown origin. Cytopathology 1999;10:195–200.

INFECTIOUS
DISEASE CLINICS
OF NORTH AMERICA

Infect Dis Clin N Am 21 (2007) 963–996

# Fever of Unknown Origin Due to Zoonoses

Dennis J. Cleri, MD[a,b,*], Anthony J. Ricketti, MD[a,b],
John R. Vernaleo, MD[c]

[a]Department of Medicine, St. Francis Medical Center, Room B-158,
601 Hamilton Avenue, Trenton, NJ 08629-1986, USA
[b]Seton Hall University, School of Graduate Medical Education, South Orange,
NJ 07079, USA
[c]Division of Infectious Diseases, Wyckoff Heights Medical Center,
374 Stockholm Street, Brooklyn, NY 11237, USA

When you have eliminated the impossible, whatever remains, however improbable, must be the truth.–Sherlock Holmes in the "The Adventure of the Blanched Soldier" from Sir Arthur Ignatius Conan Doyle's, "The Case-Book of Sherlock Holmes" first published in *Liberty* October 1926, and the *Strand Magazine,* London, November 1926.

There are 1407 species of human pathogens (excluding ectoparasites); more than half (816) are zoonotic, associated with 132 animal species. Of these, 73% (130) are zoonoses [1]. Having such a long list of suspects, coconspirators, and accomplices makes the diagnosis of zoonotic fever of unknown origin (FUO) a daunting task.

## Approach to the patient with a possible zoonotic fever of unknown origin

Look, and you will find it –what is unsought will go undetected.
–Sophocles, Greek tragic poet (c. 496–406 BC).

Mackowiak and Durack [2] classify FUOs into four categories: (1) classic, (2) nosocomial, (3) immunodeficient, and (4) HIV-related. Adding a fifth category, zoonotic FUO, necessitates combining their categories of the "classic," "immunodeficient," and "HIV-related" with the emphasis on accurate and detailed travel, dietary, and activity history.

---

* Corresponding author. Department of Medicine, St. Francis Medical Center, Room B-158, 601 Hamilton Avenue, Trenton, NJ 08629-1986.
*E-mail address:* dcleri@stfrancismedical.org (D.J. Cleri).

## Zoonotic immunodeficiency viruses: simian immunodeficiency virus

HIV infection and AIDS are the penultimate zoonotic FUOs. HIV-1 and HIV-2 are cross-species lentivirus infections. One factor facilitating cross-species transmission is the adaptability of the simian immunodeficiency virus–HIV envelope protein [3].

There are more than 40 nonhuman primate species infected with specific simian immunodeficiency viruses [4]. Sixty million years of coevolution of simian foamy virus, the oldest genus of Retroviridae, rendered the virus nonpathogenic in primates. Asymptomatic human infection has been documented in 1.8% of 231 individuals to 5.3% of 187 individuals working in primate research centers or zoos. Sources of infection were identified as chimpanzees (*Pan troglodytes*) and African green monkeys [5].

Simian immunodeficiency virus has resulted in a chronic human infection [6]. Primate handlers and those who hunt and butcher "bushmeat" (the meat of wild animals that includes chimpanzees, monkeys, and the gorilla) have detectable humoral and cell-mediated immunity to simian immunodeficiency viruses. There are at least eight documented incidents of zoonotic transfer of simian immunodeficiency viruses to humans [7].

In the proper epidemiologic setting, serologic or virologic diagnosis of simian immunodeficiency viruses should be attempted in those patients with FUO without other apparent cause. If history repeats itself, clinicians will soon appreciate a clinical syndrome associated with such transmission.

## Common zoonotic coinfections with HIV

### Visceral leishmaniasis and HIV infection

Visceral leishmaniasis (VL) is caused by several species of *Leishmania* [8]. These *Leishmania* spp infect more than 2 million people yearly in tropical and subtropical regions of all continents except Australia [9–11]. VL reported in troops returning from Operation Desert Storm (1990–1991) and Afghanistan (2002–2004) has made clinicians aware of the diagnosis, and prompted the consideration of the threat to the transfusion blood supply and the re-evaluation of the US military blood donor deferral policies [9,10].

VL is an important FUO in HIV-AIDS patients [12]. HIV infection increases *Leishmania* spp replication and uptake in HIV-infected macrophages [13]. At the same time, *Leishmania* is an "enhancer of the progression of AIDS" [14].

### Epidemiology and pathogenesis

*Leishmania donovani* is the agent for disease in India and East Africa; *L donovani* and *Leishmania infantum/chagasi* cause VL in the Mediterranean basin, the Middle East, central Asia, and western China; and *L infantum/*

*chagasi* is the predominant agent in Central and South America. Rare cases of VL are caused by *Leishmania amazonensis,* and *Leishmania tropica,* the agents of cutaneous leishmaniasis in Latin America, and the Middle East and India, respectively [8].

Humans and other mammalian hosts (canines, jackals, and rodents) harbor the leishmania amastigotes. The female sandfly (*Lutzomyia* sp, Western Hemisphere; *Phlebotomus* sp, Old World) is the vector [8]. An outbreak of canine VL was discovered in a Dutchess County, New York, kennel among 41% of the foxhounds tested [15]. Another survey of over 12,000 foxhounds and other canines, and 185 persons in 35 states and four Canadian provinces, found no human infection, but widespread infection among foxhounds. VL seemed to be limited to dog-to-dog transmission, but human infection is possible if the parasite becomes adapted to indigenous phlebotomus [16].

*Clinical presentation*

In the non–HIV-infected host, most disease is asymptomatic and self-limited. Some develop mild symptoms that resolve. The minority of patients develop VL (kala-azar) characterized by fever, weight loss, hepatosplenomegaly, neutropenia, and hypergammaglobulinemia. Malnutrition, wasting, and debilitation secondary to excess cytokine production occur as the disease progresses. Patients develop ulcers around the mouth, edema, petechiae, ecchymosis, gingival bleeding, and hepatitis, which may become fulminant [8]. VL patients may present with diarrhea. Patients exhibit marked hypergammaglobulinemia, anemia, neutropenia, thrombocytopenia, elevated bilirubin, liver enzymes, circulating immune complexes, high erythrocyte sedimentation, and rheumatoid factor [8].

Clinical progression of VL is related to host genetics, cell-mediated immune response, malnutrition, and immune suppression. VL has been associated with acquired hypogammaglobulinemia secondary to carbamazepine therapy, HIV disease, transplantation, neoplastic diseases, steroid therapy, and treatment with infliximab for rheumatoid arthritis [17–20]. Incubation periods range from 10 days to months. The onset of disease may be gradual or abrupt. Clinical disease may present itself only after immune suppression [8].

In patients coinfected with HIV, most present as previously mentioned. Fever is present in only half of the patients and splenomegaly may be absent [8,11]. Patients may present with acute abdominal pain and aplastic anemia. Many organs may be infected with amastigotes (lung, pleura, pericardium, larynx, oral mucosa, bone marrow, esophagus, stomach, small intestine, and skin) [8,21–23]. Bronchoalveolar adenoma and bronchiolitis obliterans have been reported [22]. Some HIV-infected patients may be asymptomatic, whereas others infected with *Leishmania braziliensis* (the common cause of cutaneous disease) may disseminate [8,24].

Atypical disseminated leishmaniasis and VL may present with polyarthritis and unusual or disseminated skin manifestations. In HIV patients, it may be mistaken for post–kala-azar dermal disease [25,26]. Fulminant eye disease and hypothyroidism are unusual complications [27,28]. Patients coinfected with VL and HIV may experience a chronic relapsing course not responding to VL therapy. Renal failure from secondary amyloidosis may occur [29].

Central nervous system (CNS) involvement is rare. It results from contiguous extension from the paranasal sinuses. Complications include cranial nerve dysfunction (especially the optic nerve); meningitis; ascending demyelinating disease similar to Guillain-Barré syndrome localized to the peripheral nervous system; and painful peripheral neuropathies. Amastigotes have been detected in the cerebrospinal fluid (CSF) [30].

HIV-associated immune reconstitution disease has unmasked subclinical VL. Immune reconstitution disease VL manifests itself with fever and hepatosplenomegaly within 2 weeks to the initial months of beginning highly active antiretroviral therapy (HAART) therapy. Cutaneous, mucosal, and post–kala-azar dermal leishmaniasis, leishmanial uveitis, and deterioration of cutaneous and mucosal leishmaniasis have all been reported as a consequence of immune reconstitution disease [31].

Pediatric patients (mean age, 1.7 years) not infected with HIV all presented with fever and splenomegaly. Hepatomegaly was present in 90.1%; thrombocytopenia and anemia in 70.2%; and leukopenia in 42.3% [32]. Non–HIV-infected pregnant patients present with hepatosplenomegaly. Treatment of pregnant patients with amphotericin B (five patients) resulted in no treatment failures, no congenital VL, and no congenital abnormalities [33].

*Laboratory diagnosis*

Most commonly, the diagnosis is confirmed by identifying the amastigotes in Wright-Giemsa biopsy touch preparations or in special parasite cultures. Bone marrow biopsy is positive in 66% of AIDS patients and 87% of patients without AIDS. A urine latex agglutination test has been developed and serologic tests are available [8,34]. Polymerase chain reaction is highly sensitive and specific for diagnosis, speciation, and estimation of parasite load [8].

*Differential diagnosis*

The differential diagnosis includes tropical splenomegaly from chronic malaria, hepatosplenic schistosomiasis and Katayama fever, miliary tuberculosis, histoplasmosis, brucellosis, bacterial endocarditis, infectious mononucleosis, prolonged *Salmonella* spp bacteremia and typhoid fever, amebic liver abscess, acute Chagas' disease (CD), and other bacterial and viral infections [8].

*Treatment*

Treatments for VL include liposomal amphotericin B (treatment of choice in the United States); pentavalent antimonies (sodium stibogluconate, meglumine antimonate), where there is no resistance; azoles (ketoconazole, fluconazole, itraconazole); paromomycin; and miltefosine [8]. HIV protease inhibitors (indinavir and saquinavir) display antileishmanial activity [35]. Patients with uncontrolled HIV replication or poor response to HAART have frequent VL relapses [36].

## Conclusion

In the proper epidemiologic setting, VL is an important consideration as a cause of FUO because of (1) the highly variable incubation period; (2) in some patients, presentation only after immune suppression; (3) both acute and gradual onset of disease; (4) highly variable clinical presentations; and (5) the absence of typical clinical findings in a significant minority of patients. HIV patients have atypical presentations, and immune reconstitution disease may unmask the disease.

## Chagas' disease

### Epidemiology and pathogenesis

CD infects 18 million people exclusively in North and South America [11]. CD is caused by *Trypanosoma cruzi* [37]. *T cruzi* produces lifelong infections in humans and domestic, wild, and zoo animals in endemic areas (from the southern United States to Argentina). Ten percent to 30% of human infections become symptomatic.

CD is transmitted by reduviid (kissing bugs) triatomes (*Triatoma* spp, *Rhodnius* spp, and *Panstrongylus* spp) through infected feces [37]. Transfusion, organ transplantation, laboratory accident, congenital infection, tattooing, body piercing, and ingestion of food or drink contaminated with triatome insect feces have caused infection [37,38]. One case of fatal congenital disease involving an HIV-positive mother was associated with cervical CD [39].

*Trypanosoma cruzi* infection, even asymptomatic reactivation, markedly increases HIV viral loads [40].

### Clinical manifestations

A red and indurated lesion at the parasite's entry site heralds acute disease. Romaña's sign (unilateral painless periorbital edema) is found when the entry site is the conjunctiva. With systemic spread, patients develop fever, malaise, facial and lower limb edema, hepatosplenomegaly, and lymphadenopathy. Complications of chronic disease include cardiac (cardiomegaly, left ventricular apical aneurysm, and mural thrombi); megaesophagus; dilatation and thickening of the colon (most often the sigmoid colon); parotid enlargement; and stomach and urinary tract involvement [37]. Sudden death has been associated with cardiac focal denervation, regional asynergy, compensatory adrenergic stimulus with myotoxicity, and malignant arrhythmia [37].

*Trypanosoma cruzi* may have a long silent course in HIV-infected patients or may present with acute congestive heart failure, skin lesions, spontaneous peritonitis, and acute esophageal and gastric disease [37,41,42]. Reactivation of CD (now an AIDS-defining disease) in HIV patients most commonly manifests as meningoencephalitis [43]. In immunosuppressed and HIV patients, *T cruzi* brain abscesses have occurred and may be the initial presentation of AIDS [37,44].

Whereas CNS disease is rare in CD patients, HIV-CD patients commonly exhibit CNS disease (acute fatal meningoencephalitis, mass lesions, and granulomatous encephalitis) [11,43]. Cerebral toxoplasmosis and trypanosomiasis in HIV patients may coexist [45]. Neuroimaging reveals large solitary or multiple ring-enhancing lesions with edema [44]. These may be confused with cerebral toxoplasmosis, CNS primary lymphoma, or cerebral metastases [37,46].

Parasitemia is more frequent and intense in HIV patients. Erythema nodosum, acute meningoencephalitis with parasites detectable in the CSF, and acute myocarditis have been disease presentations in HIV patients [47].

### Diagnosis

Diagnosis of disease and meningoencephalitis is made by direct observation of intracellular *T cruzi* and by PCR (of blood and CSF) [46,48]. Serologic tests may assist in the diagnosis [37,40]. Xenodiagnosis is made by examining uninfected laboratory triatomes (reduviid bugs) after feeding on patients or by blood culture [11,37].

### Treatment

Nifurtimox or benznidazole are the treatments of choice [37]. Treatment of non-HIV patients without heart failure and nonacute disease with benznidazole resulted in reduced progression of diseases, and increased seronegative conversion [49]. Immune reconstitution with HAART and benznidazol has resulted in long-term (3-year) survival [50].

### Conclusion

Fever is a sign of dissemination in acute disease. CD is transmittable by transfusion and transplantation, and known to reactivate late in the disease in HIV-infected patients. CD becomes a serious consideration as a cause of FUO in anyone even with a distant exposure history, especially in the immunocompromised or the HIV patient.

### Schistosomiasis

### Epidemiology and pathogenesis

Worldwide, 200 to 300 million people are infected with schistosomiasis. Eighty-five percent of those individuals live in sub-Saharan Africa, the area with the world's highest prevalence and total number of HIV-1–infected patients [51]. The disease is a zoonoses acquired in fresh water from free-living cercarial larvae that penetrate the skin. The adults lay eggs during their 3- to 7-year life span. The eggs migrate to venous plexuses (mesenteric venous plexus: *Schistosoma mansoni*, *Schistosoma japonicum*, *Schistosoma mekongi*, *Schistosoma intercalatum*; bladder venous plexus: *Schistosoma haematobium*) and result in liver, intestinal, kidney, and bladder disease; anemia; and growth retardation in children [51].

Human *S mansoni* infections increase the progression of AIDS by enhancing the HIV replication rates, increase immune activation, enhance selective pressure for virulent variant strains, and impair cytolytic functions of T cells and other viral-specific responses [52]. Urinary tract and genital schistosomiasis increases the risk of HIV infection in women [53].

*Clinical manifestations*

The three stages of schistosomal disease are (1) dermatitis caused by penetration of the cercaria (swimmers itch); (2) acute febrile and systemic disease; and (3) chronic disease. Human schistosoma (*S mansoni* and *S haematobium*) cause a pruritic rash with red papules within 24 hours of exposure. The acute febrile disease with systemic symptoms begins 4 to 8 weeks later coinciding with migration and maturation of the schistosomulae. This is followed by chronic disease and complications: periportal fibrosis; portal hypertension; pulmonary hypertension; cor pulmonale; CNS complications (especially seizures); ulcer formation in the bowel wall with chronic bleeding; and urinary complications (bladder neck obstruction, hydroureter, hydronephrosis, and hematuria) [51].

HIV can cause recrudescence of long-dormant disease [54]. Immune reconstitution after HAART has resulted in *S mansoni*–associated enteritis with fever, vomiting, diarrhea, abdominal pain, and eosinophilia [55].

*Diagnosis*

Diagnosis is traditionally accomplished by identification of eggs in the stool and urine. Serologic tests include indirect hemagglutination assay and ELISA [51].

In the immunosuppressed patient with CNS complications, imaging reveals solitary or multiple hyperdense lesions in the brain or spinal cord and "arborized" enhancement on MRI with surrounding edema and granuloma [56].

*Treatment*

Praziquantel treatment (the drug of choice) results in similar responses in HIV-positive and HIV-negative patients (86% and 85%, respectively). Cure rates based on circulating antibodies were found to be 31% and 52%, respectively [57].

*Conclusion*

With hundreds of millions of people infected, schistosomiasis becomes an important cause of FUO. In the otherwise normal patient, fever appears weeks to months after the initial exposure. Recrudescence is seen in HIV-infected patients. Fever and a constellation of symptoms are seen in immune reconstitution disease.

### Cryptosporidiosis

#### Epidemiology and pathogenesis

Cryptosporidium hominis and others are the etiologic agents for crypto-sporidiosis. The protozoan infects many mammals and birds [58].

The organism's lifecycle (both sexual [sporogony] and asexual [merogony]) is completed within a single host. In the normal host, the organisms are found in the microvillus layer of the epithelial cells in the distal small intestine and proximal colon. In immunocompromised patients, it may be found through-out the gastrointestinal tract, biliary tree, and the respiratory tract. Heavy infection and chronic infection in children results in villous atrophy, crypt hy-perplasia, and inflammatory cell infiltration of the mucosa [58].

The organisms have a worldwide distribution. Waterborne outbreaks have infected many individuals and the organism is the cause of chronic di-arrhea in AIDS and other immunocompromised patients. After hurricanes Katrina and Rita, Cryptosporidium spp were detected in the canals around New Orleans [59]. Infections after contact with animals, in daycare centers, and laboratory accidents have been reported. In the United States, the num-ber of infections peaks between July and September [58].

#### Clinical manifestations

Asymptomatic carriage is not uncommon. The incubation period is usu-ally 7 days (range, 1–30 days). In developing countries, it most commonly affects 5% to 10% of children. Ten percent to 15% of infected children de-velop persistent diarrhea that lasts more than 14 days (mean duration, 23.2 days). Breastfeeding makes no statistical difference in infection rates [60]. In developed countries and among travelers, adults are most often infected [58].

In all groups of patients, diarrhea (mucoid or watery) is the most common presentation. In immunocompetent patients, patients exhibit nausea, vomit-ing, and fever. Respiratory symptoms may accompany the illness. Symptoms last 5 to 10 days and diarrhea may recur days to weeks later [58,60].

In HIV patients, cryptosporidiosis is self-limited in those with more than 150 $CD4^+$ cells/$mm^3$, but relapses when the cell count falls. With more severe HIV, the disease may be mild, severe, chronic, and associated with extraintestinal disease (acalculous cholecystitis, sclerosing cholangitis, or pancreatitis) [58].

#### Diagnosis

Diagnosis may be made by biopsy, phase-contrast microscopy of stool wet mounts, and modified Ziehl-Neelsen stain of stool. Other methods include ELISA antigen testing of stool, PCR, and immunofluorescence staining combined with flow cytometry [58].

### Treatment

Treatment should include supportive therapy, HAART for AIDS patients, and immune restoration in immunocompromised patients when possible. Nitazoxanide is the preferred treatment, although it is probably not efficacious in HIV-positive patients. Paromomycin and macrolides (azithromycin, roxithromycin, and clarithromycin) have shown some efficacy [58], although in one study, spiramycin did not [61].

### Conclusion

Because cryptosporidia are ubiquitous, fever and diarrhea with or without systemic symptoms should suggest the diagnosis. Symptoms may last for many days, and diarrhea may recur. HIV-compromised patients have prolonged courses sometimes with extraintestinal complications, obfuscating the diagnosis.

## Selected zoonotic viral illnesses of interest

With the proper epidemiology, the diagnosis of avian influenza and severe acute respiratory syndrome (coronavirus) can be confirmed in due course. The viral hemorrhagic fevers (Arenaviridae, Bunyaviridae [including Hantavirus genus], Filoviridae [Ebola and Marburg viruses], and Flaviviridae [dengue and yellow fever]) have been reviewed [62].

### Monkeypox

#### Epidemiology

Monkeypox virus along with variola virus are the two Orthopoxviridae that cause systemic disease along with their vesiculopustular rash [63]. Monkeypox, a zoonoses found naturally in the Congo Basin and West Africa, was introduced into North America in 2003, with the importation of infected African rodents. The virus was transmitted to prairie dogs, and subsequently to individuals handling these animals. Human-to-human spread was also documented [64,65].

#### Clinical manifestations

Patients without lesions may present as a true FUO; patients with few lesions may be confused with other pustular diseases; patients with many lesions may be confused with smallpox; and hemorrhagic lesions present a broader differential diagnosis. The incubation period (7–17 days), prodrome (1–4 days for monkeypox, 2–4 days for smallpox, and 0–2 days for chickenpox), and symptomatology for the three pox diseases all overlap [66]. Fever is the most common manifestation (90%–100%). Other symptoms include chills (70%–90%); lymphadenopathy (60%–90%); sweats (60%–90%); headache

(70%); muscle pain (60%–90%); sore throat (58%–70%); cough (55%); nausea and vomiting (20%–50%); back pain (30%–60%); runny nose (20%–40%); abdominal pain (15%); wheezing (10%); diarrhea (10%); and dyspnea (10%). About half the patients have less than 25 lesions (55%); 32.5% have 26 to 100 lesions; 5% have 101 to 249 lesions; and 7.5% have more than 250 lesions [63]. Exposure to the virus involving bites or scratches shortens the incubation period and increases the severity of illness [63].

## Diagnosis

Although viral culture is the gold standard, PCR and microarray assay using species-specific oligonucleotide probes have been used successfully [66]. Lesions may be tested with immunohistochemical tests for orthopoxvirus antigens. PCR remains the most important modality for definitively differentiating monkeypox from other orthopoxviridae [66].

The differential diagnosis for monkeypox is the same for smallpox [67]. In endemic areas, coinfection with varicella-zoster virus has been reported [68].

Buffalopoxvirus outbreaks have been limited to individuals with direct animal contact. In 2004 and 2005, a nosocomial outbreak was reported in Karachi, Pakistan, placing this virus higher in the differential diagnosis for those patients with the proper epidemiology [69].

## Treatment

There are no licensed therapies, although the smallpox vaccine may protect or ameliorate monkeypox infection [66].

## Conclusion

Now that monkeypox has been introduced into North America, it must be part of the differential diagnosis of most if not all pustular-vesicular febrile diseases. It becomes an important consideration in FUO when it presents in the paucivesicular or hemorrhagic form.

## Colorado tick fever (coltiviruses)

### Epidemiology and pathogenesis

The agent of Colorado tick fever is one of three (double-stranded RNA) coltiviruses of the Reoviridae family transmitted to man by a tick bite. Most common hosts are the ground squirrel and hare, and smaller and larger mammals, especially deer and porcupines. The virus infects erythropoietic cell lines in the bone marrow and peripheral blood. Transfusions are documented risks for acquiring the infection. Infection from mother to child is suspected. Viremia persists for more than 4 weeks in 50% of patients, and is independent of the severity of the disease.

### Clinical manifestations

Incubation periods average 3 to 4 days (range, <1–14 or 19 days). Symptoms include a sudden onset of fever, chills, headache, myalgias, hyperesthesia, weakness, and prostration. One fifth of patients have gastro-intestinal complaints. Physical findings include infected conjunctivae and pharynx, and an enanthem. Some patients have minimum splenomegaly and lymphadenopathy. A maculopapular or petechial rash is seen in 15% of patients, which may be confused with Rocky Mountain spotted fever.

Resolution occurs in 1 week, but 50% of patients have recurrence of fever and symptoms 2 to 3 days later. Rarely, there is a third recurrence.

*Complications*

Five percent to 10% of patients have aseptic meningitis or encephalitis. Almost all cases of CNS disease occur in children under 10 years of age. Fatal cases have demonstrated encephalitis; hemorrhage; purpura; petechiae; disseminated intravascular coagulopathy; swollen endothelial cells in lymph node capillaries; hyaline membranes in alveoli; and focal necrosis of the liver, myocardium, spleen, intestines, and brain.

Coinfection with other tick-borne diseases, especially Rocky Mountain spotted fever, should be included in the differential diagnosis. The differential diagnosis includes hemorrhagic fever with renal syndrome (also endemic in Colorado tick fever endemic areas); hemorrhagic scarlet fever; leptospirosis; scrub typhus; murine typhus; hemolytic-uremic syndrome (from Coxsackie viruses A4, B2, B4; parechovirus 1; and *Escherichia coli* O157:H7); and causes of disseminated intravascular coagulopathy.

Typically, there is leukopenia and thrombocytopenia. CSF in patients with CNS complications reveals elevated protein and a monocytosis.

*Diagnosis*

Diagnosis is made by seroconversion of neutralizing antibodies, compliment fixation, immunofluorescent antibodies, or ELISA testing.

*Conclusion*

The pathophysiology, persistence, recurrence after primary infection, vertical transmission, and transmission by transfusion place Colorado tick fever among the important causes of FUOs in those with the proper exposure history [70].

*West Nile virus*

West Nile virus (WNV) is a (RNA) flavivirus of birds, transmitted between different birds and to man by *Culex* mosquitoes. The organism first appeared in New York City in 1999, spread across the continent, and has caused nearly 900 human deaths. Horses are also infected but, like humans, do not develop a significant viremia to become an intermediate or amplifying hosts [71]. In 2006, there were 4261 cases of WNV disease reported from across the United States. Of these cases, 1491 were WNV neuroinvasive disease, which was a 14% increase from 2005. Of the patients with neuroinvasive disease,

1311 (87.9%) were hospitalized and 161 (10.8%) died. Based on past serosurveys, the Centers for Disease Control and Prevention estimates there were 41,750 cases of nonneuroinvasive WNV infections in 2006 [72].

The virus infects over 300 different bird and vertebrate species. Host die-off (especially in corvids [crows, jays, magpies] and geese) facilitates the spread of the disease, allowing infected mosquitoes to bypass immune and already infected hosts [73]. The American crow population alone has been reduced by 45%.

In nonhuman mammals, horses represent most reported infections (96.9%) [71]. Peridomestic chipmunks, eastern cottontail rabbits, and fox squirrels along with the golden hamster develop high-grade viremias, are ready meal sources for domestic mosquitoes, and are important amplifying hosts [74].

WNV represents a transfusion-transmission risk, with seven cases reported since 2003 when nucleic acid amplification testing of blood was introduced [75].

Incubation period is 2 to 6 days (range, 2–21 days). Most illnesses are mild, presenting as sudden onset of fever; chills; rash; malaise; headache; backache; arthralgia; myalgia; and eye pain (15%–20%). Febrile prodromes occur for 1 to 7 days, before onset of neurologic complications, and may be biphasic.

Meningitis, encephalitis, and acute flaccid paralysis occurs in less than 1% of patients. These patients have stiff neck, headache, weakness, gastrointestinal symptoms, disorientation, tremors, seizures, and paralysis [71,76].

Diagnosis is made by PCR or serology (ELISA). Although viral cultures are the gold-standard, isolation can be difficult [71].

WNV infection is well-established in many hosts and represents a risk in most places across North America. Those who become symptomatic primarily present with fever. The disease may be biphasic, making it an important cause of FUO.

*Japanese encephalitis*

JE, like WNV, is a zoonotic flavivirus exclusive to southern Asia and the Pacific Islands [71]. JE is transmitted to humans by *Culex* with amplifying vertebrate hosts (usually cattle, swine, and birds) [77]. The flying fox seems to be the natural host for JE and enterovirus (hand-foot-and-mouth disease with neurologic and systemic complications) [76]. Endemic areas report approximately 30,000 to 50,000 cases yearly with 10,000 to 15,000 deaths. Large outbreaks occurred in northern India, and it is now an emerging infection in Nepal [77]. Congenital infections have been reported in international travelers [78].

After an incubation period of 1 to 2 weeks, JE causes a mild febrile illness with aseptic meningitis. The disease is more severe in children. Presentations include stupor, seizures, local motor impairment, parkinsonian movement disorders, infrequent cranial nerve palsy, acute flaccid paralysis, and impaired consciousness or abnormal behavior [71,77,79]. Half of all survivors have severe neuropsychiatric sequelae [77].

In children, the prodrome is short (average, 2.61 days). Findings include seizures (98.7%); hypertonia (50.6%); focal deficits (45.4%, monoparesis and hemiparesis); gastric hemorrhage (54.5%); extrapyramidal signs (31.1%); hyperpnea; thrombocytopenia; elevated liver enzymes; and elevated CSF cell counts (15.6%) [79]. Clinical cases may exceed 30% mortality [77,79]. Half of children discharged after clinical disease requiring hospitalization have neurologic sequelae (most commonly hemiparesis). Sequelae were associated with prolonged vomiting, altered sensorium, and focal neurologic deficits on admission, but 66% eventually resolved [80].

Virus is found in the lungs, liver, kidneys, myocardium, and the CNS. Viremia may last months. Fatal cases reveal neuronal necrosis, microglial nodules, perivascular inflammation, and acellular necrotic foci [71,81].

Prevention includes prevention of mosquito bites. A vaccine is available. Larvicides, insecticides, and vaccination of pigs have been unsuccessful attempts at controlling human disease. Human vaccination does not result in herd immunity [77].

Diagnosis is made by serology (IgM ELISA in serum and CSF); viral culture; and PCR. In endemic areas, JE has been confused with Nipah and Chandipura virus infections [71,77,79]. Temporal lobe involvement on MRI and CT imaging may confuse JE with herpes simplex encephalitis [82].

A single case report indicates there may be some benefit to treatment with intravenous immunoglobulin [83]. Mass vaccination campaigns in Japan, Taiwan, and Korea have reduced the incidence of disease [77].

WNV has disseminated across North America. WNV, Sindbis virus, Tahyna virus, and louping ill virus are present in Great Britain. The future spread of JE virus, along with dengue, yellow fever, Rift Valley fever, Crimean-Congo hemorrhagic fever, bluetongue, and African horse sickness, may depend on the ability to survive in changing environments in the northern latitudes as global warming progresses [84].

JE is a well-established and emerging infection in southeast and eastern Asia, and the Pacific archipelagoes. The virus disseminates, and viremia lasts for months. Large outbreaks have occurred. Presentations most frequently include fever, but additional symptoms may be mild and nonspecific or severe and variable, making it an important cause of FUO in the international traveler.

## Toscana virus (Phlebovirus genus, Bunyavirdae family)

Toscana virus is an arthropod-borne virus transmitted by sand flies (*Phlebotomus periciosus* and *Phlebotomus perfiliewi*) in the Mediterranean basin, first described in 1971. In some areas of central Italy, Toscana virus is the most frequent cause of viral meningoencephalitis, and one of the most prevalent arboviruses in Spain [85].

The most common presentation is acute meningitis and encephalitis occurring in the warmer months, usually in inhabitants and travelers from central Italy, Spain, France, and other Mediterranean countries [85]. Severe headache, nuchal rigidity, and generalized malaise are typical findings. Vomiting and electroencephalogram abnormalities are less frequent, and there are no sequelae [85].

CSF reveals an elevated white blood cell count (30–900 cells/cu mm$^3$), with lymphocytosis (60%–90%); elevated protein (669–1840 mg/L); and CSF to serum glucose ratios of 0.61 to 0.72 [85]. Diagnosis is made by detection of IgG and IgM antibodies in the serum and CSF, and by reverse transcription-nested PCR [85].

Toscana virus is the most common cause of aseptic meningitis in southern European countries. Half of the time, the disease is accompanied by fever. As with JE in travelers to southern Asia, Toscana virus is an important cause of FUO in travelers returning from the Mediterranean basin.

## Chikungunya virus

Chikungunya virus, an alphavirus (Togaviridae family), is transmitted by *Aedes albopictus* and *Aedes aegypti*. It is endemic throughout tropical Asia, Africa, and the islands of the Indian Ocean [86,87]. Peripartum mother-to-infant transmission has occurred [88].

Explosive outbreaks in 2006 on Reunion Island affecting 35% of the population (260,000 individuals over a 6-month period), and 1.4 million people in India are well documented [88]. In 2006, of the estimated 2 million cases worldwide, 1000 travelers returning to Europe and 37 cases in travelers returning to the United States were confirmed. Epidemics have been related to drought conditions and global warming [88]. *A albopictus* is now present across the United States, Central America, and parts of South America [88]. Asymptomatic viremic patients have been documented by the Centers for Disease Control and Prevention, and no doubt represent only a small number of viremic individuals [86]. To date there has been no indigenous spread of chikungunya virus in the United States, but there is always the danger of this disease becoming endemic as did WNV [86,88].

## Clinical presentation

Patients initially present with abrupt onset of fever (89%); debilitating polyarthralgia (96%); conjunctivitis; and maculopapular rash (40.1%). Almost 60% of patients presenting without fever had taken antipyretics. Distal joints and lower limbs are principally affected. Joint swelling was present in 31.8% of patients, and may persist for months to a year [86,89]. Mortality is approximately 1 per 1000 [88].

Half of the patients had pruritic maculopapular rashes that rarely affected the face. Few patients developed bullous lesions. Other findings include gastrointestinal complaints (47.1%); lymphadenopathy (cervical in most cases, 8.9%); aphthous ulcers (2.5%); and dry cough (8.9%) [89]. Bilateral macular choroiditis has been reported [90]. Hemorrhagic complications from thrombocytopenia (6.4%) and hepatic failure occur [89]. Neurologic complications (12%) include confusion (7.6%); meningoencephalitis; and rare seizures [88,89].

*Diagnosis and treatment*

Diagnosis is made by ELISA, plaque reduction neutralization, and viral cultures confirmed by PCR. Viral loads have exceeded $10^9$ viral particles/ mm$^3$ [88]. Treatment is supportive. Hepatic failure may have resulted from excess doses of acetaminophen [86,87].

Chikungunya virus is an important cause of FUO in patients returning from tropical Asia, Africa, and the Indian Ocean, especially those with arthritic symptoms.

## Rodent-associated infections

> Rats! They fought the dogs and killed the cats, And bit the babies in the cradles, And ate the cheeses out of the vats, And licked the soup from the cooks' own ladles, Split open the kegs of salted sprats, Made nests inside men's Sunday hats, And eve.
>
> –Robert Browning

Rodent-associated infections include 10 Arenaviridae, 4 Bunyaviridae, 2 Orthopoxviridae, hepatitis E virus, 15 bacteria, 6 anaplasma and rickettsiae, 2 fungi, 3 dermatophytic fungi, 18 protozoa, microsporidia, helminths, and ectoparasites. All of the viruses, bacteria, anaplasma and rickettsiae, and the fungi (not including the dermatophytes) prominently cause fever.

The ones that first come to mind when considering the differential diagnosis of zoonotic FUO are the rat-bite fevers (*Streptobacillus moniliformis* and *Spirillum minus*); plague (*Yersinia pestis*); lymphocytic choriomeningitis virus; hantaviruses; *Francisella tularensis*; *Pasteurella multocida*; *Leptospira* sp; and all of the rickettsial species. These have been reviewed with extensive references elsewhere [91–93].

What was not included in these reviews was *Salmonella enterica* serotypes typhimurium and enteritidis. These agents are still included in rodenticides (Biorat contains 1.25% *Salmonella* and 0.02% hydroxycoumarin; Ratin contains *S enteritidis* var. Danysz). Agents containing *Salmonella* species were first used in San Francisco in 1895 during the outbreak of plague. They had no effect on the rat population and caused morbidity and mortality among those handling and producing the product.

The products were discontinued in Europe in the 1960s but are still produced in Central and South America and Asia. Both products are mixed with rice or grain, may be mistaken for human food, and accidentally ingested. They are readily available and pose a threat as bioterrorism agents [94].

## Streptobacillus moniliformis

*Streptobacillus moniliformis* is a gram-negative pleomorphic aerobic and facultatively anaerobic bacterium that is difficult to culture. It is part of the normal oral pharynx and upper airway flora of most rodents; weasels; squirrels; dogs (especially greyhounds who have an appetite for rodents); cats; and pigs. Disease results from rat bites or ingestion of contaminated foods including milk.

### Clinical presentation

Haverhill fever (erythema arthriticum epidemicum) has an incubation period from 1 to 22 days, but in most cases does not exceed 10 days. In adults, the rat bite heals and there is no lymphadenopathy. In children, the rat bites may be fresh because the disease can progress rapidly to death.

Patients experience a sudden onset of fever, chills, headache, vomiting, and migratory arthritis. A nonpruritic measles-like, petechial, maculopapular, morbilliform, vesicular, pustular, or hemorrhagic pustular rash appears over the palms, soles, and extremities, sometimes with blisters or cutaneous abscesses. The rash appears 2 to 4 days after the onset of the fever and then desquamates. Rare patients have the rash limited to macules on the fingers. Arthritis usually follows the rash days later. Half of the patients have polyarthritis and some patients develop septic arthritis with the rash. Known complications include endocarditis; myocarditis; pericardial effusion; pneumonia; hepatitis; nephritis; amnionitis; anemia; subglottic mass with bilateral parotid swelling; brain, liver, spleen, kidney, and female genital tract abscess; and meningitis.

Uncomplicated untreated patients become afebrile in 3 to 5 days and have resolution of disease within 2 weeks. Untreated patients may remain sick for months and arthritis may persist for up to 2 years. The mortality in untreated patients is 7% to 10% to 10% to 13%.

### Diagnosis

Patients have periperal white blood cell count of approximately 30,000/ mm$^3$; false-positive serology for syphilis (25%); and elevated C-reactive protein, gamma-glutamyl transpeptidase, erythrocyte sedimentation rate, aspartate transaminase, and alanine transaminase. Organisms are seen in peripheral blood, pus, or joint fluid stained with Giemsa, Gram, or Wayson stains. Culture is definitive. ELISA and PCR also assist in the diagnosis.

The differential diagnosis includes viral infections, meningococcemia, enteric fever, drug reactions, Rocky Mountain spotted fever, and secondary syphilis. The arthritis suggests rheumatoid arthritis, Lyme disease, brucellosis, septic arthritis, and vasculitic disease.

### Treatment

Recommendations for uncomplicated cases include oral amoxicillin (875 mg/100 g) twice daily for 10 to 14 days, or doxycycline, 100 mg twice daily orally or intravenously. Endocarditis needs 4 weeks therapy with intravenous penicillin 20 million units daily. Alternate therapies include combination of rifampin and clindamycin, clarithromycin, tetracycline, and combination of ofloxacin and imipenem.

Prophylaxis with oral penicillin, amoxicillin-clavulanate, or doxycycline is recommended after rat bites.

## Conclusion

The ubiquitous nature of the rodent and the inability to know whether food or drink may be contaminated places *S moniliformis* in the pantheon of causes of FUO [91].

## Spirillum minus

*Spirillum minus* is a motile spiral-shaped probably gram-negative bacterium that is found in blood, peritoneal fluid, conjunctival fluid, muscle, tongue, and lung tissue of infected rodents [91]. It also infects wild and domestic cats and other carnivores that feed on infected rodents.

## Clinical presentation

Rat-bite fever from *S minus* (Sodoku or Sokosha) has an incubation period from 5 to 30 days (usually 5–10 days). The initial bite-wound heals, but in 1 to 4 weeks becomes swollen, painful, purple, and is accompanied by lymphangitis and lymphadenitis. The wound progresses to a chancre-like ulcer. Patients develop fever, chills, headache, and malaise. There is hyperreflexia, myalgia, arthralgia, hyperesthesia, and edema. The patients' temperature rises over 3 days, remains elevated for 3 days, and returns to normal for 5 to 10 days before rising again. Untreated, recurrences occur every 3 to 9 days. A red-brown to purple macular (infrequently urticarial) rash is seen over the extremities, trunk, face, and scalp.

Uncomplicated untreated cases resolve in 1 to 2 months. Some untreated cases have been symptomatic for years. Rare complications include endocarditis, myocarditis, pleurisy, hepatitis, splenomegaly, meningitis, epididymitis, conjunctivitis, anemia, and meningoencephalitis.

## Diagnosis

Half of the patients have a positive serology for syphilis. Peripheral white blood cell counts are 10,000 to 20,000/mm$^3$. Occasional patients have eosinophilia. Diagnosis is made by direct visualization of the organism in blood, pus, or nodes by Giemsa stain, Wright stain, or darkfield microscopy. Serology is not available, and the organisms cannot be cultured on artificial media. The organism multiples after intraperitoneal injection. The differential diagnoses include *Borrelia* spp, malaria, lymphoma, and other relapsing infections.

*Treatment*

High-dose intravenous penicillin G (12–24 million units daily) is the drug of choice. Uncomplicated cases are treated for 10 to 14 days. Alternate therapies include oral amoxicillin-clavulanate, 875 mg/100 mg twice daily (for 10–14 days), or oral or intravenous doxycycline, 100 mg twice daily.

*Conclusion*

Although untreated cases often resolve, occasional cases may remain symptomatic for years, becoming an important cause of FUO.

**Infections of the land and sea**

> Wouldst thou' – so the helmsman answered./Learn the secret of the sea?/ Only those who brave its dangers/Comprehend its mystery!
>                                        –Henry Wadsworth Longfellow

As occupations and recreation become more intimately associated with fresh and salt-water, other organisms must be considered zoonotic risks. *Flavobacterium xinjiangensis, Leptothrix discophora, Aeromonas, Clostridium, Klebsiella, Legionella, Listeria, Pseudomonas,* and *Vibrio* species are found in estuaries and oceans [95]. Injury from coral formations, sharks, and stingrays are a particular hazard to surfers [96]. Halophilic *Vibrio, Cytophaga-Flavobacterium-Bacteroides* group, and *Clostridium* spp, are all present on coral [95,96].

Because most shark attacks victims suffer relatively minor injuries (81% require simple primary suturing), infection accompanying trauma becomes a major concern [97]. Cultures from the mouth of a possibly still living 442-cm, 1227-kg adult male white shark (*Carcharodon carcharias*) revealed *Vibrio alginolyticus, Vibrio parahaemolyticus, Vibrio fluvialis, Pseudomonas putrefaciens, Staphylococcus* sp, *Psseudomonas* sp, *Citrobacter* sp, and *Micrococcus* sp [98]. Parenthetically, witnessed attacks by one or more great white sharks leave only floating lung tissue in the water or washed ashore. Because the cause of death from these attacks is massive trauma and not drowning, lungs remain buoyant, and finding one floating by should alert individuals to take immediate action to avoid shark-bite–related infections [99].

Thalassogenic infections from the consumption of filter-feeding shellfish (bivalves) is responsible for 4 million cases of hepatitis A and E causing 40,000 deaths and 40,000 cases of chronic liver disease. This figure is believed to be an underestimate with numbers approximately 50% higher [100].

*Vibrio parahaemolyticus*

Outbreaks of *V parahaemolyticus* have been associated with raw oyster and clam consumption. Most patients (89%) develop gastroenteritis (diarrhea, 100%; nausea, 94%; vomiting, 82%; fever, 47%; blood stools, 29%;

headache, 24%; myalgia, 24%). A small number (11%) develop sepsis and lower-extremity edema and bullae [101].

## Vibrio vulnificus

*Vibrio vulnificus* was the leading cause of food-borne illness deaths in Florida from 1981 to 1992 [102]. It has caused wound infections, sepsis with multiorgan failure, and gastroenteritis without sepsis. One half of patients with wound infections have underlying liver disease, hematopoietic disorders, chronic renal insufficiency, are receiving immunosuppressive agents, or abusing alcohol. These at-risk individuals have often handled or cleaned shellfish, and have an associated mortality of 15%. Patients with sepsis have fever, chills, prostration, rapid onset of hypotension, and 50% mortality. The onset of sepsis is often associated with eating raw oysters within the last 24 to 48 hours. Seventy percent have bullous skin lesions, which may suggest the diagnosis. Circular necrotic lesions (ecthyma gangrenosum) are also seen [102].

## Brucellosis

Brucellosis (*B abortus*, *B suis*, *B ovis*, *B melitensis*, *B canis*, *B neotomae*) is a frequently considered FUO [103]. From 0.8% to 5.2% of patients with FUO were seropositive for the disease. Males predominate and seropositivity is age-related only in males [104]. Animal handlers and consumers of fresh yogurt and goat milk have as high as a 20% seroprevalence [104]. Risk factors include laboratory handling of livestock products of conception; consumption of unpasteurized milk (especially from camels); and other unpasteurized milk products [105].

Seals, dolphins, porpoises, otters, minke whale, killer whale, and a pilot whale, including beached and stranded animals, were reported to be infected with *Brucella* sp. Thirty-three strains of *Brucella* were identified [106]. Collectively, these marine strains have been named *B maris*.

Subcutaneous lesions are present in sea mammals. The organisms were isolated from the spleen, mammary glands, uterus, testes, blood, and lymph nodes from the mandible, stomach, iliac, sublumbar, and colorectal area in these animals. The extensive nature of the infections puts animal handlers and curiosity seekers at risk for this infection [106].

In children, 70% present with arthritis, 20% with fever without localizing signs, and 10% had fever with focal signs [105]. Patients presenting with epididymo-orchitis had swollen painful testicles (unilateral or bilateral); undulant fever (96%); chills (54%); and arthralgia (23%) [107]. Fever and nonproductive cough is an unusual presentation [108]. Endocarditis is a rare complication; neuropsychiatric, adverse outcomes of pregnancy, and transplacental congenital infection have been reported [109,110].

Blood cultures are positive in only 38% of cases. Diagnosis must be made by serology or PCR [110]. With undulant fever and multiorgan presentations, in the proper epidemiologic setting, this becomes an important cause of FUO.

## Old favorites

### Malaria

Malaria is easily diagnosed and only becomes an FUO when it is not suspected. Approximately 1000 to 1500 cases are reported annually in the United States, almost all imported from endemic areas. Locally acquired mosquito-transmitted malaria clusters in the United States have been documented 63 times involving 1 to 32 cases annually, for a total of 156 cases. California has reported the most cases (27%). *Plasmodium vivax* is the most common species (*Plasmodium falciparum* 11.1%, *Plasmodium malariae* 10.6%) [111].

### Hyperreactive malarial splenomegaly

Hyperreactive malarial splenomegaly, or fulminant tropical splenomegaly (previously termed "tropical splenomegaly"), may present with fever, acute hemolysis, and splenomegaly. Hyperreactive malarial splenomegaly is diagnosed when a combination of antimalarial antibodies (IgM) are higher than 2 standard deviations above the "local mean," and in the presence of gross splenomegaly. Villous lymphocytes are seen in some hyperreactive malarial splenomegaly patients. It is postulated that hyperreactive malarial splenomegaly may be linked to splenic lymphoma. Malarial parasites are present on Giemsa-stained peripheral smears in the minority of patients. PCR may assist in confirming the diagnosis, although even that is not positive in all cases.

Hyperreactive malarial splenomegaly is associated with repeated attacks of malaria, and the use of chloroquine as a single agent for malarial treatment. Hyperreactive malarial splenomegaly is treated with antimalarial therapy. The differential diagnosis includes chronic kala-azar, typhoid, congenital hemolytic anemia, leukemia, and lymphoma [112,113].

### Conclusion

Malaria is easily diagnosed if suspected. Malaria without the typical epidemiologic history (travel or transfusion) occurs, and must be considered as a cause of FUO. Hyperreactive malarial splenomegaly, another cause of FUO, is more difficult to diagnose because the malaria parasites are seen in a minority of peripheral smears.

### Amoebae and amoebae-resistant organisms

Amoebae feed on and kill almost any bacteria [114]. Free-living amoebae are more commonly found along with their parasitizing amoeba-resistant bacteria in cooling towers and hospital water systems than natural aquatic environments [115]. These amoeba-resistant bacteria include *Legionella pneumophila*; *Legionella anisa*; *Pseudomonas* spp; *Parachlamydia* spp (possible cause of community-acquired pneumonia, especially in immunocompromised patients, and humidifier-related fever); *Simkania negevensis* (a cause of adult pneumonia and pediatric bronchiolitis); *Mycobacterium leprae*; *Mycobacterium avium*; *Mycobacterium marinum*; *Mycobacterium ulcerans*; *Mycobacterium simiae*; and other mycobacteria. Other organisms that readily survive in amoebae are Burkholderiaceae, *Coxiella burnetti*, *F tularensis*, Enterobacteriaceae, Vibrionaceae, *Listeria monocytogenes*, *Helicobacter pylori*, and *Cryptococcus neoformans* [115].

Mimivirus, a newly described large virus that was cocultured in amoeba, caused self-limited pneumonia in a laboratory worker. Seroconversion to mimivirus was found more frequently among ventilator-associated pneumonia patients than community-acquired pneumonia patients (31.6% and 10.5%, respectively). If amoebae act as an amplifying host or "Trojan horse," this agent may be added to that of zoonoses [116].

As one of the smallest members of the animal kingdom, amoeba may cause a zoonotic FUO. Approximately 85% of infections are (afebrile) amoebic keratitis in otherwise normal contact-lens wearers, granulomatous amebic encephalitis in immunocompromised patients, and disseminated acanthamebiasis [117].

The incidence of disseminated acanthamebiasis has been increasing. Six cases have been reported in solid organ transplant patients. The most recent case involved a heart transplant patient who presented with fever; skin abscesses; violaceous and ulcerated plaques; deep abscesses; and an atypical pyoderma gangrenosum (*Acanthamoeba leticulata*) [117].

Disseminated acanthamebiasis is an important although apparently unusual cause of FUO in immunocompromised patients. Amoebae as vehicles for amoebae-resistant organisms (ie, mimivirus), where amoebae act as an amplifying host, are being newly recognized.

## *Viceral larva migrans* (Toxocara canis *and* Toxocara cati)

Visceral larva migrans is typically a disease of children with pica under the age of 5 years. It is caused by migration of the round worms and is characterized by fever, malaise, myalgia, cough, abdominal discomfort, urticaria, wheezing, and hepatomegaly. Most cases are self-limited with symptoms lasting several months. Eosinophilia and hypergammaglobulinemia are common. Occasional patients develop hypereosinophilia; liver abscesses; myocarditis; pericardial tamponade; eosinophilic pleural effusion; and eye complications (diminished acuity with or without strabismus, white pupil) [118].

Asymptomatic infection is common, and one third of adults have serologic evidence of prior exposure. A study of asymptomatic seropositive adults found that 68% had single or multiple ill-defined oval, small, low-attenuating liver lesions on CT scan. Patients with liver lesions had higher eosinophil counts [118].

Adult visceral larva migrans patients have presented with fever; fatigue; headaches; eosinophilic pneumonia; myocarditis; spinal cord swelling; and cerebral vasculitis (*Toxocara canis* and *Fasciola hepatica* co-infection). Visceral larva migrans may mimic liver tumors. Biopsies reveal nonspecific granuloma with eosinophilic infiltrate [118–122].

For systemic disease, diagnosis is made by ELISA; however, ELISA is unsatisfactory for ocular disease, which must be diagnosed by funduscopic examination. Treatments include albendazole, mebendazole, diethylcarbamazine, or ivermectin. Ocular disease is treated with laser photocoagulation or local or systemic therapy [118].

Serologic evidence of visceral larva migrans is found in a significant minority of adults. Fever and eosinophilia present in both adult and pediatric symptomatic disease, making it an important cause of FUO in this clinical setting.

## Bartonella *species and cat-scratch disease*

*Bartonella* species cause a variety of zoonotic diseases with differing epidemiologies. *Bartonella bacilliformis* (female *Lutzomyia verrucarum* sandfly vector) causes Oroya fever, an acute septicemic disease of Peru and high South American rain forests. The same organism causes verruga peruana, which may or may not follow untreated Oroya fever. It is characterized by arthralgia, fevers, and crops of painless papules [123].

A new *Bartonella* species that causes sepsis, recurrent fever, insomnia, myalgia, nausea, headache, mild cough, and splenomegaly has been isolated. The patient had visited Peru, hiked, camped, and received multiple insect bites. The organism was cultured, and analysis suggests it is more closely related to *Bartonella clarridgeiae* than *B bacilliformis*. The patient responded to 5 days of oral levofloxacin [124].

*Bartonella quintana* (*Pediculus humanus corporis* louse vector) is the cause of trench fever. The disease is sometimes mild, or may be prolonged, severe, bacteremic, and complicated by endocarditis. Immunocompromised and AIDS patients have developed bacillary angiomatosis and peliosis, similar to that caused by *Bartonella henselae* [123].

*Bartonella elizabethae* (*Xenopsylla cheopis* oriental rat flea vector, *Rattus norvegicus* rat host) and *Bartonella vinsonii* (*Trombicula miroti* vole ear mite, *Ixodes scapularis* deer tick, and other unknown tick vectors) cause endocarditis [123,125]. Dogs are hosts for *B vinsonii* (subsp. *berkhoffii*). Importantly, dogs may be coinfected with *Ehrlichia*, *Babesia*, and *Bartonella* spp. In the Netherlands, *Ixodes ricinus* ticks are coinfected with *Borrelia burgdorferi* and *Bartonella* spp. In the United States, *Peromyscus leucopus* mice cosegregate *B burgdorferi*, *Babesia microti*, and *Bartonella* sp [125].

The common host and vector for *B henselae*, the cause of cat-scratch disease, bacillary angiomatosis, bacillary peliosis, neuroretinitis, optic neuritis, submacular exudates, serous retinal detachment of the macula, and osteomyelitis, are the cat and cat flea (*Ctenocephalides felis*). *Afipia felis* and *B clarridgeiae* are also believed to be causes of cat-scratch disease [123]. Seroprevalence in cats in the United States is 3.7% to 54.6%, with the highest rates in warmer areas with higher flea infestations. Feral cats, opossums, zoo animals, rodents, mountain lions, bobcats, coyotes, gray foxes, elk, black-tailed deer, and wild rabbits may also host the bacteria [125].

*Bartonella* sp has caused FUO in several clinical situations. Culture or serologic evidence of *Bartonella* infection was found (by PCR, culture or immunofluorescence assay) in 18% of 382 patients with FUO, most of whom were HIV infected [126]. Other cases have involved liver masses 2.5 years after liver transplant; pancytopenia, rash, hepatitis with bone marrow and skin granulomas; extensive granulomas of the liver and spleen; bone pain with osteomyelitis; headache and visual disturbance with neuroretinitis; and diffuse lymphadenopathy, weight loss, splenic lesions with disseminated disease, and treatment for hepatitis C [127,128]. *B henselae* has caused FUOs in children with granulomatous hepatitis without peripheral adenopathy, and mesenteric lymphadenopathy [129].

Up to 16.1% of patients with positive serology for cat-scratch disease had no lymphadenopathy. This was associated with FUO, persistent fever, or systemic complications [130]. In another study, 21% of patients with culture-negative endocarditis were found to be infected with *Bartonella* sp [131].

Only 50% of patients with encephalopathy have fever. Seizures (46%), combative behavior (40%), lethargy, facial nerve paresis, neuroretinitis, and peripheral neuropathy were noted. Recovery from neurologic disease occurred within 1 week to 3 months in 78% of patients, and all patients recovered within 1 year [132].

Although it is common to find a papule at the inoculation site, rashes are uncommon. Papuloedematous eruptions across the upper trunk have been accompanied by lymphadenopathy, arthralgia, and fever. Other cutaneous manifestations include erythema nodosum, erythema multiforme, erythema marginatum, maculopapular, petechial, and morbilliform rashes. Most, but not all, are nonpruritic [133].

Diagnosis is made by PCR, culture, ELISA, and immunoblot analysis [123,127]. Biopsy specimens of lymph nodes show necrotizing granuloma with peripheral palisading epithelioid cells, plasma cells, and lymphocytes. Stellate necroses with microabscesses are typical of cat-scratch disease [123].

Doxycycline is the treatment of choice [123,127]. Neuroretinitis has been treated with minocycline and steroids [123].

All epidemiologic and etiologic variants of *Bartonella* species diseases (Oroya fever, verruga peruana, trench fever, bacillary angiomatosis, peliosis, and cat-scratch fever) cause fever or recurrent fever. A significant minority of HIV-infected patients have serologic evidence of infection. Its varied clinical presentations and complications make it a common consideration in the FUO diagnostic work-up.

## Special populations

> All human actions have one or more of these seven causes: chance, nature,
> compulsion, habit, reason, passion, and desire.
>
> –Aristotle

### Homeless patients

Homeless people are exposed to ectoparasites and mites. These individuals are at risk for trench fever (*B quintana*); epidemic typhus (*Rickettsia prowazekii*); relapsing fever (*Borrelia recurrentis*); plague; murine typhus; cat-scratch disease; rickettsialpox (*Rickettsia akari*); and other flea-borne spotted rickettsiosis [134].

### Patients with zoophilia

In a study conducted in Pakistan, of 465 men seeking care at a sexually transmitted disease clinic, 0.5% reported having sex with animals [135]. A case-control study (psychiatric inpatients versus medical inpatients and psychiatric staff) found that actual or fantasized zoophilia was expressed by 55% versus 10% and 15% in the control groups, respectively [136]. Postconviction polygraph testing of sexual offenders revealed that 36% had engaged in sex with animals [137]. Others report zoophilia associated with bouts of depression, and dopaminergic therapy for Parkinson's disease [138].

Veterinarians and their assistants are at risk for plague pneumonia, simian foamy virus, simian immunodeficiency viruses, herpesvirus simiae (B virus), brucellosis, tuberculosis from nonhuman primates, *Echinococcus multilocularis* from domestic cats, psittacosis, *C burnetii*, tularemia, cryptosporidiosis, and avian influenza [5,6,139–141]. Occupational allergies and the risk for motorneuron diseases seem to be increased in this group [142]. There seems to be no increased risk of *Toxoplasma gondii* infection [143].

### Conclusion

Difficulty in obtaining an accurate history is typical when treating the homeless. Obtaining a history of zoophilia is unusual, because the question is rarely asked. At-risk (ie, prison and psychiatric) populations with FUOs should be queried as to their past and present sexual practices.

A complete history from veterinarians, their assistants, and zoo workers in direct contact with the animals is usually readily available. It is these histories that help direct the diagnostic work-up for FUO.

## Peripatetic zoonotic infections

> ...It is a riddle wrapped in a mystery inside an enigma: but perhaps there is
> a key.
>
> –Sir Winston Churchill (1939 radio speech commenting on Russia).

*Plague* (Yersinia pestis)

Clinical presentations of *Y pestis* infection include the following [93]:

1. Subclinical disease (positive serology in asymptomatic populations in endemic areas)
2. A mild febrile illness (pestis minor)
3. Bubonic plague
4. Septicemic plague (pestis siderans)
5. Primary inhalation plague pneumonia (demic plague)
6. Secondary hematogenous plague pneumonia (<50% of patients have lymphadenopathy)
7. Plague meningitis as a complication of bubonic or septicemic plague

*Yersinia pestis* hosts are principally 200 species of rodents. Other animals may be infected, although dogs, cats, pigs, sheep, goats, and horses are difficult to infect. Fifty-seven genera and 85 species of fleas and the *Hyalomma detritium* tick are natural vectors. Plague is endemic in the rodent population in western Canada, the western United States, and Mexico [93].

Peripatetic bubonic plague has been reported in the District of Columbia in 1990 in a mammologist who had returned from the La Paz area of Bolivia [144]. Bubonic plague was diagnosed in a husband and wife from Santa Fe County, New Mexico. They presented to a New York City emergency department with fever and unilateral inguinal adenopathy. Fleas trapped near the patients' home in New Mexico were culture positive for *Y pestis* [145].

*Francisella tularensis (rabbit fever or deer fly fever)*

Tularemia is an acute febrile illness often accompanied by an ulcer at the site of inoculation (skin or mucous membrane). Patients may develop pharyngitis, eye lesions, regional lymphadenopathy sepsis, and pneumonia. Diagnosis is made by culture and serology. On average, 124 cases are reported yearly (between 1990 and 2000) from 44 states. Disease is acquired from contact with infected animals (especially rabbits, prairie dogs, and muskrats); tick and deerfly bites (summer cases); or ingestion of contaminated meat [146].

*Bacillus anthracis (anthrax)*

Humans acquire anthrax by ingestion, contact, or inhalation of spores, causing pulmonary, cutaneous, or gastrointestinal disease. This may occur from contact with infected animals (cattle, sheep, goats, antelope, and others) or infected animal products [147].

In 2006, a resident of New York City collapsed after a 3-day history of shortness of breath, dry cough, and malaise. Radiographs revealed bilateral pneumonia and pleural effusions. The patient had become infected after handling hard-dried animal hides for making traditional African drums he had obtained from Ivory Coast. Diagnosis was made by blood culture [147].

Anthrax spores, used as a bioterrorism weapon, were sent through the US Mail. This resulted in at least 21 cases between October 3, 2001, and October 31, 2001 [148].

Inhalation disease presents with fever, chills, severe fatigue, nonproductive cough, or cough with blood-tinged sputum. Some patients complain of abdominal pain, nausea, vomiting, chest heaviness, shortness of breath, headache, myalgias, and sore throat. Peripheral white blood cell counts were minimally elevated. Chest radiographs revealed widening mediastinum, paratracheal fullness, hilar fullness, and mediastinal lymphadenopathy [147].

## Temporary petting zoos

A visit to a petting zoo is a risk for zoonotic infection. Most are temporary (67%); and although hand-washing facilities are present at most zoos, compliance is poor. Problematic behavior on the part of the public includes bringing edibles into the zoo; unsupervised animal contact with children under the age of 6 years; animal contact with very young children (including those less than 1 year of age); animal contact by pregnant women; feeding animals from ice-cream cones; feeding animals by hand; and entering animal pens not open to the public. Outbreaks of E coli O157:H7 associated with petting zoos were reported in North Carolina, Florida, and Arizona [149].

## Zoonotic agents of bioterrorism

The zoonotic organisms that are likely candidates as agents of bioterrorism are Bacillus anthracis, Burkholderia mallei, agents of brucellosis, Y pestis, C burnetii, F tularensis, Venezuelan equine encephalitis virus, and agents of viral hemorrhagic fevers. Some clues suggest a deliberate spread of pathogens: (1) large epidemic in a discrete population; (2) more severe disease than expected for the pathogen; (3) unusual routes of exposure, age groups, or attack rates and populations; (4) association with zoonotic disease outbreak; (5) a single case of an unusual disease; and (6) absence of the disease's vector in the area [150]. When used as weapons they remain zoonoses except without the usual four-legged animals.

Animals that may act as sentinels for a bioterrorist attack with a zoonotic agent include sheep and cattle (anthrax, Rift Valley fever); cats (plague); horses (Venezuelan equine encephalitis and eastern equine encephalitis); and wild birds (WNV and JE virus). Increased morbidity and mortality among animals, illness in species not normally infected by the suspect agent, lack of response to normal therapy, and disease occurrence at the "wrong time" and "wrong place," all suggest a nefarious rather than a natural vector [151].

## Summary

In theory there is no difference between theory and practice. In practice there is.

-Yogi Berra.

Physicians solve difficult diagnostic problems by comparing patterns of presentation. This involves (1) grouping findings into patterns; (2) "selection of a pivotal ... finding..."; (3) a list of possible etiologies; (4) selection of the most likely diagnosis and the differential diagnoses; and (5) confirmation of the diagnosis [152]. Histories, physical findings, rashes, and temperature curves overlap among different etiologies. Confirmatory laboratory tests, especially serology, are too numerous and may give false-positive information if not properly focused. The gold standard of positive cultures of fastidious organisms or viruses may be difficult to obtain even when a specific pathogen is suspected. Solving the diagnostic conundrum requires a thorough understanding of the patient's immune status and epidemiology.

## References

[1] Woolhouse MEJ, Gowtage-Sequeria S. Host range and emerging and reemerging pathogens. Emerg Infect Dis 2005;11:1842–7.

[2] Mackowiak PA, Durack DT. Fever of unknown origin. In: Mandell GL, Bennett JE, Dolin R, editors. Mandell, Douglas, and Bennett's principles and practice of infectious diseases, vol. 1. 6th edition. Philadelphia: Elsevier Churchill Livingston; 2005. p. 718–29.

[3] Demma LJ, Vanderford TH, Logsdon JM Jr, et al. Evolution of the uniquely adaptable lentiviral envelope in a natural reservoir host. Retrovirology 2006;3:19.

[4] Vande Woude S, Apetrei C. Going wild: lessons from naturally occurring T-lymphotropic lentiviruses. Clin Microbiol Rev 2006;19:728–62.

[5] Switzer WM, Bhullar V, Shanmugam V, et al. Frequent simian foamy virus infection in persons occupationally exposed to nonhuman primates. J Virol 2004;78:2780–9.

[6] Reynolds SJ, Bessong PO, Quinn TC. Human retroviral infections in the tropics. In: Guerrant RL, Walker DH, Weller PF, editors. Tropical infectious diseases—principles, pathogens, practice, vol. 1. 2nd edition. Philadelphia: Elsevier Churchill Livingston; 2006. p. 852–83.

[7] Peeters M, Courgnaud V, Abela B, et al. Risk to human health from a plethora of simian immunodeficiency viruses in primate bushmeat. Emerg Infect Dis 2002;8:451–7.

[8] Jeronimo SMB, De Queiroz Sousa A, Pearson RD. Leishmaniasis. In: Guerrant RL, Walker DH, Weller PF, editors. Tropical infectious diseases—principles, pathogens, practice, vol. 2. 2nd edition. Philadelphia: Elsevier Churchill Livingston; 2006. p. 1095–113.

[9] Centers for Disease Control and Prevention. Two cases of visceral leishmaniasis in U.S. military personnel—Afghanistan, 2002–2004. MMWR Morb Mortal Wkly Rep 2004;53: 265–8.

[10] Cardo LJ. Leishmania: risk to the blood supply. Transfusion 2006;46:1641–5.

[11] Harms G, Feldmeier H. The impact of HIV infection on tropical diseases. Infect Dis Clin North Am 2005;19:121–35.

[12] Cunha BA. Fever of unknown origin in HIV/AIDS patients. Drugs Today (Barc) 1999;35: 429–34.

[13] Barreto-de-Souza V, Pacheco GJ, Silva AR, et al. Increased leishmania replication in HIV-1-infected macrophages is mediated by tat protein through cyclooxygenase-2 expression and prostaglandin E2 synthesis. J Infect Dis 2006;194:846–54.

[14] Nigro L, Rizzo ML, Vancheri C, et al. CCR5 and CCR3 expression on TCD3+ lymphocytes from HIV/leishmania co-infected subjects. Med Microbiol Immunol 2007;196: 253–5 [Epub ahead of print].

[15] Gaskin AA, Schantz P, Jackson J, et al. Visceral leishmaniasis in a New York foxhound kennel. J Vet Intern Med 2002;16:34–44.

[16] Duprey ZH, Steurer FJ, Rooney JA, et al. Canine visceral leishmaniasis, United States and Canada 2000–2003. Emerg Infect Dis 2006;12:440–6.

[17] Voutsinas D, Foudoulaki L, Sofroniadou K, et al. Visceral leishmaniasis in a patient with acquired hypogammaglobulinemia. Eur J Intern Med 2001;12:127–9.

[18] Masedo Gonzalez A, Barbero Allende JM, Perez-Carreras M, et al. Intestinal leishmaniasis and Sezary syndrome: endoscopic diagnosis. Gastroenterol Hepatol 2006;29:546–50.

[19] Pittalis S, Nicastri E, Spinazzola F, et al. *Leishmania infantum* leishmaniasis in corticosteroid-treated patients. BMC Infect Dis 2006;6:177.

[20] Fabre S, Gibert C, Lechiche C, et al. Visceral leishmaniasis infection in a rheumatoid arthritis patient treated with infliximab. Clin Exp Rheumatol 2005;23:891–2.

[21] Garcia-Cordoba F, Ortuno FJ, Segovia M, et al. Fatal visceral leishmaniasis, with massive bone-marrow infection, in an immunosuppressed but HIV-negative Spanish patient, after the initiation of treatment with meglumine antimoniate. Ann Trop Med Parasitol 2005;99: 125–30.

[22] Herrejon A, Cervera A, Macia M, et al. Bronchioalveolar adenoma associated with bronchiolitis obliterans and leishmaniasis with lung involvement in acquired immunodeficiency syndrome. Arch Bronconeumol 2005;41:233–5.

[23] Mofredj A, Guerin JM, Leibinger F, et al. Visceral leishmaniasis with pericarditis in an HIV-infected patient. Scand J Infect Dis 2002;34:151–3.

[24] Cnudde F, Raccurt C, Boulard F, et al. Diffuse cutaneous leishmaniasis with visceral dissemination in an AIDS patient in Guadeloupe, West Indies. AIDS 1994;8:559–60.

[25] Boumis E, Chinello P, Della Rocca C, et al. Atypical disseminated leishmaniasis resembling post-kala-azar dermal leishmaniasis in an HIV-infected patient. Int J STD AIDS 2006;17: 351–3.

[26] Mellor-Pita S, Yebra-Bango M, Tutor de Ureta P, et al. Polyarthritis caused by *Leishmania* in a patient with human immunodeficiency virus. Clin Exp Rheumatol 2004;22:131.

[27] Meenken C, van Agtmael MA, Ten Kate RW, et al. Fulminant ocular leishmaniasis in an HIV-1 –positive patient. AIDS 2004;18:1485–6.

[28] Ranieri R, Veronelli A, Santambrogio C, et al. Subclinical hypothyroidism in a patient affected by advanced AIDS and visceral leishmaniasis. Scand J Infect Dis 2005;37:935–7.

[29] Navarro M, Bonet J, Monal J, et al. Secondary amyloidosis with irreversible acute renal failure caused by visceral leishmaniasis in a patient with AIDS. Nefrologia 2006;26:745–6.

[30] Walker M, Kublin JG, Zunt JR. Parasitic central nervous system infections in immunocompromised hosts: malaria, microsporidiosis, leishmaniasis, and African trypanosomiasis. Clin Infect Dis 2006;42:115–25 [Epub 2005 Nov 23].

[31] Posada-Vergara MP, Lindoso JA, Tolezano JE, et al. Tegumentary leishmaniasis as a manifestation of immune reconstitution inflammatory syndrome in 2 patients with AIDS. J Infect Dis 2005;192:1819–22.

[32] Cascio A, Colomba C, Antinori S, et al. Pediatric visceral leishmaniasis in western Sicily, Italy: a retrospective analysis of 111 cases. Eur J Clin Microbiol Infect Dis 2002;21:277–82.

[33] Pagliano P, Carannante N, Rossi M, et al. Visceral leishmaniasis in pregnancy: a case series and a systematic review of the literature. J Antimicrob Chemother 2005;55:229–33 [Epub 2005 Jan 13].

[34] Singh S. New developments in diagnosis of leishmaniasis. Indian J Med Res 2006;123: 311–30.

[35] Savoia D, Allice T, Tovo PA. Antileishmanial activity of HIV protease inhibitors. Int J Antimicrob Agents 2005;26:92–4.

[36] Mira JA, Corzo JE, Rivero A, et al. Frequency of visceral leishmaniasis relapses in human immunodeficiency virus-infected patients receiving highly active antiretroviral therapy. Am J Trop Med Hyg 2004;70:298–301.

[37] Kirchhoff LV. American trypanosomiasis (Chagas' disease). In: Guerrant RL, Walker DH, Weller PF, editors. Tropical infectious diseases—principles, pathogens, practice, vol. 2. 2nd edition. Philadelphia: Elsevier Churchill Livingston; 2006. p. 1082–94.

[38] De Nishioka SA, Gyorkos TW, Joseph L, et al. Tattooing and transfusion-transmitted diseases in Brazil: a hospital-based cross-sectional matched study. Eur J Epidemiol 2003;18: 441–9.

[39] Concetti H, Retegui M, Perez G, et al. Chagas disease of the cervix uteri in a patient with acquired immunodeficiency syndrome. Hum Pathol 2000;31:120–2.

[40] Sartori AM, Caiaffa-Filho HH, Berzerra RC, et al. Exacerbation of HIV viral load simultaneous with asymptomatic reactivation of chronic Chagas' disease. Am J Trop Med Hyg 2002;67:521–3.

[41] Iliovich E, Lopez R, Kum M, et al. Spontaneous chagasic peritonitis in a patient with AIDS. Medicina (B Aires) 1998;58(5 Pt 1):507–8.

[42] Sartori AM, Sotto MN, Braz LM, et al. Reactivation of Chagas disease manifested by skin lesions in a patient with AIDS. Trans R Soc Trop Med Hyg 1999;93:631–2.

[43] Rosemberg S, Chaves CJ, Higuchi ML, et al. Fatal meningoencephalitis caused by reactivation of *Trypansoma cruzi* infection in a patient with AIDS. Neurology 1992;42(3 Pt 1): 640–2.

[44] Lambert N, Mehta B, Walters R, et al. Chagasic encephalitis as the initial manifestation of AIDS. Ann Intern Med 2006;144:941–3.

[45] Yoo TW, Mlikotic A, Cornford ME, et al. Concurrent cerebral American trypanosomiasis and toxoplasmosis in a patient with AIDS. Clin Infect Dis 2004;39:e30–4 [Epub 2004 Jul 28].

[46] Pimentel PC, Handfas BW, Carmignani M. *Trypansoma cruzi* meningoencephalitis in AIDS mimicking cerebral metastases: case report. Arq Neuropsiquiatr 1996;54:102–6.

[47] Sartori AM, Neto JE, Nunes EV, et al. *Trypansoma cruzi* parasitemia in chronic Chagas disease: comparison between human immunodeficiency virus (HIV)-positive and HIV-negative patients. J Infect Dis 2002;186:872–5 [Epub 2002 Aug 9].

[48] Lages-Silva E, Ramirez LE, Silva-Vergara ML, et al. Chagasic meningoencephalitis in a patient with acquired immunodeficiency syndrome: diagnosis, follow-up, and genetic characterization of *Trypansoma cruzi*. Clin Infect Dis 2002;34:118–23 [Epub 2001 Nov 26].

[49] Viotti R, Vigliano C, Lococo B, et al. Long-term cardiac outcomes of treating chronic Chagas disease with benznidazole versus no treatment: a nonrandomized trial. Ann Intern Med 2006;144:724–34.

[50] Corti M, Yampolsky C. Prolonged survival and immune reconstitution after chagasic meningoencephalitis in a patient with acquired immunodeficiency syndrome. Rev Soc Bras Med Trop 2006;39:85–8 [Epub 2006 Feb 23].

[51] King CH. Schistosomiasis. In: Guerrant RL, Walker DH, Weller PF, editors. Tropical infectious diseases—principles, pathogens, practice. vol. 2. 2nd edition. Philadelphia: Elsevier Churchill Livingston; 2006. p. 1341–8.

[52] Secor WE. Interactions between schistosomiasis and the infection with HIV-1. Parasite Immunol 2006;28:597–603.

[53] Kjetland EF, Ndhlovu PD, Gomo E, et al. Association between genital schistosomiasis and HIV in rural Zimbabwean women. AIDS 2006;20:593–600.

[54] Payet B, Chaumentin G, Boyer M, et al. Prolonged latent schistosomiasis diagnosed 38 years after infestation in a HIV patient. Scand J Infect Dis 2006;38:572–5.

[55] de Silva S, Walsh J, Brown M. Symptomatic *Schistosoma mansoni* infection as an immune restoration phenomenon in a patient receiving antiretroviral therapy. Clin Infect Dis 2006; 42:303–4.

[56] Walker M, Zunt JR. Parasitic central nervous system infections in immunocompromised hosts. Clin Infect Dis 2005;40:1005–15 [Epub 2005 Mar 2].

[57] Kallestrup P, Zinyama R, Gomo E, et al. Schistosomiasis and HIV in rural Zimbabwe: efficacy of treatment of schistosomiasis in individuals with HIV coinfection. Clin Infect Dis 2006;42:1781–9.

[58] White AC Jr. Cryptosporidiosis (Cryptosporidium hominis, Cryptosporidium parvum) and other species. In: Mandell GL, Bennett JE, Dolin R, editors. Mandell, Douglas, and Bennett's principles and practice of infectious diseases, vol. 2. 6th edition. Philadelphia: Elsevier Churchill Livingston; 2005. p. 3215–28.

[59] Sinigalliano CD, Gidley ML, Shibata T, et al. Impacts of hurricanes Katrina and Rita on the microbial landscape of the New Orleans area. Proc Natl Acad Sci USA 2007;104: 9029–34 [Epub 2007 May 8].

[60] Tumwine JK, Kekitinwa A, Nabukeera N, et al. Cryptosporidium parvum in children with diarrhea in Mulago Hospital, Kampala, Uganda. Am J Trop Med Hyg 2003;68:710–5.

[61] Abubakar I, Aliyu SH, Arumugam C, et al. Treatment of cryptosporidiosis in immunocompromised individuals: systematic review and meta-analysis. Br J Clin Pharmacol 2007;63: 387–93 [Epub 2007 Mar 1].

[62] Cleri DJ, Ricketti AJ, Porwancher RB, et al. Viral hemorrhagic fevers: current status of endemic disease and strategies for control. Infect Dis Clin North Am 2006;20:359–93.

[63] Reynolds MG, Yorita KL, Kuehnert MJ, et al. Clinical manifestations of human monkeypox influenced by route of infection. J Infect Dis 2006;194:773–80 [Epub 2006 Aug 8].

[64] Hutson CL, Lee KN, Abel J, et al. Monkeypox zoonotic associations: insights from laboratory evaluation of animals associated with multi-state US outbreak. Am J Trop Med Hyg 2007;76:757–68.

[65] Cunha BE. Monkeypox in the United States: an occupational health look at the first cases. AAOHN J 2004;52:164–8.

[66] Nalca A, Rimoin AW, Bavari S, et al. Reemergence of monkeypox: prevalence, diagnostics, and countermeasures. Clin Infect Dis 2005;41:1765–171 [Epub 2005 Nov 11].

[67] Cleri DJ, Porwancher RB, Ricketti AJ, et al. Smallpox as a bioterrorist weapon: myth or menace? Infect Dis Clin North Am 2006;20:329–57.

[68] Rimoin AW, Kisalu N, Kebela-Ilunga B, et al. Endemic human monkeypox, Democratic Republic of Congo, 2001–2004. Emerg Infect Dis 2007;13:934–7.

[69] Zafar A, Swanepoel R, Hewson R, et al. Nosocomial buffalopoxvirus infection, Karachi, Pakistan. Emerg Infect Dis 2007;13:902–4.

[70] Cleri DJ, Ricketti AJ, Vernaleo JR. Colorado tick fever. Infectious Disease Practice for Clinicians 2007;31:573–6.

[71] Watts DM, Granwehr BP, Shope RE, et al. Japanese encephalitis and West Nile and other flavivirus infections. In: Guerrant RL, Walker DH, Weller PF, editors. Tropical infectious diseases—principles, pathogens, practice, vol. 1. 2nd edition. Philadelphia: Elsevier Churchill Livingston; 2006. p. 823–30.

[72] Centers for Disease Control and Prevention. West Nile virus activity—United States, 2006. MMWR Morb Mortal Wkly Rep 2007;56:556–9.

[73] Foppa IM, Spielman A. Does reservoir host mortality enhance transmission of West Nile virus? Theor Biol Med Model 2007;4:17 [Epub ahead of print].

[74] Platt KB, Tucker BJ, Halbur PG, et al. West Nile virus in eastern chipmunks (Tamias striatus) sufficient for infecting different mosquitoes. Emerg Infect Dis 2007;13:831–7.

[75] Stamer SL. Current risks of transfusion-transmitted agents: a review. Arch Pathol Lab Med 2007;131:702–7.

[76] Solomon T. Exotic and emerging viral encephalitides. Curr Opin Neurol 2003;16:411–8.

[77] Solomon T. Control of Japanese encephalitis. N Engl J Med 2006;355:869–71.

[78] McGovern LM, Boyce TG, Fischer PR. Congenital infections associated with international travel during pregnancy. J Travel Med 2007;14:117–28.

[79] Kumar R, Tripathi P, Singh S, et al. Clinical features in children hospitalized during the 2005 epidemic of Japanese encephalitis in Uttar Pradesh, India. Clin Infect Dis 2006;43: 123–31 [Epub 2006 Jun 9].

[80] Rayamajhi A, Singh R, Prasad R, et al. Clinico-laboratory profile and outcome of Japanese encephalitis in Nepali children. Ann Trop Paediatr 2006;26:293–301.

[81] German AC, Myint KS, Mai NT, et al. A preliminary neuropathological study of Japanese encephalitis in humans and a mouse model. Trans R Soc Trop Med Hyg 2006;100:1135–45, [Epub 2006 Jun 30].

[82] Handique SK, Das RR, Barman K, et al. Temporal lobe involvement in Japanese encephalitis: problems in differential diagnosis. AJNR Am J Neuroradiol 2006;27:1027–31.

[83] Caramello P, Canta F, Balbiano R, et al. Role of intravenous immunoglobulin administration in Japanese encephalitis. Clin Infect Dis 2006;43:1620–1.

[84] Gould EA, Higgs S, Buckley A, et al. Potential arbovirus emergence and implications for the United Kingdom. Emerg Infect Dis 2006;12:549–55.

[85] Di Nicuolo G, Pagliano P, Battisti S, et al. Toscana virus central nervous system infections in southern Italy. J Clin Microbiol 2005;43:6186–8.

[86] Centers for Disease Control and Prevention. Update: Chikungunya fever diagnosed among international travelers—United States, 2006. MMWR Morb Mortal Wkly Rep 2007;56: 276–7.

[87] Pialoux G, Gauzere BA, Jaureguiberry S, et al. Chikungunya, an epidemic arbovirosis. Lancet Infect Dis 2007;7:319–27.

[88] Charrel RN, de Lamballierie X, Raolt D. Chikungunya outbreaks—the globalization of vectorborne diseases. N Engl J Med 2007;356:769–71.

[89] Borgherini G, Poubeau P, Staikowsky F, et al. Outbreak of chikungunya on Reunion Island: early clinical laboratory features in 157 adult patients. Clin Infect Dis 2007;44: 1401–7 [Epub 2007 Apr 18].

[90] Chanana B, Azad RV, Nair S. Bilateral macular choroiditis following chikungunya virus infection. Eye 2007;21:1020–1 [Epub ahead of print].

[91] Shenk SH, Ricketti AJ, Muddasir SM, et al. Rat-bite fevers: *Steptobacillus moniliformis* and *Spirillum minus*. Infectious Disease Practice for Clinicians 2006;30:509–13.

[92] Shenk SH, Ricketti AJ, Muddasir SM, et al. Rodent associated infectious diseases. Infectious Disease Practice for Clinicians 2006;30:527–40.

[93] Cleri DJ, Ricketti AJ, Panesar M, et al. Plague (*Yersinia pestis*)—parts I. and II. Infectious Disease Practice for Clinicians 2004;28:259–65, 271–5.

[94] Painter JA, Molbak K, Sonne-Hansen J, et al. Salmonella-based rodenticides and public health. Emerg Infect Dis 2004;10:985–7.

[95] Eilers H, Pernthaler J, Glockner FO, et al. Culturability and *in situ* abundance of pelagic bacteria from the North Sea. Appl Environ Microbiol 2000;66:3044–51.

[96] Taylor KS, Zoltan TB, Achar SA. Medical illnesses and injuries encountered during surfing. Curr Sports Med Rep 2006;5:262–7.

[97] Woolgar JD, Cliff G, Nair R, et al. Shark attack: review of 86 consecutive cases. J Trauma 2001;50:887–91.

[98] Buck JD, Spotte S, Gadbaw JJ Jr. Bacteriology of the teeth from a great white shark: potential medical implications for shark bite victims. J Clin Microbiol 1984;20:849–51.

[99] Byard RW, James RA, Heath KJ. Recovery of human remains after shark attack. Am J Forensic Med Pathol 2006;27:256–9.

[100] Shuval H. Estimating the global burden of thalassogenic diseases: human infectious diseases caused by wastewater pollution of the marine environment. J Water Health 2003;1: 53–64.

[101] Centers for Disease Control and Prevention. Outbreak of *Vibrio parahaemolyticus* infection associated with eating raw oysters and clams harvested from Long Island Sound—Connecticut, New Jersey, and New York. 1998. MMWR Morb Mortal Wkly Rep 1999;48: 48–51.

[102] Hlady WG, Mullen RC, Hopkin RS. Vibrio vulnificus from raw oysters: leading cause of reported deaths from foodborne illness in Florida. J Fla Med Assoc 1993;80:536–8.

[103] Samra Y, Shaked Y, Hertz M, et al. Brucellosis: difficulties in diagnosis and a report on 38 cases. Infection 1983;11:310–2.

[104] Baba MM, Sarkindared SE, Brisibe F. Serological evidence of brucellosis among predisposed patients with pyrexia of unknown origin in the north eastern Nigeria. Cent Eur J Public Health 2001;9:158–61.

[105] Shaalan MA, Memish ZA, Mahmoud SA, et al. Brucellosis in children: clinical observations in 115 cases. Int J Infect Dis 2002;6:182–6.

[106] Foster G, MacMillan AP, Godfroid J, et al. A review of *Brucella* sp. infection of sea mammals with particular emphasis on isolates from Scotland. Vet Microbiol 2002;90:563–80.

[107] Memish ZA, Venkatesh S. Brucellar epididymo-orchitis in Saudi Arabia: a retrospective study of 26 cases and review of the literature. BJU Int 2001;88:72–6.

[108] Wiesli P, Flepp M, Greminger P. Fever and dry cough in a construction worker from Portugal. Schweiz Rundsch Med Prax 1997;86:1215–9.

[109] Giannacopoulos I, Eliopoulou MI, Ziambaras T. Transplacentally transmitted congenital brucellosis due to *Brucella abortus*. J Infect 2002;45:209–10.

[110] Gotuzzo E. Brucellosis. In: Guerrant RL, Walker DH, Weller PF, editors. Tropical infectious diseases—principles, pathogens, practice, vol. 1. 2nd edition. Philadelphia: Elsevier Churchill Livingston; 2006. p. 463–70.

[111] Centers for Disease Control and Prevention. Locally acquired mosquito-transmitted malaria: a guide for investigations in the United States. MMWR Morb Mortal Wkly Rep 2006;55(RR13):1–9.

[112] Puente S, Rubio JM, Subirats M, et al. The use of PCR in the diagnosis of hyper-reactive malarial splenomegaly (HMS). Ann Trop Med Parasitol 2000;94:559–63.

[113] Singh RK. Hyperreactive malarial splenomegaly in expatriates. Travel Med Infect Dis 2007;5:24–9 [Epub 2006 May 18].

[114] Greub G, LaScola B, Raoult D. Amoebae-resisting bacteria isolated from human nasal swabs by amoebal coculture. Emerg Infect Dis 2004;10:470–7.

[115] Greub G, Raoult D. Microorganisms resistant to free-living amoebae. Clin Microbiol Rev 2004;17:413–33.

[116] Raoult D, La Scola B, Birtles R. The discovery and characterization of mimivirus, the largest known virus and putative pneumonia agent. Clin Infect Dis 2007;45:95–102.

[117] Barete S, Combes A, de Jonckheere JF, et al. Fatal disseminated *Acanthamoeba lenticulata* infection in a heart transplant patient. Emerg Infect Dis 2007;13:736–8.

[118] Kravetz JD, Federman DG. Cat-associated zoonoses. Arch Inern Med 2002;162:1945–52.

[119] Abe K, Shimokawa H, Kubota T, et al. Myocarditis associated with visceral larva migrans due to *Toxocara canis*. Intern Med 2002;41:706–8.

[120] Umehara F, Ookatsu H, Hayashi D, et al. MRI studies of spinal visceral larva migrans syndrome. J Neurol Sci 2006;249:7–12 [Epub 2006 Jul 3].

[121] Oujamaa L, Sibon I, Vital A, et al. Cerebral vasculitis secondary to *Toxocara canis* and *Fasciola hepatica* co-infestation. Rev Neurol (Paris) 2003;159:447–50.

[122] Rey P, Bredin C, Carrere C, et al. Toxocariasis mimicking liver tumor. Presse Med 2005;34:1715–6.

[123] Walker DH, Maguina C, Minnick M. Bartonelloses. In: Guerrant RL, Walker DH, Weller PF, editors. Tropical infectious diseases—principles, pathogens, practice, vol. 1. 2nd edition. Philadelphia: Elsevier Churchill Livingston; 2006. p. 454–62.

[124] Eremeeva ME, Gerns HL, Lydy SL, et al. Bacteremia, fever, and splenomegaly caused by a newly recognized *Bartonella* species. N Engl J Med 2007;356:2381–7.

[125] Breitschwerdt EB, Kordick DL. *Bartonella* infection in animals: carriership, reservoir potential, pathogenicity, and zoonotic potential for human infection. Clin Microbiol Rev 2000;13:428–38.

[126] Koehler JE, Sanchez MA, Tye S, et al. Prevalence of *Bartonella* infection among human immunodeficiency virus-infected patients with fever. Clin Infect Dis 2003;37:559–66.

[127] Thudi KR, Kreikemeier JT, Phillips NJ, et al. Cat scratch disease causing hepatic masses after liver transplant. Liver Int 2007;27:145–8.

[128] Keynan Y, Yakirevitch E, Shusterman T, et al. Bone marrow and skin granulomatosis in a patient with *Bartonella* infection. J Med Microbiol 2007;56:133–5.

[129] Malatack JJ, Jaffe R. Granulomatous hepatitis in three children due to cat-scratch disease without peripheral adenopathy: an unrecognized cause of fever of unknown origin. Am J Dis Child 1993;147:949–53.

[130] Tsuneoka H, Tsukahara M. Analysis of data in 30 patients with cat scratch disease without lymphadenopathy. J Infect Chemother 2006;12:224–6.

[131] Werner M, Fournier PE, Andersson R, et al. *Bartonella* and *Coxiella* antibodies in 334 prospectively studied episodes of infective endocarditis in Sweden. Scand J Infect Dis 2003;35: 724–7.

[132] Silver BE, Bean CS. Cat scratch encephalopathy. Del Med J 1991;63:365–8.

[133] Daye S, McHenry JA, Roscelli JD. Pruritic rash associated with cat scratch disease. Pediatrics 1988;81:559–61.

[134] Brouqui P, Raoult D. Arthropod-borne diseases in homeless. Ann N Y Acad Sci 2006;1078: 223–35.

[135] Rehan N. Profile of men suffering from sexually transmitted infections in Pakistan. J Pak Med Assoc 2006;56:S60–5.

[136] Alvarez WA, Freinhar JP. A prevalence study of bestiality (zoophilia) in psychiatric in-patients, medical in-patients, and psychiatric staff. Int J Psychosom 1991;38:45–7.

[137] English K, Jones L, Patrick D, et al. Sexual offender containment: use of the postconviction polygraph. Ann N Y Acad Sci 2003;989:411–27 [discussion 441–445].

[138] Jimenez-Jimeniz FJ, Sayed Y, Garcia-Soldevilla MA, et al. Possible zoophilia associated with dopaminergic therapy in Parkinson disease. Ann Pharmacother 2002;36:1178–9.

[139] Cleri DJ, Vernaleo JR, Lombardi LJ, et al. Plague pneumonia disease caused by *Yersinia pestis*. Semin Respir Infect 1997;12:12–23.

[140] Centers for Disease Control and Prevention. Tuberculosis in imported nonhuman primates—United States, June 1990–May 1993. MMWR Morb Mortal Wkly Rep 1993; 42:572–6.

[141] Myers KP, Setterquist SF, Capuano AW, et al. Infection due to 3 avian influenza subtypes in the United States veterinarians. Clin Infect Dis 2007;45:4–9.

[142] Seward JP. Occupational allergy to animals. Occup Med 1999;14:285–304.

[143] Shuhaiber S, Koren G, Boskovic R, et al. Seroprevalence of *Toxoplasma gondii* infection among veterinary staff in Ontario, Canada (2002): implications for teratogenic risk. BMC Infect Dis 2003;3:8.

[144] Centers for Disease Control and Prevention. Epidemiologic notes and reports imported bubonic plague—District of Columbia. MMWR Morb Mortal Wkly Rep 1990;39:895.

[145] Centers for Disease Control and Prevention. Imported plague—New York City. 2002. MMWR Morb Mortal Wkly Rep 2003;52:725–8.

[146] Centers for Disease Control and Prevention. Tularemia—United States, 1990–2000. MMWR Morb Mortal Wkly Rep 2002;51:181–4.

[147] Centers for Disease Control and Prevention. Inhalation anthrax associated with dried animal hides—Pennsylvania and New York City, 2006. MMWR Morb Mortal Wkly Rep 2006;55:280–2.

[148] Centers for Disease Control and Prevention. Update: investigation of bioterrorism-related inhalation anthrax—Connecticut, 2001. MMWR Morb Mortal Wkly Rep 2001;50: 1049–51.

[149] Weese JS, McCarthy L, Mossop M, et al. Observation of practices at petting zoos and the potential impact on zoonotic disease transmission. Clin Infect Dis 2007;45:10–5.

[150] Woods JB, editor. USAMRID's medical management of biological casualties handbook. 6th edition. Fort Detrick, Frederick, (MD): US Army Medical Research Institute of Infectious Diseases; 2005 . p. 7–9, 16–105.

[151] Rabinowitz P, Gordon Z, Chudnov D, et al. Animals as sentinals of bioterrorism agents. Emerg Infect Dis 2006;12:647–52.

[152] Eddy DM, Clanton CH. The art of diagnosis: solving the clinicopathological exercise. N Engl J Med 1982;306:1263–8.

ELSEVIER
SAUNDERS

INFECTIOUS
DISEASE CLINICS
OF NORTH AMERICA

Infect Dis Clin N Am 21 (2007) 997–1011

# Fever of Unknown Origin Due to Rickettsioses

## Elisabeth Botelho-Nevers, MD[a], Didier Raoult, MD, PhD[a],*

[a]Unité des Rickettsies, CNRS UMR 6020, IFR 48, Faculté de Médecine, Université de la Méditerranée, 27 Boulevard Jean Moulin, 13385 Marseille cedex 5, France

Fever of unknown origin (FUO) can be classified into four diagnostic categories: infections, which remain the most important category; tumors; noninfectious inflammatory diseases; and miscellaneous [1]. Nowadays, FUO are defined as (1) an illness of at least 3 weeks' duration, (2) measured temperatures greater than 38.3°C on several occasions, and (3) no diagnosis after at least three outpatient visits or at least 3 days in hospital [2]. At one time, all fevers were of unknown etiology. By the mid twentieth century, most had been unmasked by science. Such is the case of Rickettsioses (Q fever, ehrlichioses, and diseases caused by rickettsiae) and of Bartonellosis. These bacteria infect humans incidentally and are mainly agents of zoonoses. They are emerging infectious diseases, most of which have been described in the past 15 years [3]. Some of these diseases (eg, ehrlichiosis, bartonellosis) are considered causes of emerging FUO [1,4].

Causes of FUO are variable according to regional infectious epidemiologic factors. Concerning Rickettsioses, the same notion of variable geographic distribution also applies [3]. A rickettsiosis seldom responsible for FUO in one geographic area may be frequent in another geographic area. This is true of Q fever, rare in some countries, but a common cause of FUO in Spain [5,6], and of scrub typhus and murine typhus, common causes of acute fever in Laos and Thailand [7,8], also considered a cause of FUO [4]. Rickettsial infections are also responsible for FUO in returned travelers, in which they represent the third most common vector-borne disease acquired during international travel [9] and represent from 0.5% to 3.3% of cases of fever after travel [2,9,10]. History of travel and animal and insect

---

* Corresponding author.
*E-mail address:* Didier.raoult@medecine.univ-mrs.fr (D. Raoult).

0891-5520/07/$ - see front matter © 2007 Elsevier Inc. All rights reserved.
doi:10.1016/j.idc.2007.08.002
*id.theclinics.com*

exposure should be an emphasis in exploration of FUO. In these conditions, infections occur usually within the month of return or arrival and are managed most frequently without hospitalization [10], not filling the criteria of FUO but being responsible for undifferentiated acute fever. In other conditions, depending on geographic area, these etiologies are rarer; however, diagnosis could be made within 3 days of investigation [11].

Few rickettsioses fill the strict criteria of FUO described previously. This article discusses the rickettsioses as causes of acute fever or of intermediate duration and underlines those that are the cause of real FUO.

## Rickettsioses

Rickettsioses represent three families of diseases: (1) diseases caused by rickettsiae, (2) ehrlichioses, and (3) Q fever. Geographic repartition is described in Table 1.

### Rickettsial diseases

*Rickettsia* sp are small gram-negative, obligately intracellular bacteria that grow within eukaryotic cells (eg, endothelial cells in humans). Among rickettsiae, two subgroups, typhus group and spotted fever group, were identified on the basis of growth conditions and antigenicity. Rickettsiae from both groups can have as vector an insect (louse or flea) or an acarid (tick or mite). These bacteria are distributed worldwide with specific disease in specific geographic area, mainly determined by their vectors. The geographic and temporal distribution helps in the diagnosis of FUO caused by these microorganisms.

### Ehrlichioses

The *Ehrlichia* have been reclassified into four genera, mainly on the basis of 16S ribosomal RNA-derived phylogenetic analysis [3]. Two are the tick-associated genera *Ehrlichia* and *Anaplasma*. One is a helminthic-associated genus, *Neorickettsia*, including *N sennetsu*. The fourth is *Wolbachia pipientis*, a bacterium associated with fertility bias in arthropods and in helminth worms (mainly filarial). Ehrlichiae multiply exclusively in vacuoles of their eukaryotic cell host, in whom they form clusters also termed "morulae." Their target cells differ among species. Ehrlichiosis, especially American human monocytic ehrlichiosis (HME) caused by *Ehrlichia chaffensis*, can be a cause of FUO [1,12].

### Q fever

The disease caused by *Coxiella burnetii* is a worldwide zoonosis; however, its incidence is variable. In some geographic areas, such as Spain, it is

Table 1
Geographic repartition of rickettsioses and bartonellosis

| | North America | Central and South America | Central Asia | Middle East North Africa | Europe and Russia | Sub-Saharan Africa | India | China and Japan | Australia and New Zealand |
|---|---|---|---|---|---|---|---|---|---|
| Tick-borne rickettsiosis | *R rickettsii*<br>*R parkeri*<br>*R akari*<br>(mouse mite) | *R rickettsii*<br>*R parkeri*<br>*R africae*<br>(West Indies) | *R helvetica* (?)<br>*R conorii indica*<br>*R honei*<br>*R sibirica*<br>*R heilongjiangensis* | *R conorii*<br>*conorii*<br>*R conorii*<br>*israeli* | *R conorii*<br>(*conorii*,<br>*caspia, israeli*)<br>*R helvetica*<br>*R slovaca*<br>*R sibirica*<br>*mongolitimonae*<br>*R aeschlimannii*<br>*R massiliae* | *R africae*<br>*R conorii*<br>*conorii*<br>*R aeschlimannii* | | *R heilongjiangensis*<br>*R japonica*<br>*R sibirica*<br>*siribica*<br>*R siribica*<br>*mongolitimonae*<br>*R helvetica* | *R honei*<br>*R australis* |
| Flea-transmitted rickettsiosis | *R typhi*<br>*R felis* | *R typhi*<br>*R felis* | *R felis*<br>*R typhi* | *R typhi*<br>*R felis* +++ | *R typhi*<br>(Southern Europe)<br>*R felis* | *R typhi* | *R typhi* | *R typhi* | *R typhi*<br>*R felis* |
| Louse-borne rickettsiosis | *R prowazekii* | *R prowazekii*<br>(Peru and Mexico) | | *R prowazekii* | *R prowazekii* | *R prowazekii*<br>+++<br>(war, refugees camps) | ? | *R prowazekii* | |
| Scrub typhus | | *O tsutsugamushi* | *O tsutsugamushi* | | | | *O tsutsugamushi* | *O tsutsugamushi* | *O tsutsugamushi* |
| Ehrlichiosis | *E chaffensis*<br>*A phagocytophila*<br>*E ewingii* | | | | *A phagocytophila* | | | | |
| *Bartonella* spp. | *B henselae*<br>*B quintana*<br>*B elizabethae* | *B henselae*<br>*B quintana*<br>*B baciliformis*<br>(« *verruga*<br>*zone* ») | *B henselae*<br>*B quintana* | *B henselae*<br>*B quintana* | *B henselae*<br>*B quintana* | *B henselae*<br>*B quintana* | *B henselae*<br>*B quintana* | *B henselae*<br>*B quintana* | *B henselae*<br>*B quintana* |
| Q fever | Worldwide distribution +++ with foci of endemic disease | | | | | | | | |

considered a common cause of FUO [5,6] and represents 21% of the cases of fever of intermediate duration in the southwest of Spain [6]. Cattle, sheep, and goats are the most important reservoirs for human infection. A desiccation-resistant form of *C burnetii* is shed in extremely high concentrations in placental and amniotic fluids, and also in urine, feces, and milk of these ruminants. It infects birds and ticks. *Coxiella* survive in the environment and can spread far by wind [3]. Aerosol transmission is the primary route of transmission to humans; less frequently, infection occurs with milk products. It is usually an occupational disease, especially among ranchers, veterinarians, and abattoir workers. Rarely, interhuman infections have been reported [3]. The bacterium is a gram-negative bacterium that naturally infects its host's monocytes and multiplies in acidic vacuole (phagolysosome). In vitro *C burnetti* in vitro generates a deleted, avirulent mutant also named phase II, after repeated passage of phase I virulent organisms that exist in nature.

## Bartonellosis

Infections caused by *Bartonella* spp have been associated with human disease and are considered as emerging diseases. The bacteria are facultative intracellular, gram-negative rods belonging to the α2 subgroup of proteobacteria. Cat-scratch disease (CSD), caused by *Bartonella henselae*, is an etiology of FUO in children [13]. *B henselae* and *Bartonella quintana* are also causes of hepatic and splenic abscesses, bacillary peliosis hepatic, chronic bacteremia, and culture-negative endocarditis, all responsible for FUO [4,14,15].

## Fever of unknown origin caused by rickettsioses associated with rash

### Rocky Mountain spotted fever

Rocky Mountain spotted fever (RMSF) is the most severe of the rickettsioses, caused by *Rickettsia rickettsii*, which belongs to the spotted fever group of rickettsiae. It is responsible for acute fever in America occurring mainly after the bite of *Dermacentor* species ticks [16], although other ticks also transmit the disease [16,17]. The seasonal distribution of RMSF parallels tick activity (April–September) [16]. The bite is painless and frequently goes unnoticed.

Two to 14 days after the tick bite, the disease starts with high fever (> 38.8°C), headaches, and unspecific symptoms. The rash, the major diagnostic sign, appears usually on day 4 of the illness [18] and occurs in 84% to 91% of cases. The classic triad of fever, headache, and rash is present in only 44% of confirmed cases [3]. An eschar at the site of the tick bite is rarely observed. The rash is macular and typically begins around the wrists and ankles and then generalizes: this centripetal spread is a hallmark of RMSF and helps in FUO diagnosis [18]. Spots evolve from pink to purpuric. Rocky Mountain "spotless" fever occurs in about 34% of cases and more often in older and black patients [16]. The involvement of palms and soles, although frequently lacking, is considered characteristic and theoretically differentiates the typhuses. Skin necrosis or gangrene may develop on the digits, limbs, or scrotum [18]. The disease is associated in various degrees with general manifestations, such as neurologic, renal, heart, pulmonary, liver, intestinal tract, and ocular involvements [3,16], which can lead to a multiple organ dysfunction syndrome. Biologically, data are relatively nonspecific and include thrombocytopenia; anemia; hyponatremia; hypocalcemia; and increased concentrations of serum lactate dehydrogenase, creatinine kinase, and other enzymes [16]. The evolution of RMSF depends strongly on the timing of diagnosis and of antibiotic treatment. Diagnosis of RMSF should be based on clinical and epidemiologic findings (acute unexplained fever in a patient with a history of tick exposure in an endemic area), leading to early use of doxycycline. Spontaneous evolution of RMSF is frequently fatal, and without treatment death occurs in 8 to 15 days. The overall fatality rate with antibiotic treatment was 1.4% in the last epidemiologic study in United States [19]. Fulminant cases of RMSF are more often observed in patients with glucose-6-phosphate dehydrogenase deficiency.

### Mediterranean spotted fever

This rickettsiosis is caused by *Rickettsia conorii* and belongs to the spotted fever group of rickettsiae. Many names are given to the infection caused by *R conorii*, associated with different but closely related serotypes in different geographic areas (see Table 1). Mediterranean spotted fever (MSF) or boutonneuse fever is found around the Mediterranean Sea and is caused by *R conorii*. The disease is transmitted by the brown dog tick, *Rhipicephalus sanguineus*. Only one eschar is found in 50% to 80% of cases. Cases occur mainly in warm months with peak incidence in July, August, and September in many Mediterranean locations. The typical clinical presentation is an association of fever, rash, and a "tache noire." The symptoms appear after a mean incubation of 7 days, associated with myalgia and headache. The rash is papular involving the palms and soles. In 5% to 10% of cases, the disease occurs as a malignant form [16], including purpuric rash, shock, and multiple organ dysfunction syndrome, mainly described in patients with underlying conditions, such as alcoholism, diabetes mellitus, old age, glucose-6-phosphate dehydrogenase deficiency, or debilitated patients. In France, Israel, and Spain, the death rate among hospitalized patient ranges from 1.4% to 5.6%, similar to that of RMSF [20]; however, a recent study in Portugal showed a case fatality rate of 32.3% in hospitalized patients [21]. Like RMSF, MSF does not fill the strict criteria of FUO because of its acute course; however, epidemiologic and clinical findings should lead to use of doxycycline early in the course of acute fever of unknown etiology. Israel tick bite fever and Astrakhan fever seem milder than typical MSF and "tache noire" is frequently lacking.

In RMSF and MSF, diagnosis is based on serology. Confirmation of diagnosis includes a fourfold change or a seroconversion in antibody titers between two serum samples tested. Direct detection of bacteria can be realized by polymerase chain reaction (PCR) of a skin lesion, or culture, restricted to specialized laboratories. The treatment duration with doxycycline probably could be stopped 3 days after apyrexia in RMSF and severe MSF. In MSF, a single-day treatment (200 mg of doxycycline) is often efficient [3]. Other rickettsioses cause diseases resembling MSF in other geographic areas (see Table 1).

### Murine typhus or endemic typhus

This disease is caused by *Rickettsia typhi*, which belong to the typhus group of rickettsioses. Humans are infected by inoculation of infective rats' flea feces in bite wounds. The disease is widely distributed in tropical and subtropical areas, particularly in port cities and costal regions with rodents [7,22]. The incubation period ranges from 8 to 16 days [3]. The clinical presentation is nonspecific, with fever, constitutional symptoms, and an often poorly visible maculopapular exanthema on the trunk, usually not involving the face, palms, and soles, as its main features. Lung and digestive involvement can be observed. Neurologic symptoms range from confusion to coma in severe forms. Murine typhus is frequently misdiagnosed. It is a major cause of FUO in Southeast Asia [4]. Most cases are mild, but the fatality rate may be as high as 4% [23], especially in older patients and those with glucose-6-phosphate dehydrogenase deficiency. Diagnosis is based on serology; even skin and blood samples for culture or PCR may be valuable. *R typhi* cross-reacts with *Rickettsia prowazekii* in serology.

### Flea-borne spotted fever caused by Rickettsia felis

This is a murine typhus-like rickettsiosis caused by *Rickettsia felis*, a spotted fever group *rickettsia*. It is found in patients who have not visited typical areas of endemicity. Rash seems to be more frequent than in murine typhus [3]. The vector seems to be the cat flea *Ctenocephalides felis*, cosmopolitan, suggesting a worldwide distribution [22]. The rickettsia is very common in cat and dog fleas. Most cases have been reported from North Africa.

### Exanthematic typhus or epidemic louse-borne typhus

Human body louses are prevalent during times of war, in poor countries, and in the homeless population of wealthy countries. Recent outbreaks of epidemic typhus [24,25] attest to the persistence of this agent and indicate the potential for large epidemics. Humans are the mains reservoirs of *R prowazekii* and lice are the vectors. The patient is usually contaminated by infected feces, through aerosol or by skin autoinoculation after scratching. Typhus begins abruptly, with fever, headaches, and myalgias. Cough and neurologic involvement, reflected as stupor (tuphos), are common. A rash, observed in 20% to 80% of the patients, usually macular, starts in the axilla and then spreads. In severe cases, shock and multiple organ dysfunction syndrome are observed. Spontaneously, the fatality rate is 10% to 20% [26]. This diagnosis should be considered when grouped cases of high fever with confusion are observed in patients exposed to lice. In tropical countries it can be confused with typhoid, malaria, hemorrhagic fever, and dengue. In Brill-Zinsser disease, occurring in patients who recover, the bacteria persist in a dormant form and under stressing conditions the disease can relapse. The rash is then often lacking and the prognosis is good because clinical manifestations are mild. During this relapsing form, a bacteremia occurs and may allow a new outbreak if a patient is bitten by lice. The diagnosis should be clinical and is confirmed by serology. Culture and PCR are valuable and lice, which are red when infected, are good diagnostic tools. Single-day treatment with doxycycline, 200 mg, saves the patient.

## Fever of unknown origin caused by rickettsioses associated with an eschar

### African tick bite fever

*Rickettsia africae* may be responsible for most of the tick-borne rickettsioses worldwide. It is prevalent throughout sub-Saharan Africa.

The vector ticks, *Amblyomma* species are present in Africa and in the West Indies [27]. It is the only tick-transmitted rickettsiosis in which several inoculation eschars are observed in a high proportion of cases [27]. *R africae* is often observed in patients who have hunted or traveled in the bush. The tick attacks typically generate in grouped cases in safari visitors, important information to emphasize in a history. The disease differs from MSF: it is milder; fever is frequently absent; and rash may be vesicular, maculopapular, sparse, or even absent in more than half of the patients. Distinctive features include frequent regional lymphadenopathy that drains the region of the eschars, usually found on lower limbs and, in a small portion of patients, aphthous stomatitis. The infection is very common among native Africans in whom it is frequently suspected to be malaria or typhoid fever. Its acute course, however, does not fill the criteria of FUO. The serologic response is later than RMSF or MSF and late serum samples are recommended.

*Rickettsia slovaca* causes a disease common in Europe (Hungary, France, Spain) [28]. The bacterium is transmitted to humans most often by the bite of *Dermacentor* species ticks during cold months. The illness, called TIBOLA, is characterized by an erythematous eschar, typically on the scalp, associated with enlarged and tender draining cervical lymph nodes. Patients may exhibit rarely fever and rash, although the eschar site may have persistent alopecia. *R slovaca* confers a weak serologic response, possibly because of its lack of general infection.

*Rickettsia sibirica mongolitimonae* causes a disease also named lymphangitis-associated rickettsia [29] and can exhibit specific clinical features including one or several "tache noire," a groin lymphadenopathy, and a lymphangitis joining these two lesions [3].

## Rickettsialpox

*Rickettsia akari* is transmitted by the bite of a mouse mite. Ten days after the mite bite, the beginning of the illness is marked by fever, headache, and myalgia. A careful examination reveals an inoculation eschar and a draining lymphadenopathy. Two to 6 days later, a rash appears, macular then papular and with vesicular spots. The disease is usually mild. Rickettsialpox is infrequently reported and underdiagnosed at present; however, a high prevalence of antibodies (16%) to *R akari* was detected among inner-city intravenous drug users in Baltimore [3].

## Scrub typhus

This is one of the most common infectious diseases of rural south and southeastern Asia and the western Pacific [7]. One billion people are exposed and approximately 1 million suffer annually from the disease. It is caused by *Orientia Tsutsugamushi* and is transmitted by the bite of trombiculid mite larvae. The larvae typically bite humans on the lower extremities or in the genital region. Patients present with sudden fever and a generalized lymphadenitis and more than 50% have an inoculation eschar [7,23]. Many cases are mild, but if left untreated pneumonitis, meningoencephalitis, disseminated intravascular coagulation, or renal failure are commonly seen. The fatality rate of scrub typhus ranges from 1% to 35%, depending on the virulence of the infecting strain, host factors, and treatment [23]. Relapses may occur. A diagnosis of infectious mononucleosis has been frequently considered in these patients and the disease could be considered a cause of FUO [4]. The bacterium can be detected by culture or PCR in blood and biopsies. Serology is also possible. The currently recommended regimen is doxycycline, 200 mg daily for 7 days.

## Fever of unknown origin caused by rickettsioses and bartonellosis associated with lymphadenopathy

In some rickettsioses, such as *R africae*, *R slovaca*, *R sibirica mongolitimonae*, and scrub typhus, lymphadenopathy can be present but most often drained an eschar of inoculation.

## Cat-scratch disease

*Bartonella henselae* is the etiologic agent of CSD. Cats are probably the most important vertebrate host of *B henselae* and infect humans, mainly children, by scratching or biting. CSD is typically a self-limiting disease and manifests in otherwise healthy persons as prolonged regional lymphadenopathy usually preceded by an erythematous papule at the inoculation site. Lymph nodes draining the site of inoculation become enlarged and tender and suppuration can appear. Low-grade fever and malaise are seen in approximately 30% of patients [14]. It spontaneously resolves in 2 to 6 months. CSD complicated or not is associated with FUO in children [13]. Complicated forms of CSD, such as Parinaud's oculoglandular syndrome and hepatic and splenic abscesses, can occur even in immunocompetent patients and can cause FUO [14]. Other complications can occur in association with CSD, including neurologic, pulmonary, musculoskeletal manifestations, and osteomyelitis [14].

## Sennetsu neorickettsiosis

Described in the Far East, the disease resembles mononucleosis with fever, headache, myalgia, and lymphadenopathy. The incubation period is 14 days. Fever lasts for 2 weeks unless treated effectively. Absolute lymphocytosis is observed with atypical lymphocytes [30]. Treatment with doxycycline results in defervescence after 1 to 2 days.

## Fever of unknown origin caused by rickettsioses and bartonellosis associated with specific patient's condition

### Immunocompromised patients

#### Bartonella henselae

Patients with AIDS, chronic alcoholism, and immunosuppression tend to have a systemic disease that could become life-threatening. Bacillary angiomatosis, diagnosed as reddish vascular papules or nodules, is one manifestation. It can be associated with fever, chills, malaise, headache, anorexia, and weight loss [14] and can fill the criteria of FUO [4]. It also may involve lymph nodes, respiratory and gastrointestinal mucosa, heart, liver, spleen, bone marrow, and muscles. Bacillary peliosis hepatis is a common extracutaneous presentation of bacillary angiomatosis. It may occur as an isolated condition or in the course of disseminated disease. Symptoms include fever, nausea, vomiting, diarrhea, and abdominal distention. Hepatosplenomegaly is usually present on physical examination. Culture-negative endocarditis caused by bacteremia can occur in patients, who usually present with fatigue, anorexia, and fever without an obvious focus of infection, and represents a cause of FUO [4,14].

## Ehrlichia ewingii

This is the agent of canine granulocytic ehrlichioses and the most recently discovered ehrlichial species shown to be pathogenic to humans. Few cases of human infection have been reported [22]. In most cases, it seems to be an opportunistic infection of immunocompromised individuals. This pathogen has not yet been adapted to continuous cell culture, and infection can be confirmed only by using molecular methods.

## Homelessness

### Bartonella quintana

The bacterium is best known as the agent of trench fever and is restricted to human hosts and louse vectors. It is now recognized as a re-emerging pathogen among homeless populations in American and European cities [15]. Trench fever is characterized by attacks of fever that last 1 to 3 days; are associated with headache, shin pain, and dizziness; and recur every 4 to 6 days, although each succeeding attack is usually less severe. The incubation period typically varies from 15 to 25 days. Although trench fever often results in prolonged disability, no deaths have been reported [15]. Chronic bacteremia has long been associated with *B quintana* infection and can persist up to 8 years after initial infection [15]. Culture-negative endocarditis caused by *B quintana* is also observed and is a cause of FUO [4,15]. Methods of diagnosis of infections caused by bartonellosis include PCR suitable for clinical samples, serology, and culture [14,15]. On indirect immunofluorescence, immunoglobulin G titers greater than 1:800 predict endocarditis [15]. Bacteria of the genus *Bartonella* are susceptible to a wide range of agents; however, only aminoglycosides have a bactericidal effect [31]. For systemic diseases caused by *Bartonella* spp, treatment should be prolonged and should include gentamicin in endocarditis [31].

## Patients with cardiac valve lesions, vascular prosthesis, or pregnancy

### Chronic Q fever

Following a primary infection, after months to years, 0.2% to 0.5% of patients with these conditions develop a chronic infection. This form of the disease has a variety of manifestations, such as endocarditis, the prime manifestation of chronic Q fever; infection of a vascular prosthesis and aneurysm; osteomyelitis; hepatitis; interstitial pulmonary fibrosis; and purpuric eruptions [32]. Thirty percent to 50% of patients with heart valve lesions or vascular lesions who develop acute Q fever may experience chronic endocarditis within 2 years [3]. Patients with Q fever endocarditis present with low-grade fever or no fever, progressive degradation of valve function, and heart failure. Blood cultures are negative and vegetations are frequently absent on echocardiography. Marked clubbing of the fingers and hyperglobulinemia are frequently found. Splenomegaly and hepatomegaly are found in more than 50% of patients. These forms of the disease could be responsible for FUO [4]. In pregnant women, symptomatic or not, Q fever compromises the pregnancy, resulting in abortions, fetal death, and prematurity depending on the trimester of infection [33]. The disease should be considered in pregnant women with FUO. Cotrimoxazole during the entire pregnancy improves the outcome of pregnancy [33] but not the development of chronic infection. For endocarditis and other chronic conditions, a bactericidal treatment is necessary. The recommended treatment is a combination of doxycycline (200 mg daily) and hydroxychloroquine (600 mg/day, then adjusted to reach 1 mg/mL plasma concentration), which increases the pH of infectious vacuoles and restores the bactericidal effect of doxycycline [34]. This regimen is prescribed for 18 to 36 months according to serologic results.

## Fever of unknown origin caused by rickettsioses and bartonellosis associated with leucopenia and increased in serum hepatic transaminases

### American human monocytic ehrlichiosis

HME is caused by *E chaffensis* and has been observed mainly in the United States. Several lines of evidence suggest that the Lone Star tick, *Amblyomma americanum*, is the primary vector [22] of the disease and the white-tailed deer is the mammalian reservoir. Individuals participating in recreational hobbies, such as sports, hiking, or camping, may be exposed to vector ticks and *E chaffeensis* during the course of these activities. The incidence increases from April to September. In immunocompetent patients, the disease is of mild to severe multisystemic illness with a median duration of 23 days [30] and fills the criteria of FUO [4,12]. The median incubation period is 7 days. At onset, symptoms include fever, chills, headache, myalgia, and malaise. Later in the course, patients develop anorexia, vomiting, and weight loss. Fewer than half of patients have a rash, which is maculopapular and may be petechial. Untreated patients worsen and may require intensive care. Severe complications include adult respiratory distress syndrome, acute renal insufficiency, neurologic involvement, coagulopathy, and even death. Important laboratory findings are mild to moderate leukopenia (caused by both lymphopenia and neutropenia); thrombocytopenia; and elevations of serum hepatic transaminases. A virulent form of HME occurs in immunocompromised patients often associated with fatality. The prognosis in HME depends on early antibiotic treatment, but the fatality rate is still high at 2.5%. Careful examination of blood smears or cerebrospinal fluid smears may help to identify typical morulae. Diagnosis can be confirmed by a serology or by culture in specialized laboratories. PCR is more practical with a confirmatory PCR using a second target gene. Treatment should be started in any suspected case and is the same as that in rickettsial disease, based on doxycycline. The treatment is usually prescribed for 2 weeks [30].

*Human granulocytic ehrlichiosis*

The disease is found in America and in Eastern Europe, and is caused by *A phagocytophila*. It is transmitted by *Ixodes* species ticks [30]. The temporal distribution, parallel to nymph tick activity, peaks in spring and in autumn. The disease resembles HME but is often milder. The evolution is favorable in most cases, even without specific therapy [35]; however, in some cases, the disease may evolve to multiple organ dysfunction syndrome. Patients with underlying conditions are more at risk of dying. Laboratory findings are the same as in HME. Ehrlichial morulae are identified in peripheral blood neutrophils in 20% to 80% of patients, which is rare in circulating mononuclear cells in HME [36].

*Acute Q fever*

After contamination by *C burnetii*, 60% of patients seroconvert without apparent disease, 38% experience a self-limited disease, and only 2% require an exhaustive diagnostic procedure, sometimes within the framework of FUO. Isolated prolonged fever was observed in 14% of more than 1000 patients [37] and nonfocalized febrile syndrome lasting from 7 to 28 days was the most frequent presentation in Spain [6]. Pneumonia was found in 37% but this percentage may vary according to the place of study. In most cases, pneumonia is an incidental finding in a patient with a febrile illness. Hepatitis is found in 60% of cases, isolated in 40%, and is the most common manifestation of Q fever in France [37,38]. It is usually diagnosed by the association of fever and moderate increase in transaminases. In patients with FUO related to Q fever, the typical "doughnut granuloma" is seen on liver biopsy [38]. Patients can rarely develop neurologic manifestations [39], pericarditis, and myocarditis [37]. Rash is infrequently found in Q fever. Evolution is usually favorable even without treatment except in special hosts. Nonspecific laboratory findings, such as leukopenia, thrombocytopenia, and increases in hepatic enzymes, are frequent. Circulating anticoagulant associated with antiphospholipid antibodies may be observed as anti–smooth muscle antibodies during hepatitis.

It is important to note that in most systemic rickettsioses, leucopenia and mild increase in liver transaminases are present but are not a clue in diagnosis, such as epidemic louse-borne typhus and scrub typhus [7].

## Fever of unknown origin after travel caused by rickettsioses and bartonellosis

Among travelers, systemic febrile illness without localizing findings occurred disproportionately among those returning from sub-Saharan Africa or Southeast Asia [40]. Rickettsial diseases represent 3.1% of febrile returning travelers [40] and 5.6% from sub-Saharan Africa travelers [40]. Murine typhus is reported in more than 50 travelers returning from Asia, Africa, and Europe [23]. MSF has been reported in more than 35 travelers from northern Europe and North America. Most individuals are infected in southern Europe and Africa [23]. About 20 cases of travel-associated scrub typhus have been reported from Europe, North America, and Japan in patients returning mainly from Asia [23,41]. With more than 350 imported cases reported from Europe, North and South America, Asia, and Oceania during the past few years, African tick bite fever is without comparison currently the most commonly encountered rickettsiosis in travel medicine [23,27]. Q fever can occur in travelers worldwide, with incubation often greater than 14 days [41].

## Summary

Most common rickettsioses do not fulfill the FUO criteria, with fever often inferior to 1 week. Q fever, scrub typhus, murine typhus, HME, and bartonellosis can fill these criteria, notably in uncommon presentations. Moreover, in patients returning from tropical areas or from geographic endemic areas for rickettsiosis, or in patients in contact with animals or ticks, theses etiologies should be kept in mind by the physician challenged to diagnose the cause of a fever. Some of these infections can also be life-threatening. In this context, even without confirmation of diagnosis, treatment with doxycycline should be used. Some authors ponder the use of doxycycline as empirical treatment for fever of intermediate duration [42].

## References

[1] Knockaert DC, Vanderschueren S, Blockmans D. Fever of unknown origin in adults: 40 years on. J Intern Med 2003;253(3):263–75.

[2] Mackowiak PA, Durack DT. Fever of unknown origin. In: Mandell GL, Bennett JE, Dolin R, editors. Principles and practice of infectious diseases. 6th edition. Philadelphia: Churchill Livingstone; 2005. p. 718–29.

[3] Raoult D. Rickettsioses. In: Goldman L, Ausiello D, editors. Cecil textbook of medicine. 22nd edition. Philadelphia: Elsevier Health Sciences; 2004. p. 1946–56.

[4] Arnow PM, Flaherty JP. Fever of unknown origin. Lancet 1997;350(9077):575–80.

[5] Barbado FJ, Vazquez JJ, Pena JM, et al. Fever of unknown origin: a survey on 133 patients. J Med 1984;15(3):185–92.

[6] Alarcon A, Villanueva JL, Viciana P, et al. Q fever: epidemiology, clinical features and prognosis. A study from 1983 to 1999 in the south of Spain. J Infect 2003;47(2):110–6.

[7] Phongmany S, Rolain JM, Phetsouvanh R, et al. Rickettsial infections and fever, Vientiane, Laos. Emerg Infect Dis 2006;12(2):256–62.

[8] Suttinont C, Losuwanaluk K, Niwatayakul K, et al. Causes of acute, undifferentiated, febrile illness in rural Thailand: results of a prospective observational study. Ann Trop Med Parasitol 2006;100(4):363–70.

[9] O'Brien D, Tobin S, Brown GV, et al. Fever in returned travelers: review of hospital admissions for a 3-year period. Clin Infect Dis 2001;33(5):603–9.

[10] Bottieau E, Clerinx J, Schrooten W, et al. Etiology and outcome of fever after a stay in the tropics. Arch Intern Med 2006;166(15):1642–8.

[11] Goto M, Koyama H, Takahashi O, et al. A retrospective review of 226 hospitalized patients with fever. Intern Med 2007;46(1):17–22.

[12] Carpenter CF, Gandhi TK, Kong LK, et al. The incidence of ehrlichial and rickettsial infection in patients with unexplained fever and recent history of tick bite in central North Carolina. J Infect Dis 1999;180(3):900–3.

[13] Jacobs RF, Schutze GE. *Bartonella henselae* as a cause of prolonged fever and fever of unknown origin in children. Clin Infect Dis 1998;26(1):80–4.

[14] Anderson BE, Neuman MA. *Bartonella* spp. as emerging human pathogens. Clin Microbiol Rev 1997;10(2):203–19.

[15] Foucault C, Brouqui P, Raoult D. Bartonella quintana characteristics and clinical management. Emerg Infect Dis 2006;12(2):217–23.

[16] Walker DH, Raoult D. Rickettsia rickettsii and other spotted fever group rickettsiae (Rocky Mountain spotted fever and other spotted fevers). In: Mandell GL, Bennett JE, Dolin R, editors. Principles and practice of infectious diseases. 6th edition. Philadelphia: Churchill Livingstone; 2005. p. 2287–95.

[17] Demma LJ, Traeger MS, Nicholson WL, et al. Rocky Mountain spotted fever from an unexpected tick vector in Arizona. N Engl J Med 2005;353(6):587–94.

[18] Drage LA. Life-threatening rashes: dermatologic signs of four infectious diseases. Mayo Clin Proc 1999;74(1):68–72.

[19] Chapman AS, Murphy SM, Demma LJ, et al. Rocky Mountain spotted fever in the United States, 1997–2002. Vector Borne Zoonotic Dis 2006;6(2):170–8.

[20] Raoult D, Zuchelli P, Weiller PJ, et al. Incidence, clinical observations and risk factors in the severe form of Mediterranean spotted fever among patients admitted to hospital in Marseilles 1983–1984. J Infect 1986;12(2):111–6.

[21] de Sousa R, Nobrega SD, Bacellar F, et al. Mediterranean spotted fever in Portugal: risk factors for fatal outcome in 105 hospitalized patients. Ann N Y Acad Sci 2003;990:285–94.

[22] Comer JA, Paddock CD, Childs JE. Urban zoonoses caused by bartonella, coxiella, ehrlichia, and rickettsia species. Vector Borne Zoonotic Dis 2001;1(2):91–118.

[23] Jensenius M, Fournier PE, Raoult D. Rickettsioses and the international traveler. Clin Infect Dis 2004;39(10):1493–9.

[24] Raoult D, Roux V, Ndihokubwayo JB, et al. Jail fever (epidemic typhus) outbreak in Burundi. Emerg Infect Dis 1997;3(3):357–60.

[25] Tarasevich I, Rydkina E, Raoult D. Outbreak of epidemic typhus in Russia. Lancet 1998; 352(9134):1151.

[26] Raoult D, Woodward T, Dumler JS. The history of epidemic typhus. Infect Dis Clin North Am 2004;18(1):127–40.

[27] Raoult D, Fournier PE, Fenollar F, et al. *Rickettsia africae*, a tick-borne pathogen in travelers to sub-Saharan Africa. N Engl J Med 2001;344(20):1504–10.

[28] Raoult D, Lakos A, Fenollar F, et al. Spotless rickettsiosis caused by rickettsia slovaca and associated with dermacentor ticks. Clin Infect Dis 2002;34(10):1331–6.

[29] Fournier PE, Gouriet F, Brouqui P, et al. Lymphangitis-associated rickettsiosis, a new rickettsiosis caused by *Rickettsia ibirica mongolotimonae*: seven new cases and review of the literature. Clin Infect Dis 2005;40(10):1435–44.

[30] Walker DH, Dumler JS. *Ehrlichia chaffeensis* (human monocytotropic ehrlichiosis), *Anaplasma phagocytophilum* (human granulocytotropic anaplasmosis), and other ehrlichieae. In: Mandell GL, Bennett JE, Dolin R, editors. Principles and practice of infectious diseases. 6th edition. Philadelphia: Churchill Livingstone; 2005. p. 2310–8.

[31] Rolain JM, Brouqui P, Koehler JE, et al. Recommendations for treatment of human infections caused by bartonella species. Antimicrob Agents Chemother 2004;48(6):1921–33.

[32] Brouqui P, Dupont HT, Drancourt M, et al. Chronic Q fever: ninety-two cases from France, including 27 cases without endocarditis. Arch Intern Med 1993;153(5):642–8.

[33] Raoult D, Fenollar F, Stein A. Q Fever during pregnancy: diagnosis, treatment, and follow-up. Arch Intern Med 2002;162(6):701–4.

[34] Rolain JM, Mallet MN, Raoult D. Correlation between serum doxycycline concentrations and serologic evolution in patients with *Coxiella burnetii* endocarditis. J Infect Dis 2003; 188(9):1322–5.

[35] Bakken JS, Dumler JS. Human granulocytic ehrlichiosis. Clin Infect Dis 2000;31(2):554–60.

[36] Bakken JS, Krueth J, Wilson-Nordskog C, et al. Clinical and laboratory characteristics of human granulocytic ehrlichiosis. JAMA 1996;275(3):199–205.

[37] Raoult D, Tissot-Dupont H, Foucault C, et al. Q Fever 1985–1998: clinical and epidemiologic features of 1,383 infections. Medicine (Baltimore) 2000;79(2):109–23.

[38] Marrie TJ, Raoult D. *Coxiella burnetii*. In: Mandell GL, Bennett JE, Dolin R, editors. Principles and practice of infectious diseases. 6th edition. Philadelphia: Churchill Livingstone; 2005. p. 2296–303.

[39] Bernit E, Pouget J, Janbon F, et al. Neurological involvement in acute Q Fever: a report of 29 cases and review of the literature. Arch Intern Med 2002;162(6):693–700.

[40] Freedman DO, Weld LH, Kozarsky PE, et al. Spectrum of disease and relation to place of exposure among ill returned travelers. N Engl J Med 2006;354(2):119–30.

[41] Ryan ET, Wilson ME, Kain KC. Illness after international travel. N Engl J Med 2002;347(7): 505–16.

[42] Sanchez-Tejero E, Garcia-Sanchez E. [Empirical treatment with doxycycline for fever of intermediate duration?]. Enferm Infecc Microbiol Clin 2004;22(6):365–6 [in Spanish].

ELSEVIER
SAUNDERS

INFECTIOUS
DISEASE CLINICS
OF NORTH AMERICA

Infect Dis Clin N Am 21 (2007) 1013–1032

# Fever of Unknown Origin in HIV/AIDS Patients

Arnaud Hot, MD[a],
Laura Schmulewitz, BSc, MB, ChB[a],
Jean-Paul Viard, MD[a],
Olivier Lortholary, MD, PhD[a,b,*]

[a]*Université Paris V, Service des Maladies Infectieuses et Tropicales,
Centre d'Infectiologie Necker-Pasteur, Hôpital Necker-Enfants Malades, 149 rue de Sèvres,
75743 Paris Cedex 15, France*
[b]*Centre National de Référence Mycologie et Antifongiques, CNRS URA3012,
Institut Pasteur, 25 rue du Dr Roux, 75724 Paris Cedex 15, France*

Fever of unknown origin (FUO) in adults is defined as a temperature greater than 38.3°C (100.9°F) lasting for more than 3 weeks with no obvious source, despite appropriate investigation. The four categories of FUO are (1) classical, (2) nosocomial, (3) immune deficiency–associated, and (4) HIV-related [1], and the differential diagnoses can be subcategorized into infections, malignancies, autoimmune conditions, and miscellaneous causes [2,3]. A thorough history, physical examination, and standard laboratory testing form the basis of the initial evaluation of the patient with FUO, although newer diagnostic modalities play an important role in assessment.

Fever, either continuous or recurrent, is a common finding in patients infected with HIV and is often accompanied by significant morbidity, prolonged hospitalization, and extensive evaluation [4]. Before highly active antiretroviral therapy (HAART) was introduced, patients with HIV experienced FUO with relative frequency, in most cases caused by opportunistic infections, such as tuberculosis, infection with *Mycobacterium avium* complex (MAC), and in the Middle East and Mediterranean regions of Europe visceral leishmaniasis. The use of HAART has reduced the frequency of HIV-associated FUO, although the etiologic spectrum remains largely

* Corresponding author. Université Paris V, Service des Maladies Infectieuses et Tropicales, Centre d'Infectiologie Necker-Pasteur, Hôpital Necker-Enfants Malades, 149 rue de Sèvres, 75743 Paris Cedex 15, France.

*E-mail address:* olivier.lortholary@nck.aphp.fr (O. Lortholary).

unchanged [5]. It remains a common problem in those poorer countries where HAART is less universally available. This article provides a review of the causes of FUO in HIV-infected patients and a rational approach to their diagnostic and therapeutic evaluation.

## Definition and epidemiology

A consensus definition of FUO in the setting of HIV infection is lacking. Many authors use the criteria proposed by Durack and Street [6]: temperature greater than or equal to $38°3C$ ($100.9°F$) on multiple occasions; fever of greater than or equal to 4 weeks' duration for outpatients or more than 3 days for inpatients, including at least 2 days' incubation of microbiologic cultures; and a diagnosis that remains uncertain after 3 days despite appropriate investigation. This definition has remained unchanged in the era of HAART [6]. It has been suggested that this period of 4 weeks proposed by Durack and Street [6] may, however, be too lengthy in the context of immunocompromised individuals, such as those infected with HIV.

FUO in HIV-infected individuals is not uncommon. The range reported in the literature is variable (3.4%–21% in previous studies) [7–10] probably reflecting rigorous inclusion criteria for FUO diagnosis not always being applied, differential inclusion of outpatient and inpatient populations, and the criteria used for admission to hospital and geographic variation. Most case series of HIV-associated FUO include only patients in the pre-HAART era.

Long-lasting fever in HIV with no recognizable cause is characteristic of the more advanced stages of HIV infection, in patients with a profound loss of their $CD4^+$ T lymphocytes, when the inflammatory reaction responsible for the clinical and radiologic focal signs is impaired because of severe immunosuppression. One series reported 77% of FUO-HIV patients having fewer than 100 $CD4^+$ lymphocytes/$mm^3$ and 66% with fewer than 50 [7]. The median $CD4^+$ cell count in previous reports has ranged from 40 to 94/$mm^3$ [7,9–17]. As a consequence, most documented cases were caused by infection (over 72% of cases) with malignancies and drug effects providing the major noninfectious causes, a classification that reflects the classic studies of Petersdorf and Beeson [18].

The spectrum of causes may be affected by prophylactic medication against opportunistic infection, although few reviews record these data. One study documented those patients on prophylaxis, finding that the percentage of patients diagnosed with MAC and receiving rifabutin prophylaxes (27%) was not significantly lower than those with an etiology other than MAC (35%) or no diagnosis (34%). The percentage with *Pneumocystis jiroveci* pneumonia on prophylaxis (40%) was statistically lower, however, than that of patients with another etiology (85%) or no diagnosis (71%) [7,11].

The widespread use of HAART and antimicrobial prophylaxis has dramatically reduced morbidity and mortality in the setting of HIV infection caused by a reduction in viral load, an increase in $CD4^+$ cell counts [12], and a marked decrease in the incidence of opportunistic infection through a maintenance of immune function [8,19]. Pre-HAART, the incidence of MAC and tuberculosis was approximately three and two cases per 100 person years of follow-up, respectively, with a marked decrease in tuberculosis, and to a larger extent MAC, among HIV-patients since the introduction of HAART. A further series found a substantial reduction in the occurrence of bacteremia in HIV-infected individuals in the post-HAART era [20]. It seems, however, that whereas HAART has significantly reduced the frequency of FUO in HIV, it has not dramatically altered its etiologic spectrum [11].

## Causes of HIV-associated fever of unknown origin

### Mycobacterial infection

Infectious diseases remain the predominant cause of FUO in HIV-infected persons worldwide, both pre- and post-HAART, accounting for 82.2% and 90.6% in the United States and Europe, respectively [9–12, 14,16,17,21]. These are often infective agents common in the setting of non-immunocompromised hosts, but manifesting clinically as protracted fever in the context of HIV [7]. All series have demonstrated that mycobacterial infection is the most common cause of FUO in the setting of HIV infection. *Mycobacterium tuberculosis* is the primary cause of FUO in HIV worldwide, especially in areas of high prevalence, such as southwest Europe and developing countries. The global HIV epidemic has created a large population of individuals, including children, who are highly susceptible to disease from *M tuberculosis* and it is estimated that 4 in 10 people are co-infected with HIV and *M tuberculosis* [22].

HIV alters the clinical presentation of tuberculosis, with an increased proportion of cases having extrapulmonary or disseminated disease, an effect that becomes more pronounced as HIV disease advances [23]. Pulmonary tuberculosis remains the commonest presentation, although the proportion is lower than for HIV-negative patients and the diagnosis may be delayed because the radiologic findings are often atypical [24]. In addition, in a study of HIV patients, sputum smears were positive in 40% to 76% of patients in whom the clinical suspicion of tuberculosis was high. The proportion of cases with smear-negative pulmonary tuberculosis ranged from 24% to 61% [25]. Tuberculous lymphadenitis is a more common finding in HIV-positive patients with FUO. Clinically, this can be difficult to diagnose because only abdominal lymph nodes may be involved and fever is often the sole feature of the disease. Abdominal CT and lymph node biopsy are frequently indicated, allowing for microscopic examination (which may show caseation or granuloma); staining for acid-fast bacilli; and cytologic examination and culture [26].

Blood culture is an extremely useful tool in the diagnosis of tuberculosis in HIV-positive persons, especially those with disseminated infection. Tissue nucleic acid amplification by polymerase chain reaction (PCR) should also be performed, especially in those with less than 200 $CD4^+/mm^3$ where sputum smears are frequently negative and there is clinical suspicion of an atypical mycobacterial infection [27]. In resource-limited settings, sputum smear and sputum culture remain the gold standard [28].

Disseminated MAC is the leading cause of HIV-associated FUO in northern Europe and the United States (31% of cases in the study by Armstrong and coworkers [11]), highlighting that the relative frequencies of individual infectious diseases accounting for FUO in HIV varies markedly depending on local prevalences. A single positive blood culture is considered evidence for disseminated MAC infection and mycobacteria recovered from other normally sterile body tissue sites including bone marrow, liver, lymph nodes, cerebral spinal fluid, or brain tissue should also be interpreted as indicative of disseminated disease. The yield of bone marrow aspiration for cultures is high in this setting and should be performed in cases of negative blood cultures [29].

## Pneumocystis jiroveci pneumonia

Pneumocystis jiroveci pneumonia accounts for between 5% and 13% of cases of FUO in HIV, depending on regional variations in its prevalence. In patients with very low $CD4^+$ counts, P jiroveci pneumonia often presents as prolonged fever before the onset of specific respiratory symptoms [14], whereas those with a relatively preserved $CD4^+$ repertoire generally experience early shortness of breath [30]. Fever with a paucity of respiratory symptoms is characteristic of P jiroveci pneumonia as a cause of FUO in the late stages of HIV-AIDS. Diagnosis relies on demonstrating P jiroveci in induced sputum, bronchoalveolar lavage fluid, or in some cases transbronchial or open lung biopsy tissue [4,31]. In the era of HAART and antimicrobial prophylaxis, the mortality rate of P jiroveci pneumonia remains high (25%), whereas mortality in those not receiving antiretroviral therapy is 63% [32].

## Cytomegalovirus infection

Cytomegalovirus (CMV) accounts for 5% of cases of prolonged, undifferentiated fever in HIV patients [4]. CMV is the most common HIV-associated viral opportunistic infection, typically manifesting when latent virus reactivates in patients with $CD4^+$ counts less than $100/mm^3$. Patients may be asymptomatic, have nonspecific constitutional symptoms including isolated fever, or display localized end-organ disease [33]. Chorioretinitis remains the most common initial presentation, reported to occur in 30% of AIDS patients during the course of their illness [34]; other presentations that should alert physicians to the possible diagnosis of CMV infection, even if the features are subtle, include hepatitis, enterocolitis, meningitis, radiculitis, myelitis, encephalitis, and pneumonia.

A variety of laboratory techniques are available for the rapid and reliable diagnosis of CMV infection including blood culture, detection of pp65 antigenemia, and PCR. Detection of CMV DNA in plasma [35] or whole blood [36] at the time of initial diagnosis of retinitis has been shown to be associated with a higher risk of mortality than a high HIV viral load. Similarly, asymptomatic patients with CMV DNA detectable in plasma at the initiation of HAART therapy had a significantly increased risk of developing subsequent CMV end-organ disease [37]. Furthermore, plasma CMV viremia is a stronger predictor of CMV disease and death than CD4-cell count or plasma HIV RNA concentration [38].

In HIV-infected patients with FUO and CMV viremia, it may be difficult to differentiate whether fever is caused by CMV reactivation. The decision to treat a patient for CMV solely on the basis of a positive plasma PCR result implies unnecessarily treating every third to fourth HIV-infected patient with CMV viremia. Therapy with antiviral drugs is associated with severe side effects and toxicity, such as myelosuppression, which may be particularly detrimental in patients with advanced HIV-infection. Consequently, isolated CMV viremia should only be treated after other causes have been carefully eliminated [39].

*Endemic mycoses*

Disseminated histoplasmosis caused by *Histoplasma capsulatum* var. *capsulatum* accounts for 7% of cases of HIV FUO in the United States, but very few cases have been documented in Europe [11]. Histoplasmosis is the first AIDS-defining event in 60% of cases in the United States [40]. The clinical symptoms (fever, malaise, weight loss) are nonspecific and common in HIV patients [41] and often clinically indistinguishable from that of disseminated MAC infection. Histoplasmosis should be considered in HIV-infected individuals with any unexplained febrile illness in endemic areas and in those with a previous history of travel to an endemic area, however long ago [42]. Markedly elevated lactate dehydrogenase levels may provide a clue to the diagnosis [43] but the highest yield is culture of blood or bone marrow, and bone marrow biopsy often allows rapid identification before culture or serologic results are available. In a series of 36 adult patients with AIDS and disseminated histoplasmosis, examination of bone marrow aspirates or biopsies resulted in rapid identification in one third of infected patients and also identified infections in some whose cultures were negative [44]. Blood culture remains a method limited by slow growth (2–4 weeks) [45] and serologic testing often lacks sensitivity in immunocompromised hosts. Detection of circulating *H capsulatum* polysaccharide antigen in urine and serum is available, but has false-positive rates in cases of other endemic mycoses caused by dimorphic fungi. PCR assay for histoplasmosis is not currently commercially available for routine use but is being investigated as a rapid method of identification.

Other endemic mycoses, such as coccidioidomycosis, may present as FUO in HIV-infected patients, particularly when the CD4$^+$ cell count is below 250/mm$^3$. A multivariate analysis identified black race and a history of oropharyngeal or esophageal candidiasis to be associated with an increased risk of coccidioidomycosis, and HIV protease inhibitor or azole therapy was associated with a reduced risk [46]. There are multiple manifestations of coccidioidomycosis in HIV infection including symptoms similar to those of pneumocystosis with dyspnea, fever, and night sweats, radiologically manifesting as diffuse reticulonodular pneumonia or focal primary pneumonia. Disseminated coccidioidomycosis, defined as disease that has spread beyond the thoracic cavity [47], is also common in HIV and some patients present with prolonged fever, weight loss, and no clear organ involvement [48]. Diagnosis is based on serologic analysis, culture, and histopathologic identification [49].

*Visceral leishmaniasis*

This opportunistic infection accounts for fewer than 5% of cases of HIV-FUO, although the prevalence of visceral leishmaniasis in HIV is increasing in developing countries. As the AIDS pandemic spreads to rural regions and leishmaniasis becomes more common in suburban areas, there is an ever-greater degree of overlap between the geographic distributions of the two diseases and, as a result, increasing rates of leishmania-HIV coinfection. Such cases have been reported in 35 countries around the world, most in southwest Europe with a total of 1911 cases detected in Spain, France, Italy, and Portugal. The incidence is expected to continue to rise in eastern Africa and fall in southwest Europe, where increasing numbers have access to HAART. At diagnosis most patients with visceral leishmaniasis-HIV coinfection have fewer than 200 CD4$^+$ cells and 50% meet AIDS-defining criteria. Fever, pancytopenia, and hepatosplenomegaly are found in 75% of cases. Only 40% to 50% of those coinfected have positive antileishmania antibodies [50] making diagnosis difficult, and antileishmania antibodies in HIV-positive patients are indeed 50 times lower than in HIV-negative patients [51], resulting in a number of false-negative results. The direct examination of amastigotes in spleen and bone marrow aspirates is the investigation of choice. Amastigotes appear in the peripheral blood in 50% of cases, with improved sensitivity using Novy-McNeal-Nicolle culture media [52]. Detection of *Leishmania* antigens by urine Western blot is currently being investigated, as are rk39 strips with a sensitivity and specificity close to 95% [53]. PCR on blood and tissue samples is increasingly used in clinical practice, and nested PCR assays have a sensitivity of 95% in peripheral blood and 100% in bone marrow [54].

*Other infectious agents*

Cryptoccocosis and aspergillosis have both been implicated in FUO-HIV [55]. Although cryptococcosis may present as isolated FUO, concomitant meningoencephalitis is frequent (83%). Fungemia is seen in 40% of these cases, whereas urine culture is positive in 25% [56]. Mortality rate remains high despite HAART. A series demonstrated that mortality per 100 person-years was 63.8 in the pre-HAART era and 15.3 since the introduction of HAART, although early mortality did not differ between the two periods [57]. Although rare, aspergillosis is a serious complication in the advanced stage of AIDS (CD4$^+$ <50/mm$^3$). The diagnosis should be considered in those patients presenting with a new pulmonary cavity on chest radiograph [58] but can present as FUO.

In Asia, *Penicillium marneffei* is an important cause of FUO in HIV patients and may present as an emergent opportunistic infection in HIV-positive travelers to endemic regions [59]. Clinical signs include fever (99%); anemia (78%); weight loss (76%); generalized lymphadenopathy (58%); and hepatomegaly (51%). Skin lesions, most commonly papules with central necrotic umbilication, are seen in only 70% of HIV patients with FUO caused by disseminated *P marneffei* infection [60]. Diagnosis is by demonstration of the organism in blood cultures, antigen detection, or serologic analysis. HIV-positive patients tend to have lower serum antibody levels as a result of underlying immune defects. Their serum antigen levels are generally markedly higher, however, presumably because of a higher fungal load secondary to immune defects [61].

Toxoplasmosis has been demonstrated as a cause of HIV-associated FUO [55]. Isolated fever has been observed in severely immunocompromised HIV patients with extracerebral toxoplasmosis receiving trimethoprim-sulfamethoxazole as primary prophylaxis. PCR was positive for *Toxoplasma gondii* and fever resolved with high-dose toxoplasmosis treatment [62].

Physicians should maintain a high index of suspicion for *Bartonella* infection in HIV because recurrent fever occurs in 86% of cases. Recent data indicate that its prevalence among HIV-infected individuals may be much greater than previously reported [63]. The associated cutaneous lesions of bacillary angiomatosis are rarely present in the context of HIV infection [64]. Diagnosis is achieved through PCR or blood culture, and bartonellosis is usually easily treatable even in immunocompromised patients with late-stage HIV disease.

Infective endocarditis may present as FUO in the context of HIV and must be considered, especially in intravenous drug users. Small numbers of case reports implicate other infective agents in FUO of HIV-infected patients: nocardiasis in 2% of one series [8], *Rhodococcus equi* found in splenic microabscesses [13], babesiosis [65], and neurosyphilis [8]. The spectrum of infectious agents involved in HIV-associated FUO is wide, varies markedly from that of the normal host, and reflects the geographic distribution of pathogens.

## Neoplasia

Malignancies are a common and well-described cause of classic FUO in immunocompetent patients. In sharp contrast, malignancies represent only about 8% of cases of FUO in HIV. Only lymphomas, especially non-Hodgkin's lymphoma, are highly represented, with incidences of 4% to 7% in case series [7,8,11,44,66]. Although most studies note a significant decrease in the global incidence of AIDS-related lymphoma in the HAART era, recent studies have found a threefold higher risk of Hodgkin's disease in HIV-infected persons treated with HAART compared with those not treated [67]. In addition, the incidence of non-Hodgkin's lymphoma has decreased less than other AIDS-defining illnesses and aggressive B-cell lymphoma has emerged as a common AIDS-defining illness [68]. Bone marrow involvement is frequently found in AIDS-related lymphoproliferative diseases (46%), and bone marrow biopsy may be helpful diagnostically [69].

FUO caused primary by central nervous system lymphoma and Kaposi's sarcoma is less commonly encountered. Cases of prolonged fever associated with disseminated visceral Kaposi's sarcoma account for 1% of cases [4], although Kaposi's sarcoma with fever may be associated with Castleman disease. The incidence of Kaposi's sarcoma has also decreased in the era of HAART [70]. Other cancers, such as primary lung and liver cancer, are increasingly found among HIV-AIDS patients [69] and may present as FUO, even in those receiving HAART [71].

## Drug fever

Drug fever is an important consideration for FUO-HIV because drug allergy in HIV-positive individuals remains a major problem. The frequency of drug hypersensitivity in HIV-infected patients ranges from 3% to 20% and drug-related rashes have been estimated to be 100 times more common in HIV-positive patients than in the general population. The typical reaction of maculopapular pruritic rash, with or without fever, accounts for 17% of all adverse drug reactions and isolated fever is responsible for 1.7% [9]. Intake of multiple drugs including antiretrovirals and prophylactic-curative anti-infective therapy, in conjunction with high dosing regimens, changes in drug metabolism and interactions, immune hyperactivation, and oxidative stress, all in the context of advanced HIV disease, are risk factors for adverse reactions [70]. Hypereosinophilia is a clue to a drug hypersensitivity reaction but the diagnosis is established by withdrawal of the most likely offending drug, with most patients responding in 24 to 48 hours [72].

The drugs involved in hypersensitivity reactions have changed over the years. In the 1980s the commonest drugs responsible were the antimicrobials used for prophylaxis of opportunistic infections, commonly trimethoprim-sulfamethoxazole, isoniazid, rifampicin, pyrazinamide, β-lactam antibiotics, sulphonamides, and dapsone. The rate of adverse drug reactions to trimethoprim-sulfamethoxazole was reported at 25% to 50%, with hypersensitivity reactions occurring in 30% of HIV-infected patients at prophylactic doses and in 50% at full therapeutic treatment doses (versus 1%–3% in HIV-negative patients) [73]. With the advent of HAART, adverse reactions to the antiretrovirals themselves have become increasingly important. A number of antiretroviral agents can cause hypersensitivity reactions but few are associated with fever more commonly than rash.

Abacavir, a nucleoside reverse transcriptase inhibitor, has been associated with severe hypersensitivity reactions in 3% to 5% of patients [72]. The reaction generally occurs after 9 days of treatment and is characterized by fever (80% of cases) and systemic symptoms with a rash occurring later in some patients. Such cases require termination of the drug. Rechallenge, which can be rapidly fatal, should not be attempted. Zidovudine-induced prolonged fever has also been documented [74] as has fever with nevirapine (15%) and amprenavir (7%) and anecdotally with virtually all antiretroviral drugs, but in most cases with an associated rash making them less likely etiologic agents in sole FUO. Enfuvirtide, which is administered subcutaneously, is generally responsible for local cutaneous reactions at the site of injection but can also provoke systemic symptoms, such as fever. The Swiss HIV Cohort Study found the use of combination antiretroviral treatment with two protease inhibitors and no non nucleoside reverse transcriptase inhibitors to be associated with greater risk of fever (and diarrhea) than alternative antiretroviral combinations [75].

*HIV*

Genne and colleagues [14] reported HIV itself as the cause of FUO in 27% of their series, a result not in keeping with the results of cohort studies. Primary HIV infection is associated with a nonspecific mononucleosis-like syndrome characterized by fever, rash, and lymphadenopathy in 40% to 70% of patients. The symptoms of primary HIV infection generally resolve spontaneously within 2 weeks, however, making it rarely the exclusive cause of the FUO. In HIV-infected patients presenting with FUO as their initial clinical manifestation of the HIV virus, coexisting opportunistic infection or malignancy are generally reported as responsible for the pyrexia [7,8,14].

**Immune reconstitution inflammatory syndrome**

In the initial period of HAART therapy, immune reconstitution may be complicated by adverse clinical phenomena (immune reconstitution inflammatory syndrome [IRIS]) where either previously latent infections are unmasked or pre-existing opportunistic infections apparently deteriorate.

This is seen in around 25% to 35% of HIV-positive patients. Most cases occur within the first 60 days of initiating treatment but the onset of IRIS may be seen for up to 2 years post-HAART initiation, predominantly in patients with low pre-HAART CD4$^+$ cell counts. Fever is a common finding and cases of FUO attributed to IRIS have been reported [5]. IRIS is often associated with more specific, infection-associated signs, however, such as respiratory symptoms or inflammatory adenopathies in tuberculosis or raised intracranial pressure in cryptococcosis [51], focusing the diagnosis. Various infectious agents have been reported in the literature in association with IRIS, and Box 1 summarizes the pathogens. Mycobacteria are frequently implicated, accounting for around 30% to 40% of reported cases of IRIS. Shelburne and colleagues [76] described patients with prolonged fever in the context of IRIS associated with both underlying MAC infection and *M tuberculosis*. A further report presented a case of prolonged fever caused by a lymphoid interstitial pneumonitis during early IRIS after HAART initiation [77]. In addition, sarcoidosis has been reported as a cause of FUO after the onset of the HAART [78]. Treatment with interleukin-2 or interferon-$\alpha$ may be a risk factor for its development.

## Miscellaneous causes

In smaller numbers of cases, HIV-associated FUO is caused by other noninfectious pathologies. Multicentric Castleman disease is a polyclonal lymphoplasmacytic and vascular proliferation prominent in lymphoid tissues and associated with constitutional symptoms and prominent fever. Cases have presented as FUO in HIV [11]. There is a prominent role for human herpes virus-8 and cytokine dysregulation in this disorder and it remains a challenging clinical problem in the HIV-infected population. Cases of FUO-HIV caused by systemic lupus erythematosus and Reiter's

---

**Box 1. Opportunistic infectious diseases implicated in IRIS**

Bacterial
    Tuberculosis
    Atypical mycobacterium
Fungal
    Cryptococcosis
    Histoplasmosis
    Coccidioidomycosis
Viral
    Cytomegalovirus
Parasitic
    Toxoplasmosis

syndrome have been reported [79]. In contrast with classic FUO, however, autoimmune and inflammatory conditions constitute a small percentage of cases. Single cases of FUO-HIV caused by neuralgic amyotrophy [7] and subacute thyroiditis [80] exist in the literature, as do a limited number of episodes of factitious fever presenting as FUO in HIV [9].

**Multiple etiologies or no cause found**

A cause of FUO in HIV is elucidated in around 80% of cases [31]. Immunocompromised individuals are vulnerable to a wide variety of infectious agents and multiple etiologies are responsible for between 8% and 19% of individual cases of FUO, a situation not commonly seen in classical FUO. One series found 12.5% of patients with a diagnosis of two etiologic processes and 3.3% with three. Should fever persist despite adequate treatment for a diagnosed entity, further studies should be performed to rule out coexisting conditions.

The cause of HIV-associated FUO remains unidentified in 6% to 14% of reported series, a proportion apparently unaltered in the era of HAART. This is more frequently seen in the very latest stages of HIV infection, where an exhaustive investigation is more complicated given the risks of invasive diagnostic procedures. In the absence of a diagnosis, nonsteroidal anti-inflammatory drugs or corticosteroids can be used as antipyretic agents and empirical antimycobacterial therapy should be initiated.

**Evaluation of the patient with fever of unknown origin in the context of HIV**

Physicians confronted with an HIV-infected patient with FUO should take into account the relative frequencies of causative agents as previously discussed and the geographic setting of the patient, including any history of travel. Initially, a detailed medical history should be obtained and a thorough physical examination performed including ophthalmologic examination for CMV retinitis, which may suggest a likely etiology. Review the patient's previous isolates because some microorganisms are chronic colonizers of the respiratory and digestive tracts. Attention should also be directed to the patient's medications. If the fever started in the 10 to 14 days following a change or addition of a drug, drug fever must be considered, especially when accompanied by a rash or gastrointestinal symptoms.

Noninvasive investigations should follow. Appropriate blood cultures remain the most important investigation in determining the cause of FUO in HIV patients, useful in diagnosing disseminated tuberculosis; disseminated MAC [81]; disseminated histoplasmosis; and a variety of bacterial and fungal pathogens including *Cryptococcus neoformans*, *Bartonella* sp, *R equi*, and *P marneffei* [13]. Blood cultures should ideally be incubated in DuPont Isolator (Wampole Laboratories, Cranbury, Jew Jersey) or Bactec (Becton

Dickinson Diagnostic Instrument Systems, Sparks, Maryland) medium and held for a sufficient time period of time to demonstrate pathogens. Blood should be stained for acid-fast bacilli and fungi. Examination of the blood smear without culture may demonstrate such organisms as *Leishmania infantum* and *H capsulatum* in Europe or *Leishmania donovani* in India [82]. The latex agglutination test for *Cryptococcus* detection has high sensitivity and specificity for disseminated cryptococcosis including meningitis [56]. CMV can be detected by pp65 antigenemia or PCR on a blood sample. Antibody detection is of little value in diagnosing FUO in patients with less than 200 CD4$^+$ lymphocytes/mm$^3$. The test for anti-*Toxoplasma* antibodies has only a high negative predictive value, although in severely immunocompromised hosts, a negative test does not exclude active toxoplasmosis [37]. Other noninvasive methods include analysis of sputum for *P jiroveci* and *M tuberculosis*. Urine and stool culture are of little value unless there are relevant symptoms. Abdominal and thoracic CT should be performed early because they have a high diagnostic yield and may assist in the identification of two of the most common causes of FUO: mycobacterial infection and lymphoproliferative disorders. Cerebral CT may be useful in anti-*Toxoplasma* antibody carriers with a low CD4$^+$ cell count.

*Nuclear imaging*

Fluorodeoxyglucose positron emission tomography scanning is commonly used in the investigation of FUO in immunocompetent hosts and has an emerging role as a rapid whole-body assessment in FUO in HIV, although availability and cost limits its widespread use. O'Doherty and colleagues [83] first reported its use in FUO in HIV in 1997, where 29 patients presented with moderate or high uptake of fluorodeoxyglucose, the scans successfully localizing tumor in those with non-Hodgkin's lymphoma in soft tissue, nodal, and bone sites. Positron emission tomography allows accurate and rapid localization of malignant and infectious diseases in patients enabling biopsy of specific sites to be performed. In some cases, however, it may be difficult to distinguish malignancy from inflammatory causes (Fig. 1). The use of $^{67}$Ga-citrate has not been shown to be superior to fluorodeoxyglucose positron emission tomography in the only available study to date [84].

*Bone marrow examination*

Bone marrow aspiration or biopsy and culture are a high-yield procedure in HIV-positive patients with FUO [85]. Benito and colleagues [86] investigated such a group, reporting specific diagnoses by means of culture and histopathologic examination in 38% of those biopsied. The diagnostic yield reported in other studies ranges from 25% to 34% [87,88]. Diagnoses elicited by bone marrow biopsy include extranodal non-Hodgkin's

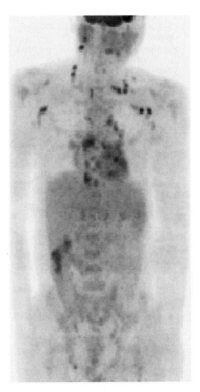

Fig. 1. Immune reconstitution inflammatory syndrome demonstrated on fluorodeoxyglucose positron emission tomography scanning in a 39-year-old HIV-positive man with tuberculosis 1 month after initiating antituberculous therapy. Lymphadenitis with fluorodeoxyglucose uptake in multiple areas.

lymphoma; mycobacterial infection (although blood culture is more sensitive in identifying MAC infection); drug-induced changes; and Castleman disease.

*Liver biopsy*

The overall diagnostic yield of liver biopsy in HIV-associated FUO is 45% [4], increasing to 80% in disseminated mycobacterial disease [89]. In a study performed pre-HAART, 26.8% of HIV patients with FUO underwent percutaneous liver biopsy as part of the diagnostic work-up and the biopsy was diagnostic in 43% of cases and contributory in a further 22.4% [90]. The presence of hepatosplenomegaly and lone splenomegaly has a high predictive value of a positive liver biopsy, and raised serum alkaline phosphatase levels are a clinical marker of the usefulness of liver biopsy in cases of tuberculosis [91]. Liver biopsy should be performed in the context of a raised alkaline phosphatase level or hepatosplenomegaly after exhaustive, nonconfirmatory, noninvasive investigations [92].

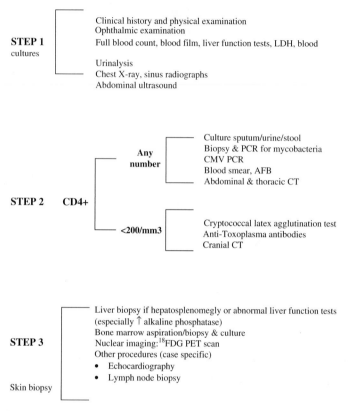

Fig. 2. Diagnostic algorithm for evaluating the HIV patient with FUO. AFB, acid-fast bacilli; CMV, cytomegalovirus; FDG, fluorodeoxyglucose; LDH, lactate dehydrogenase; PCR, polymerase chain reaction; PET, positron emission tomography.

## Biopsy of skin lesions or peripheral lymphadenopathy

If skin lesions or peripheral lymphadenopathy are new or altering in size or number, biopsies should be obtained. Lymph node biopsy has a high diagnostic yield and may aid in the detection of lymphomas, disseminated mycobacterial disease, and toxoplasmosis. Skin lesions are more often a clue to drug hypersensitivity reactions or disseminated infection as opposed to localized infection [31].

## Other investigations

Transthoracic echocardiography (sensitivity 63%, specificity 98%) and transesophageal echocardiography (sensitivity 100%, specificity 98%) may allow early detection of valvular vegetations in the context of infective endocarditis [93]. These tests should be high priority in HIV-infected intravenous drug users where FUO may be the sole clinical feature of infective endocarditis [94].

## Diagnostic approach

Diagnosing FUO in HIV-infected patients requires attention to detail, and although no formal protocol exists [4,10], a systematic approach using all available investigative methods is advised. Fig. 2 represents a proposed algorithm for the diagnostic work-up of HIV-associated FUO. Empirical treatments are best avoided but therapeutic attempts with antibiotics, anti-mycobacterial agents, or corticosteroids may be indicated in cases of clinical deterioration or when both clinical suspicion is high and the risks derived from a delay in the initiation of therapy are significant. Tuberculosis remains a paradigm of this situation [95]. Stopping empirically introduced antimicrobial agents is advised if cultures remain negative and if clinical states fail to improve.

## Summary

FUO in HIV-AIDS patients remains a challenge. HAART has contributed to a decrease in its incidence but has not altered the spectrum of causes. It is a common cause of admission to hospitals and is associated with substantial cost and significant mortality. In most cases FUO in the context of HIV is a result of occult opportunistic infection and physicians should take into consideration differing geographic prevalences of infectious pathogens. If no infectious cause can be demonstrated, AIDS-related lymphoproliferative diseases and drug fever should be considered along with a number of less common etiologies. The diagnostic work-up is initially directed toward infection, which remains the single leading etiology. The single most important early investigation is blood culture. Bone marrow examination, liver biopsy, and newer nuclear imaging techniques are useful further diagnostic modalities. An algorithm for the diagnostic approach and management of patients with HIV-associated FUO is presented.

## References

[1] Arnow PM, Flaherty JP. Fever of unknown origin. Lancet 1997;350(9077):575–80.
[2] Lortholary O, Guilletin L, Blétry O, et al. Fever of unknown origin: a retrospective multicentric study of 103 cases, 1980–1988. Eur J Intern Med 1992;1(3):109–20.
[3] Vanderschueren S, Knockaert D, Adriaenssens T, et al. From prolonged febrile illness to fever of unknown origin: the challenge continues. Arch Intern Med 2003;163(9):1033–41.
[4] Mayo J, Collazos J, Martinez E. Fever of unknown origin in the HIV-infected patient: new scenario for an old problem. Scand J Infect Dis 1997;29(4):327–36.
[5] Lozano F, Torre-Cisneros J, Santos J, et al. Impact of highly active antiretroviral therapy on fever of unknown origin in HIV-infected patients. Eur J Clin Microbiol Infect Dis 2002; 21(2):137–9.
[6] Durack DT, Street AC. Fever of unknown origin: reexamined and redefined. Curr Clin Top Infect Dis 1991;11:35–51.
[7] Bissuel F, Leport C, Perronne C, et al. Fever of unknown origin in HIV-infected patients: a critical analysis of a retrospective series of 57 cases. J Intern Med 1994;236(5):529–35.

[8] Lozano F, Torre-Cisneros J, Bascunana A, et al. Prospective evaluation of fever of unknown origin in patients infected with the human immunodeficiency virus. Grupo Andaluz para el Estudio de las Enfermedades Infecciosas. Eur J Clin Microbiol Infect Dis 1996;15(9):705–11.

[9] Miller RF, Hingorami AD, Foley NM. Pyrexia of undetermined origin in patients with human immunodeficiency virus infection and AIDS. Int J STD AIDS 1996;7(3):170–5.

[10] Miralles P, Moreno S, Perez-Tascon M, et al. Fever of uncertain origin in patients infected with the human immunodeficiency virus. Clin Infect Dis 1995;20(4):872–5.

[11] Armstrong WS, Katz JT, Kazanjian PH. Human immunodeficiency virus-associated fever of unknown origin: a study of 70 patients in the United States and review. Clin Infect Dis 1999;28(2):341–5.

[12] Palella FJ Jr, Delaney KM, Moorman AC, et al. Declining morbidity and mortality among patients with advanced human immunodeficiency virus infection. HIV Outpatient Study Investigators. N Engl J Med 1998;338(13):853–60.

[13] Bernabeu-Wittel M, Villanueva JL, Pachon J, et al. Etiology, clinical features and outcome of splenic microabscesses in HIV-infected patients with prolonged fever. Eur J Clin Microbiol Infect Dis 1999;18(5):324–9.

[14] Genne D, Chave JP, Glauser MP. [Fever of unknown origin in a cohort of HIV-positive patients]. Schweiz Med Wochenschr 1992;122(47):1797–802 [in French].

[15] Carbonell Biot CEMJ, Pasquau Liano F, Badia Ferrando P, et al. Fiebre de origen desconocido en pacientes infectados por el virus de la immunodeficiencia humana. Rev Clin Esp 1996;196(1):4–8.

[16] Knobel H, Supevia A, Salvado M, et al. [Fever of unknown origin in patients with human immunodeficiency virus infection: study of 100 cases]. Rev Clin Esp 1996;196(6):349–53 [in Spanish].

[17] Riera M, Altes J, Homar F, et al. [Fever of unknown origin in patients with HIV infection]. Enferm Infecc Microbiol Clin 1996;14(10):581–5 [in Spanish].

[18] Larson EB, Featherstone HJ, Petersdorf RG. Fever of undetermined origin: diagnosis and follow-up of 105 cases, 1970–1980. Medicine (Baltimore) 1982;61(5):269–92.

[19] Mocroft A, Ledergerber B, Katlama C, et al. Decline in the AIDS and death rates in the EuroSIDA study: an observational study. Lancet 2003;362(9377):22–9.

[20] Meynard JL, Guiguet M, Fonquernie L, et al. Impact of highly active antiretroviral therapy on the occurrence of bacteraemia in HIV-infected patients and their epidemiologic characteristics. HIV Med 2003;4(2):127–32.

[21] Carbonell Biot C, Ena Munoz J, Pasquau Liano F, et al. [Fever of unknown origin in patients infected with the human immunodeficiency virus]. Rev Clin Esp 1996;196(1):4–8 [in Spanish].

[22] Dye C, Scheele S, Dolin P, et al. Consensus statement. Global burden of tuberculosis: estimated incidence, prevalence, and mortality by country. WHO Global Surveillance and Monitoring Project. JAMA 1999;282(7):677–86.

[23] Havlir DV, Barnes PF. Tuberculosis in patients with human immunodeficiency virus infection. N Engl J Med 1999;340(5):367–73.

[24] Mayo J, Collazos J, Martinez E. Fever of unknown origin in the setting of HIV infection: guidelines for a rational approach. AIDS Patient Care STDS 1998;12(5):373–8.

[25] Getahun H, Harrington M, O'Brien R, et al. Diagnosis of smear-negative pulmonary tuberculosis in people with HIV infection or AIDS in resource-constrained settings: informing urgent policy changes. Lancet 2007;369(9578):2042–9.

[26] Navarro V, Guix J, Bernacer B, et al. [Tuberculosis and human immunodeficiency virus infection: a prospective study of 215 patients]. Rev Clin Esp 1993;192(7):315–20 [in Spanish].

[27] Barnes PF, Lakey DL, Burman WJ. Tuberculosis in patients with HIV infection. Infect Dis Clin North Am 2002;16(1):107–26.

[28] Dheda K, Lampe FC, Johnson MA, et al. Outcome of HIV-associated tuberculosis in the era of highly active antiretroviral therapy. J Infect Dis 2004;190(9):1670–6.

[29] Karstaedt AS, Pantanowitz L, Omar T, et al. The utility of bone-marrow examination in HIV-infected adults in South Africa. QJM 2001;94(2):101–5.

[30] Jani K, Mehta NJ. *Pneumocystis carinii* pneumonia presenting as a fever of unknown origin in a patient without AIDS. Heart Lung 2002;31(1):50–2.

[31] Cunha BA. Fever or unknown origin in HIV/AIDS patients. Drugs Today (Barc) 1999; 35(6):429–34.

[32] Morris A, Kingsley LA, Groner G, et al. Prevalence and clinical predictors of *Pneumocystis* colonization among HIV-infected men. AIDS 2004;18(5):793–8.

[33] Gerard L, Leport C, Flandre P, et al. Cytomegalovirus (CMV) viremia and the CD4+ lymphocyte count as predictors of CMV disease in patients infected with human immunodeficiency virus. Clin Infect Dis 1997;24(5):836–40.

[34] Sullivan M, Feinberg J, Bartlett JG. Fever in patients with HIV infection. Infect Dis Clin North Am 1996;10(1):149–65.

[35] Jabs DA, Van Natta ML, Kempen JH, et al. Characteristics of patients with cytomegalovirus retinitis in the era of highly active antiretroviral therapy. Am J Ophthalmol 2002;133(1): 48–61.

[36] Bowen EF, Sabin CA, Wilson P, et al. Cytomegalovirus (CMV) viraemia detected by polymerase chain reaction identifies a group of HIV-positive patients at high risk of CMV disease. AIDS 1997;11(7):889–93.

[37] Nokta MA, Holland F, De Gruttola V, et al. Cytomegalovirus (CMV) polymerase chain reaction profiles in individuals with advanced human immunodeficiency virus infection: relationship to CMV disease. J Infect Dis 2002;185(12):1717–22.

[38] Deayton JR, Prof Sabin CA, Johnson MA, et al. Importance of cytomegalovirus viraemia in risk of disease progression and death in HIV-infected patients receiving highly active antiretroviral therapy. Lancet 2004;363(9427):2116–21.

[39] Smith IL, Macdonald JC, Freeman WR, et al. Cytomegalovirus (CMV) retinitis activity is accurately reflected by the presence and level of CMV DNA in aqueous humor and vitreous. J Infect Dis 1999;179(5):1249–53.

[40] Antinori S, Magni C, Nebuloni M, et al. Histoplasmosis among human immunodeficiency virus-infected people in Europe: report of 4 cases and review of the literature. Medicine (Baltimore) 2006;85(1):22–36.

[41] Couppie P, Sobesky M, Aznar C, et al. Histoplasmosis and acquired immunodeficiency syndrome: a study of prognostic factors. Clin Infect Dis 2004;38(1):134–8.

[42] Wheat LJ, Connolly-Stringfield PA, Baker RL, et al. Disseminated histoplasmosis in the acquired immune deficiency syndrome: clinical findings, diagnosis and treatment, and review of the literature. Medicine (Baltimore) 1990;69(6):361–74.

[43] Corcoran GR, Al-Abdely H, Flanders CD, et al. Markedly elevated serum lactate dehydrogenase levels are a clue to the diagnosis of disseminated histoplasmosis in patients with AIDS. Clin Infect Dis 1997;24(5):942–4.

[44] Akpek G, Lee SM, Gagnon DR, et al. Bone marrow aspiration, biopsy, and culture in the evaluation of HIV-infected patients for invasive mycobacteria and histoplasma infections. Am J Hematol 2001;67(2):100–6.

[45] Kauffman CA. Histoplasmosis: a clinical and laboratory update. Clin Microbiol Rev 2007; 20(1):115–32.

[46] Woods CW, McRill C, Plikaytis BD, et al. Coccidioidomycosis in human immunodeficiency virus-infected persons in Arizona, 1994–1997: incidence, risk factors, and prevention. J Infect Dis 2000;181(4):1428–34.

[47] Maubon D, Simon S, Aznar C. Histoplasmosis diagnosis using a polymerase chain reaction method: application on human samples in French Guiana, South America. Diagn Microbiol Infect Dis 2007;58:441–4.

[48] Arguinchona HL, Ampel NM, Dols CL, et al. Persistent coccidioidal seropositivity without clinical evidence of active coccidioidomycosis in patients infected with human immunodeficiency virus. Clin Infect Dis 1995;20(5):1281–5.

[49] Fish DG, Ampel NM, Galgiani JN, et al. Coccidioidomycosis during human immunodeficiency virus infection: a review of 77 patients. Medicine (Baltimore) 1990;69(6):384–91.

[50] Rosenthal E, Marty P, Poizot-Martin I, et al. Visceral leishmaniasis and HIV-1 co-infection in southern France. Trans R Soc Trop Med Hyg 1995;89(2):159–62.

[51] Singh N, Perfect JR. Immune reconstitution syndrome associated with opportunistic mycoses. Lancet Infect Dis 2007;7(6):395–401.

[52] Medrano FJ, Jimenez-Mejias E, Calderon E, et al. An easy and quick method for the diagnosis of visceral leishmaniasis in HIV-1-infected individuals. AIDS 1993;7(10):1399.

[53] Maurya R, Singh RK, Kumar B, et al. Evaluation of PCR for diagnosis of Indian kala-azar and assessment of cure. J Clin Microbiol 2005;43(7):3038–41.

[54] Antinori S, Calattini S, Longhi E, et al. Clinical use of polymerase chain reaction performed on peripheral blood and bone marrow samples for the diagnosis and monitoring of visceral leishmaniasis in HIV-infected and HIV-uninfected patients: a single-center, 8-year experience in Italy and review of the literature. Clin Infect Dis 2007;44(12):1602–10.

[55] Murata M, Furusyo N, Otaguro S, et al. HIV infection with concomitant cerebral toxoplasmosis and disseminated histoplasmosis in a 45-year-old man. J Infect Chemother 2007;13(1): 51–5.

[56] Dromer F, Mathoulin-Pelissier S, Launay O, et al. Determinants of disease presentation and outcome during cryptococcosis: The CryptoA/D Study. PLoS Med 2007;4(2):e21.

[57] Lortholary O, Poizat G, Zeller V, et al. Long-term outcome of AIDS-associated cryptococcosis in the era of combination antiretroviral therapy. AIDS 2006;20(17):2183–91.

[58] Lortholary O, Meyohas MC, Dupont B, et al. Invasive aspergillosis in patients with acquired immunodeficiency syndrome: report of 33 cases. French Cooperative Study Group on Aspergillosis in AIDS. Am J Med 1993;95(2):177–87.

[59] Duong TA. Infection due to *Penicillium marneffei*, an emerging pathogen: review of 155 reported cases. Clin Infect Dis 1996;23(1):125–30.

[60] Supparatpinyo K, Khamwan C, Baosoung V, et al. Disseminated *Penicillium marneffei* infection in southeast Asia. Lancet 1994;344(8915):110–3.

[61] Wong SS, Wong KH, Hui WT, et al. Differences in clinical and laboratory diagnostic characteristics of penicilliosis marneffei in human immunodeficiency virus (HIV)- and non-HIV-infected patients. J Clin Microbiol 2001;39(12):4535–40.

[62] Zylberberg H, Robert F, Le Gal FA, et al. Prolonged isolated fever due to attenuated extracerebral toxoplasmosis in patients infected with human immunodeficiency virus who are receiving trimethoprim-sulfamethoxazole as prophylaxis. Clin Infect Dis 1995;21(3):680–1.

[63] Koehler JE, Sanchez MA, Tye S, et al. Prevalence of *Bartonella* infection among human immunodeficiency virus-infected patients with fever. Clin Infect Dis 2003;37(4):559–66.

[64] Tea A, Alexiou-Daniel S, Arvanitidou M, et al. Occurrence of *Bartonella henselae* and *Bartonella quintana* in a healthy Greek population. Am J Trop Med Hyg 2003;68(5):554–6.

[65] Falagas ME, Klempner MS. Babesiosis in patients with AIDS: a chronic infection presenting as fever of unknown origin. Clin Infect Dis 1996;22(5):809–12.

[66] Sepkowitz KA, Telzak EE, Carrow M, et al. Fever among outpatients with advanced human immunodeficiency virus infection. Arch Intern Med 1993;153(16):1909–12.

[67] Clifford GM, Polesel J, Rickenbach M, et al. Cancer risk in the Swiss HIV Cohort Study: associations with immunodeficiency, smoking, and highly active antiretroviral therapy. J Natl Cancer Inst 2005;97(6):425–32.

[68] Lim ST, Levine AM. Recent advances in acquired immunodeficiency syndrome (AIDS)-related lymphoma. CA Cancer J Clin 2005;55(4):229–41, 260–1, 264.

[69] Ciaudo M, Doco-Lecompte T, Guettier C, et al. Revisited indications for bone marrow examinations in HIV-infected patients. Eur J Haematol 1994;53(3):168–74.

[70] Jacobson LP, Kirby AJ, Polk S, et al. Changes in survival after acquired immunodeficiency syndrome (AIDS): 1984–1991. Am J Epidemiol 1993;138(11):952–64.

[71] Goedert JJ, Cote TR, Virgo P, et al. Spectrum of AIDS-associated malignant disorders. Lancet 1998;351(9119):1833–9.

[72] Carr A, Cooper DA. Adverse effects of antiretroviral therapy. Lancet 2000;356(9239): 1423–30.

[73] Cribb AE, Lee BL, Trepanier LA, et al. Adverse reactions to sulphonamide and sulphonamide-trimethoprim antimicrobials: clinical syndromes and pathogenesis. Adverse Drug React Toxicol Rev 1996;15(1):9–50.

[74] Jacobson MA, McGrath MS, Joseph P, et al. Zidovudine-induced fever. J Acquir Immune Defic Syndr 1989;2(4):382–8.

[75] Fellay J, Boubaker K, Ledergerber B, et al. Prevalence of adverse events associated with potent antiretroviral treatment: Swiss HIV Cohort Study. Lancet 2001;358(9290):1322–7.

[76] Shelburne SA, Visnegarwala F, Darcourt J, et al. Incidence and risk factors for immune reconstitution inflammatory syndrome during highly active antiretroviral therapy. AIDS 2005;19(4):399–406.

[77] Ingiliz P, Appenrodt B, Gruenhage F, et al. Lymphoid pneumonitis as an immune reconstitution inflammatory syndrome in a patient with CD4 cell recovery after HAART initiation. HIV Med 2006;7(6):411–4.

[78] Foulon G, Wislez M, Naccache JM, et al. Sarcoidosis in HIV-infected patients in the era of highly active antiretroviral therapy. Clin Infect Dis 2004;38(3):418–25.

[79] Davis P, Stein M. Human immunodeficiency virus-related connective tissue diseases: a Zimbabwean perspective. Rheum Dis Clin North Am 1991;17(1):89–97.

[80] Friedman ND, Spelman DW. Subacute thyroiditis presenting as pyrexia of unknown origin in a patient with human immunodeficiency virus infection. Clin Infect Dis 1999;29(5):1352–3.

[81] Pacios E, Alcala L, Ruiz-Serrano MJ, et al. Evaluation of bone marrow and blood cultures for the recovery of mycobacteria in the diagnosis of disseminated mycobacterial infections. Clin Microbiol Infect 2004;10(8):734–7.

[82] Deniau M, Canavate C, Faraut-Gambarelli F, et al. The biological diagnosis of leishmaniasis in HIV-infected patients. Ann Trop Med Parasitol 2003;97(Suppl 1):115–33.

[83] O'Doherty MJ, Barrington SF, Campbell M, et al. PET scanning and the human immunodeficiency virus-positive patient. J Nucl Med 1997;38(10):1575–83.

[84] Meller J, Sahlmann CO, Scheel AK. 18F-FDG PET and PET/CT in fever of unknown origin. J Nucl Med 2007;48(1):35–45.

[85] Kilby JM, Marques MB, Jaye DL, et al. The yield of bone marrow biopsy and culture compared with blood culture in the evaluation of HIV-infected patients for mycobacterial and fungal infections. Am J Med 1998;104(2):123–8.

[86] Benito N, Nunez A, de Gorgolas M, et al. Bone marrow biopsy in the diagnosis of fever of unknown origin in patients with acquired immunodeficiency syndrome. Arch Intern Med 1997;157(14):1577–80, Fluorodeoxyglucose.

[87] Engels E, Marks PW, Kazanjian P. Usefulness of bone marrow examination in the evaluation of unexplained fevers in patients infected with human immunodeficiency virus. Clin Infect Dis 1995;21(2):427–8.

[88] Ker CC, Hung CC, Huang SY, et al. Comparison of bone marrow studies with blood culture for etiological diagnosis of disseminated mycobacterial and fungal infection in patients with acquired immunodeficiency syndrome. J Microbiol Immunol Infect 2002;35(2):89–93.

[89] Prego V, Glatt AE, Roy V, et al. Comparative yield of blood culture for fungi and mycobacteria, liver biopsy, and bone marrow biopsy in the diagnosis of fever of undetermined origin in human immunodeficiency virus-infected patients. Arch Intern Med 1990;150(2):333–6.

[90] Garcia-Ordonez MA, Colmenero JD, Jimenez-Onate F, et al. Diagnostic usefulness of percutaneous liver biopsy in HIV-infected patients with fever of unknown origin. J Infect 1999; 38(2):94–8.

[91] Cavicchi M, Pialoux G, Carnot F, et al. Value of liver biopsy for the rapid diagnosis of infection in human immunodeficiency virus-infected patients who have unexplained fever and elevated serum levels of alkaline phosphatase or gamma-glutamyl transferase. Clin Infect Dis 1995;20(3):606–10.

[92] Roger PM, Mondain V, Saint Paul MC, et al. Liver biopsy is not useful in the diagnosis of mycobacterial infections in patients who are infected with human immunodeficiency virus. Clin Infect Dis 1996;23(6):1302–4.

[93] Erbel R, Rohmann S, Drexler M, et al. Improved diagnostic value of echocardiography in patients with infective endocarditis by transoesophageal approach: a prospective study. Eur Heart J 1988;9(1):43–53.

[94] Gebo KA, Burkey MD, Lucas GM, et al. Incidence of, risk factors for, clinical presentation, and 1-year outcomes of infective endocarditis in an urban HIV cohort. J Acquir Immune Defic Syndr 2006;43(4):426–32.

[95] Anglaret X, Saba J, Perronne C, et al. Empiric antituberculosis treatment: benefits for earlier diagnosis and treatment of tuberculosis. Tuber Lung Dis 1994;75(5):334–40.

ELSEVIER
SAUNDERS

INFECTIOUS
DISEASE CLINICS
OF NORTH AMERICA

Infect Dis Clin N Am 21 (2007) 1033–1054

# Fever of Unknown Origin in Solid Organ Transplant Recipients

Emilio Bouza, MD, PhD*, Belén Loeches, MD,
Patricia Muñoz, MD, PhD

*Division of Clinical Microbiology and Infections, Universidad Complutense de Madrid,
Hospital General Universitario Gregorio Marañón, Dr. Esquerdo 46, 28007 Madrid, Spain*

The improvement of prognosis in transplantation can be traced to the introduction of new immunosuppressive agents such as azathioprine and corticosteroids, in 1960, or cyclosporine, in 1980. But the biggest revolution has been the advent of tacrolimus, mycophenolate mofetil, sirolimus, everolimus, and the new monoclonal antibody therapy.

Fever is a common clinical manifestation in transplant patients, and it may be due to many different reasons, including the underlying disease of the patient, the surgical intervention, rejection episodes, drugs administered, or intercurrent infections. In the general population, infections and malignancies as causes of fever of unknown origin (FUO) have decreased over time, whereas inflammatory diseases and undiagnosed fevers have increased [1–3].

This article reviews FUO in transplant patients, despite there being no clear and widely accepted definition of FUO for such patients. Petersdorf and Beeson [4] defined FUO as fever that was prolonged (≥3 weeks) because, by the end of that period, most common fevers had been identified or had self-resolved. At present, this long evolution period cannot be witnessed passively (ie, without intervention) in most circumstances and in immunosuppressed transplant patients in particular. The methodology of diagnosis has also been accelerated and made more accurate, not only for the imaging diagnosis but also for microbiology. Durak and Street [5] offered new definitions for different subsets of populations with FUO (Table 1) as follows: classic FUO, nosocomial FUO, neutropenic FUO, and HIV-associated FUO. Most unfortunately, transplant patients were not included, and the situation remains that way today.

---

* Corresponding author.
*E-mail address:* ebouza@microb.net (E. Bouza).

Table 1
Diagnostic criteria for fever of unknown origin in different population groups

Classic FUO
  Fever of or more than 38.3°C (101°F) on several occasions
  Fever of more than 3-wk duration
  Diagnosis uncertain despite appropriate investigations, after at least 3 outpatient visits
    or at least 3 d in hospital
Nosocomial FUO
  Fever of or more than 38.3°C (101°F) on several occasions in a hospitalized patient receiving
    acute care
  Infection not present or incubating on admission
  Diagnosis uncertain after 3 d despite appropriate investigation, including at least
    2 d of incubation of microbiologic cultures
Neutropenic FUO
  Fever of or more than 38.3°C (101°F) on several occasions
  Patient has less than 500 neutrophils/μL in peripheral blood or expected to fall below
    within 1–2 d
  Diagnosis uncertain after 3 d, despite appropriate investigation, including at least
    2 d of incubation of microbiologic cultures
HIV-associated FUO
  Fever of or more than 38.3°C (101°F) on several occasions
  Confirmed positive serology for HIV infection
  Fever of more than 4-wk duration for outpatients or more than 3-d duration in hospital
  Diagnosis uncertain after 3 d, despite appropriate investigation, including at least 2 d of
    incubation of microbiologic cultures

*From* Durack DT, Street AC. Fever of unknown origin: re-examined and redefined. In: Remington JS, Swartz MN, editors. Current clinical topics in infectious diseases 11. Boston: Blackwell Scientific Publications; 1991. p. 35–51; with permission.

The term "FUO" in transplant patients should be used only for prolonged fevers that do not result in an obvious cause after 3 consecutive outpatient visits or after 3 days of hospital evaluation, provided that commonly used imaging and microbiologic tests are reported negative by that time. In transplant recipients, fever has been defined as an oral temperature of 37.8°C or greater on at least two occasions during a 24-hour period [6]. Antimetabolite immunosuppressive drugs, mycophenolate mofetil, and azathioprine are associated with significantly lower maximum temperatures and leukocyte counts [7].

Consideration should be given to the specific type of transplant patient, to the results of the physical examination, and to the epidemiologic antecedents. After that, an approach that considers different syndromes, followed by an etiologically oriented differential diagnosis, is pertinent.

## Incidence of fevers in different transplant patients

The precise incidence of fever in different transplant patients is not well known. In a prospective evaluation of febrile episodes in liver transplant recipients, Chang et al [8] reported that fever was due to infections in 78% of the episodes and to noninfectious causes in 22%. The predominant sources of fever were bacterial (62%) and viral infections (6%), whereas rejection accounted for only 4% of the episodes. Nevertheless, 40% of the infections were unaccompanied by fever, particularly fungal diseases. Overall, six of the seven febrile viral infections were due to viruses other than cytomegalovirus, of which human herpesvirus-6 (HHV-6) was the predominant pathogen, a cause particularly prone to infections that meet the present authors' definition of FUO in transplant patients. Episodes of fever in liver transplant recipients were most likely to occur within 12 weeks (58%) or 1 year (29%) after transplantation. In the latter case, 100% were due to episodes of recurrent hepatitis or malignancy, or were related to chronic hemodialysis.

The incidence of infection after heart transplantation (HT) ranges from 30% to 60% (with a related mortality of 4%–15%), and the rate of infectious episodes per patient is 1.73 in a recent series [9]. Infections are more frequent and severe than those occurring in renal transplant recipients, but less frequent than those occurring after liver or lung transplantation. The authors were unable, however, to find reports on the incidence of febrile episodes in those patients and, particularly, on the frequency in which febrile episodes present clinically as FUOs. In any case, episodes of prolonged FUO are distinctly uncommon in HT patients. Reports include cases with infections such as visceral leishmaniasis [10], intestinal tuberculosis [11], or respiratory syncytial virus pneumonia [12]. Everolimus has been reported in one occasion as a presumptive cause of a long-term fever in a heart transplant recipient [13].

In kidney transplantation, fever is no longer a frequent presentation of rejection, and prolonged FUO episodes are uncommon. Nevertheless, different infectious diseases can present with FUO in renal transplant patients (Box 1).

Noninfectious causes of prolonged fever in kidney transplant patients include drug fever caused by mycophenolate [33], sirolimus [34], systemic lupus erythematosus [17], and hemaphagocytic syndrome [35].

## A syndrome approach to transplant patients with fevers of unknown origin

Fever in most transplant recipients should be considered an emergency. Risk factors for infection should be carefully sought in all solid organ transplant (SOT) patients. The pre-transplantation history (eg, serologic status against microorganisms such as cytomegalovirus [CMV], hepatitis virus, *Toxoplasma*, etc) may yield valuable information. Previous infections or colonization, exposure to tuberculosis, contact with animals, raw food ingestion, gardening, prior antimicrobial therapy or prophylaxis, vaccines or immunosuppressors, and contact with contaminated environment or persons should be recorded [36,37]. History of residence or travel to endemic areas of regional mycosis [38] or tropical destinations must be considered in these patients because of potential emerging pathogens causing FUO such as dengue virus [39,40] *or Strongyloides stercoralis* [41]. Exposure to

---

**Box 1. Infectious diseases that can present with fevers of unknown origin in renal transplant patients**

- Herpes simplex virus with or without esophagitis [14,15]
- Cytomegalovirus (CMV) disease, particularly cases with ischemic colitis [16,17]
- Bacillary angiomatosis [18]
- Nocardiosis [19]
- Tuberculosis [20–23]
- Visceral leishmaniasis [24–29]
- Disseminated microsporidiosis [30]
- *Aspergillus* thyroiditis [31]
- Disseminated strongyloidiasis [32]

---

ticks may be essential to diagnose entities such as human monocytic ehrlichiosis, which may be potentially lethal in immunosuppressed patients [42].

A basic tenet of the management of an SOT with fever is that physical examination data should be directly obtained by the identifying consultant; one should not rely on second-hand information. This may be more useful than many expensive and time-consuming tests.

The oral cavity is frequently forgotten and may disclose previously unnoticed herpetic gingivo-stomatitis or ulcers. Within the exploration of the thoracic area, the consultant should visualize the entry sites of all intravascular devices, even if they "have just been cleansed." The presence of inflammatory signs is suggestive of infection, although their absence does not exclude infection. Fever and sepsis, without local signs, may be the initial sign of postsurgical mediastinitis in HT recipients. Although unusual after SOT, cardiac auscultation and echography may help to detect endocarditis [43], and physical examination may occasionally disclose the existence of pneumonia or empyema before abnormal radiologic signs become evident.

The abdominal examination is always essential, especially in orthotopic liver transplantation (OLT) recipients. The surgical wound is also a common site of infection and a cause of fever.

The possibility of colonic perforation in steroid-treated patients or gastrointestinal CMV disease should always be considered in intra-abdominal infections. It is important to remember that even severe intestinal CMV disease may occur in patients with negative blood antigen, especially in patients on mycophenolate mofetil [44].

Finally, skin and retinal examination are "windows" through which the physician may look and obtain useful information on the possible etiology of a previously unexplained febrile episode. The authors have analyzed the value of ocular lesions in the diagnosis and prognosis of patients with tuberculosis, bacteremia, and sepsis [45,46]. Cutaneous or subcutaneous lesions are a valuable source of information and frequently allow a rapid diagnosis.

Viral and fungal infections are the leading causes of skin lesions in this setting. The biopsy of nodules, subcutaneous lesions, or collections may lead to the immediate diagnosis of invasive mycoses and infections caused by *Nocardia* or *Mycobacteria*, among others.

Several syndromes deserve a particular mention.

## Pneumonia

Pneumonia accounts for 30% to 80% of infections suffered by SOT recipients and for a great majority of episodes of fever [47]. Pneumonia is among the leading causes of infectious mortality in this population. The incidence of pneumonia is higher in the early postoperative period, especially in patients who require prolonged ventilation.

The incidence of bacterial pneumonia is highest in recipients of heart–lung (22%) and liver transplants (17%), intermediate in HT recipients (5%), and lowest in renal transplant patients (1%–2%). The crude mortality of bacterial pneumonia in solid organ transplantation has exceeded 40% in most series [48].

Pneumonia is the most common infection following HT. Gram-negative pneumonia in the early post-transplant period is associated with significant mortality. In a recent multicentric prospective study performed in Spain, the incidence of pneumonia after HT was 15.6 episodes/100 HT [49]. Most cases occurred in the first month after transplantation. Etiology could be established in 61% of the cases: bacteria caused 91% of the cases, fungi 9%, and virus 6%. Bacterial pathogens caused early pneumonias gram-negative rods (median 9 days) and gram-positive cocci (11 days), whereas fungi (80 days), *M tuberculosis* and *Nocardia* spp (145 days), and virus (230 days) were detected later. *Legionella* should always be included in the differential diagnosis [50–53]. Pneumonia increases the risk of mortality after HT (odds ratio [OR] 3.7, CI 95% 1.5–8.1, $P<.01$).

Lung infections are common in lung and heart–lung transplant recipients. In fact, the anastomosis site is especially vulnerable to invasion with opportunistic pathogens, including gram-negative rods (*Pseudomonas*), *Staphylococci*, or fungus. Lung transplant recipients with underlying cystic fibrosis may be prone to suffer infections caused by multiresistant microorganisms such as *Burkholderia cepacia*. Pathogens transmitted from the donor may also cause pneumonia in this setting.

Pneumonia is less common after renal transplantation (8%–16%), although it remains a significant cause of morbidity [54–57].

## Postsurgical infections

Complications in the proximity of the surgical area must always be investigated in SOT patients with fever. In the early post-transplantation period, renal and pancreas transplant recipients may develop perigraft hematomas, lymphoceles, and urinary fistula. Liver transplant recipients are at risk for portal vein thrombosis, hepatic vein occlusion, hepatic artery thrombosis, and biliary stricture formation and leaks. HT recipients are at risk for mediastinitis and infection at the aortic suture line, with resultant mycotic aneurysm. Lung transplantation recipients are at risk for disruption of the bronchial anastomosis.

Hepatic abscess is frequently associated with hepatic artery thrombosis [58]. A tuberculous liver abscess was reported in a renal transplant recipient, and must be considered in the differential diagnosis [59]. Clinical presentation of hepatic abscess includes fever; however, with today's imaging technology, it rarely becomes a cause of FUO.

In heart–lung transplant recipients, the possibility of mediastinitis (2%–9%) should be considered. HT patients have a higher risk of postsurgical mediastinitis and sternal osteomyelitis than other heart surgical patients [60]. Mediastinitis may initially appear merely as fever or bacteremia of unknown origin. Mycoplasma, mycobacteria, and other less common pathogens should be suspected in "culture-negative" wound infections [61,62].

## Urinary tract infections

Urinary tract infections are the most common form of bacterial complication affecting renal transplant recipients [63,64]. The incidence in patients not receiving prophylaxis has been reported to vary from 5% to 36% in a recent series [65]. However, it is not a common cause of FUO.

## Gastrointestinal infections

Gastrointestinal symptoms are present in up to 51% of HT patients in a recent series, although only 15% are significant enough to warrant endoscopic, radiologic, or surgical procedures.

Peritonitis, intra-abdominal infections, and *Clostridium difficile* colitis accounted for 5% of all febrile episodes in OLT in the ICU [66]. Abdominal pain and/or diarrhea is detected in up to 20% of organ transplant recipients [67,68]. CMV and *C difficile* are the most common causes of infectious diarrhea in SOT patients [69–72].

CMV may involve the whole gastrointestinal tract, although the duodenum and stomach are the most frequent sites involved [73] and may occasionally behave as an FUO or as gastrointestinal bleeding. Differential diagnosis should include diverticulitis, intestinal ischemia, cancer, and lymphoproliferative disorders associated with Epstein-Barr virus. A particular gastric lymphoma, called "mucosa-associated lymphoid tissue" lymphoma, may develop in renal transplant patients. It usually responds to the eradication of *Helicobacter pylori* [74].

*C difficile* should be suspected in patients who present with nosocomial diarrhea and occasionally may present with fever and leukocytosis without evident diarrhea [75–78]. Most episodes of diarrhea associated with *C diffi-cile* in SOT patients occur early after transplantation, but they meet criteria of FUO only anecdotally. Hypogammaglobulinemia has been found to be an independent risk factor for CDAD in the HT population [79,80].

Immunosuppressive drugs, such as mycophenolate mofetil, cyclosporine A, tacrolimus, and sirolimus, are all known to be associated with diarrhea and occasionally with fever.

## Focal neurologic manifestations

The detection of central nervous system (CNS) symptoms in a SOT recipient should immediately arouse the suspicion of an infection [81,82]. Some causes of CNS infections in these patients, which are very uncommon in the general population, can present as a FUO (Table 2). Noninfectious causes include immunosuppressive-, toxic-, or metabolic-associated leukoencephalopathy; stroke; and malignancies [82,83].

The most common cause of meningoencephalitis in organ transplant recipients is herpes viruses, followed by *Listeria monocytogenes, Cryptococcus neoformans,* and *Toxoplasma gondii.*

In a recent review, HHV-6 encephalitis occurred a median of 45 days (range = 10 days to 15 months) after transplantation. Mental status changes, ranging from confusion to coma (92%), seizures (25%), and headache (25%), were the predominant clinical presentations. Focal neurologic findings were present in only 17% of the patients. Only 25% of the patients had fever, occasionally reaching 40°C, but the criteria of FUO are rarely met [84–91].

Citomegalovirus infection of the CNS is quite uncommon in SOT recipients and rarely meets FUO criteria if proper diagnostic methodology is used.

Among causes of encephalitis, West Nile virus has been described as causing outbreaks of febrile illness and encephalitis in North America over the past few years, with particular incidence in SOT patients [92–102].

*L monocytogenes* infections can occur at almost any time after transplantation, although the most common period is 2 to 6 months post-transplant

Table 2
Causes of central nervous system infections in transplant recipients

| Syndrome | Common etiologies in transplantation |
| --- | --- |
| Acute meningitis | *Listeria monocytogenes* |
| | *Cryptococcus neoformans* |
| Acute-chronic meningitis | *Mycobacterium tuberculosis* |
| | *Coccidioides immitis* |
| | *Histoplasma capsulatum* |
| Focal brain infection | *Aspergillus fumigatus* |
| | *Nocardia asteroides* |
| | *L monocytogenes* |
| | *Toxoplasma gondii* |
| Progressive dementia | Progressive multifocal leukoencephalopathy (JC virus) |

[103–108]. Patients with listeriosis commonly have fever but not a prolonged undiagnosed FUO if proper etiologic work-up is performed.

Cryptococcosis is mostly a cause of meningitis, pneumonia, and skin lesions in transplant recipients, but rarely causes FUO [109–119].

Focal brain lesions may be caused by *Listeria, T gondii*, fungi (*Aspergillus*, Mucoraceae, phaeohyphomycetes, or dematiaceous fungi), post-transplantation lymphoproliferative disease, or *Nocardia* [120–126], but modern technology and approach avoid the evolution of these diseases as causes of FUOs.

Although bartonellosis is a rare infection in liver transplant recipients, it should always be included in the differential diagnosis of patients presenting with fever, CNS symptoms, and skin lesions [127].

Toxoplasmosis was more prevalent when prophylaxis with cotrimoxazole was not provided [128,129]. The incidence is higher in HT recipients. It may behave as a prolonged FUO if not clinically suspected and if proper microbiologic tests are not performed [130–134].

*Bloodstream infections, catheter-related infections, and infective endocarditis*

Bloodstream infections are common among SOT—particularly during their postoperative period or during episodes requiring intensive care—but obviously they do not constitute a cause of FUO. Infective endocarditis is a rare event in the SOT population (1.7%–6%), but it may be an underappreciated sequela of hospital-acquired infection in transplant patients [43]. The spectrum of organisms causing infective endocarditis is clearly different in transplant recipients than in the general population; 50% of the infections are due to *A fumigatus* or *S aureus*, and only 4% to viridans streptococci. FUO may be a form of presentation in patients with infective endocarditis caused by microorganisms not easily recovered in blood, as is the case with *Aspergillus* [43,135–139]. Toxoplasma and parvovirus B19 may cause myocarditis in this population behaving as FUOs.

**Etiologic approach to fever of unknown origin in transplant patients**

*Viruses*

Most life-threatening viral infections occur within the first 3 months post-transplantation. CMV is the most common pathogen after SOT. When no prophylaxis is given, 30% to 90% of patients will show laboratory data of "CMV infection," and 10% to 50% may develop associated clinical manifestations (CMV disease). CMV may involve the whole gastrointestinal tract, although duodenum and stomach are the most frequent sites involved [52,73,140]. Differential diagnosis should include diverticulitis, intestinal ischemia, cancer, and lymphoproliferative disorders associated with

Epstein-Barr virus. Fever is a common manifestation of CMV disease, but nowadays infrequently causes FUO [16,141,142].

Herpes simplex [143,144] and varizella-zoster virus [145] may cause soft-tissue infections and pneumonia in the transplant population. HHV-6 is a neurotropic, ubiquitous virus known to cause febrile syndromes and exanthema subitum in children. HHV-6 has been reported to cause diverse clinical symptoms such as fever, skin rash, pneumonia, bone marrow suppression, encephalitis, hepatitis, and rejection [85,87]. A growing body of evidence suggests that the more important effect of HHV-6 and HHV-7 reactivation on the outcome of liver transplantation may be mediated indirectly by their interactions with CMV [146,147]. HHV-6 viremia is an independent predictor of invasive fungal infection [148].

Owing to the lack of familiarity with HHV-6 and the unavailability of diagnostic methods in many institutions, HHV-6 may present as prolonged or unexplained fevers [84,86,149].

Both Hepatitis B virus and Hepatitis C virus are very common in transplant patients but are not a cause of FUO.

Community-acquired respiratory viruses, particularly influenza, parainfluenza, adenoviruses, and respiratory syncytial virus and human metapneumovirus, are important pathogens in the transplant patient, but again, almost never behave as FUOs [94,150–158].

In a recent study, 11 transplant recipients with naturally acquired West Nile encephalitis were identified (4 kidney, 2 stem cell, 2 liver, 1 lung, 2 kidney/pancreas). Nine of the 11 patients survived infection, but 3 had significant residual deficits. This viral infection should be considered in all transplant recipients who present with a febrile illness associated with neurologic symptoms. Fever in this situation is usually transient [159–161].

Papovaviruses may be implicated in a variety of clinical syndromes in transplant patients. Papillomaviruses may cause warts and squamous cell carcinomas of the skin. The JC virus causes progressive leukoencephalopathy, and the BK virus causes transplant nephropathy in kidney recipients [162–168]. None of them are common causes of FUO.

## Bacteria

Bacteria are the most common causes of infection in transplant patients, with the pathogenesis and microbial etiology quite similar to those observed in the general population. Owing to the acuteness of most bacterial diseases and the simplicity of bacterial isolation, the vast majority of bacterial diseases in transplant patients do not present clinically as FUOs.

*Mycobacterium tuberculosis* is a well-known cause of FUO both in normal and in immunocompromised patients, including solid organ transplantation. In transplant patients living in areas of high-level endemicity, *M tuberculosis* might reach up to 15% [22,23,169]. Although there is a large regional variability, the incidence of tuberculosis in the SOT population is 20 to 74 times higher than in the general population, with a mortality rate of up to 30%. The most frequent form of acquisition of tuberculosis after transplantation is the reactivation of latent tuberculosis in patients with previous exposure. Tuberculosis develops a mean of 9 months after transplantation (0.5–13 months). Risk factors for early onset are nonrenal transplant, allograft rejection, immunosuppressive therapy with OKT3 or anti-T cell antibodies, and previous exposure to *M tuberculosis*. Clinical presentation is frequently atypical and diverse, with unsuspected and elusive sites of involvement. A large series of tuberculosis in transplant recipients described pulmonary involvement in 51% of patients, extrapulmonary tuberculosis in 16%, and disseminated infection in 33% [169]. Manifestations include FUO, allograft dysfunction, gastrointestinal bleeding, peritonitis, or ulcers. In transplant patients, *M tuberculosis* infection was also described in skin, muscle, osteoarticular system, CNS, genitourinary tract, lymph nodes, larynx, adrenal glands, and thyroid [169,170]. Ocular lesions may be an early way to detect dissemination [45].

## Fungal infections

Fungal infections should be aggressively pursued in colonized patients and in patients with risk factors. Early stages of fungal infection may be very difficult to detect [171,172]. Isolation of *Candida* or *Aspergillus*, even from superficial sites, may indicate infection and should be considered with caution. Retinal examination, blood and respiratory cultures, and *Aspergillus* and *Cryptococcus* antigen detection tests must be performed.

Different types of transplantations imply differences in fungal infections [173]. A recent series prospectively collected in Spain reported incidences of invasive aspergillosis in different types of SOT recipients and ranged from 0.3% in kidney transplant to 3.9% in pancreas recipients [174].

*Aspergillus* brain abscesses usually occur in the early post-transplantation period. Most of the patients present with simultaneous lung lesions that allow for an easier diagnostic. Thyroiditis caused by *Aspergillus* usually presents with focal abscesses, hemorrhagic lesions, or diffuse infiltration [31]. Overall, disseminated *Aspergillus* disease has been described in 9% to 36% of kidney recipients, 15% to 20% of lung recipients, 20% to 35% of heart recipients, and 50% to 60% of liver recipients with *Invasive Aspergillosis* [172,175].

*Scedosporium* and *Blastoschyzomyces* species are increasingly recognized as significant pathogens, particularly in immunocompromised hosts. These fungi now account for approximately 25% of all non-*Aspergillus* mold infections in organ transplant recipients [176–181].

*Pneumocystic jiroveci* (formerly *P carinii*) is now rarely seen in SOT receiving prophylaxis. Before prophylaxis, incidence was around 5%, although it has been described as reaching up to 80% in lung transplant recipients [54,182–184].

Incidence of cryptococcosis after organ transplantation is 0.3% to 6% [114,119,185–187]. *Cryptococcus* is mostly a cause of meningitis, pneumonia, and skin lesions [110,112,113,116,118,119,188–190]. However, more uncommon sites of infection have also been described in immunocompromised patients, such as hepatic cryptococcosis in an HT recipient [113]. Once more, fungal opportunistic infections rarely present as FUO in the SOT population. Histoplamosis can present as a prolonged febrile illness with subacute pulmonary symptoms in these patients, despite the absence of a regional outbreak [191–194].

## Parasites

Parasitic infections are uncommon, but toxoplasmosis and leishmaniasis should be especially considered in SOT patients. Serology or bone marrow cultures usually provide the diagnosis. The possibility of a *Toxoplasma* primary infection should be considered when a seronegative recipient receives an allograft from a seropositive donor. HT recipients are more susceptible to toxoplasmosis, which may be transmitted with the allograft and occasionally requires ICU admission. The risk of primary toxoplasmosis (R−D+) is greater than 50% in HT, 20% after liver transplantation, and less than 1% after kidney transplantation. Allograft-transmitted toxoplasmosis is more often associated with acute disease (61%) than with reactivation of latent infection (7%). Lethal cases associated with hemophagocytic syndrome have been described [195].

Leishmaniasis is another parasitic infection that should be excluded, though it is uncommon after SOT. It may present as fever, pancytopenia, and splenomegaly. Other parasitic infections such as Chagas disease, neurocysticercosis, schistosomiasis, and strongyloidiasis are exceedingly less common [196].

## Noninfectious causes of fever

Both infectious and noninfectious causes of fever should be considered when approaching a febrile SOT patient. In a recent series, 87% of the febrile episodes detected in OLT in the ICU were due to infections and 13% were noninfectious [66]. Rejection, malignancy, adrenal insufficiency, and drug fever were the most common noninfectious causes.

Fever is common in the first 48 hours after surgery and after certain procedures. If it is not persistent or accompanied by other signs or symptoms, it should not trigger any diagnostic action. Acute rejection accounts for 4% to 17% of the noninfectious febrile episodes [8]. It is usually related to an impairment of the allograft function and requires histologic confirmation. It is more common in the first 6 months, especially in the first 16 days after transplantation in one study [197]. Acute adrenal insufficiency should be excluded in SOT patients admitted to an ICU because of sepsis or surgery, mainly when corticosteroids have been withdrawn and drugs that accelerate the degradation of cortisol (phenytoin, rifampin) are administered [198]. Occasionally, lymphoproliferative disease may present with adrenal insufficiency after liver transplantation [199].

Malignancy—mainly lymphoproliferative disease—is relatively common after SOT and may initially present as a febrile episode (80%) [200]. It usually occurs at a later time after transplantation. The possibility of collagen–vascular diseases, giant cell arteritis, rheumatoid arthritis, and other vasculitides should also be considered.

Drugs such as OKT3 monoclonal antibodies, anti-thymocyte globulin, everolimus [201], sirolimus [34], antimicrobials, interferon, anticonvulsants, antihypertensive, antiarrhythmic drugs, and others may also cause fever in the SOT population [13]. The temporal relationship with the drug is usually a diagnostic clue. New induction therapies, such as basiliximab, are related to fewer side effects and fewer CMV infections [202].

Other causes of noninfectious fever are shown in Box 2.

Noncardiogenic pulmonary edema (pulmonary reimplantation response) is a common finding after lung transplantation (50%–60%) and may occasionally lead to a differential diagnosis with pneumonia [203].

### Management and outcome

Fever is not harmful by itself, and accordingly it should not be systematically eliminated. In fact, it has been demonstrated that fever enhances several host defense mechanisms (chemotaxis, phagocytosis, opsonization) [68,204]. Besides, antibiotics may be more active at higher body temperatures. If provided, antipyretic drugs should be administered at regular intervals to avoid recurrent shivering and an associated increase in metabolic demand.

After obtaining the previously mentioned samples, empiric antibiotics should be promptly started in all transplant patients suspected of infection and in a toxic or unstable situation. Empiric antibiotics are also recommended if a focus of infection is apparent, in the early posttransplant setting in

---

**Box 2. Other causes of noninfectious fever**

- Thromboembolic disease
- Hematoma reabsortion
- Pericardial effusions
- Tissue infarction
- Hemolytic uremic syndrome
- Transfusion reaction
- Pheocromocytoma
- Hyperthyroidism
- Subacute thyroiditis

which nosocomial infection is very common, or when there has been a recent increase of immunosuppression. In a stable patient without a clear source of infections, further diagnostic testing should be carried out and noninfectious causes determined.

## References

[1] Knockaert DC, Vanneste LJ, Bobbaers HJ. Fever of unknown origin in elderly patients. J Am Geriatr Soc 1993;41(11):1187–92.

[2] Vanderschueren S, Knockaert D, Adriaenssens T, et al. From prolonged febrile illness to fever of unknown origin: the challenge continues. Arch Intern Med 2003;163(9):1033–41.

[3] Bleeker-Rovers CP, Vos FJ, de Kleijn EM, et al. A prospective multicenter study on fever of unknown origin: the yield of a structured diagnostic protocol. Medicine (Baltimore) 2007; 86(1):26–38.

[4] Petersdorf RO, Beeson PB. Fever of unexplained origin: report on 100 cases. Medicine (Baltimore) 1961;40:1–30.

[5] Durack DT, Street AC. Fever of unknown origin–reexamined and redefined. In: Remington JS, Swartz MN, editors. Current clinical topics in infectious diseases. Volume 20. Cambridge: Blackwell Scientific Publications; 1991. p. 35–51.

[6] Singhal S, Mehta J. Reimmunization after blood or marrow stem cell transplantation. Bone Marrow Transplant 1999;23(7):637–46.

[7] Sawyer RG, Crabtree TD, Gleason TG, et al. Impact of solid organ transplantation and immunosuppression on fever, leukocytosis, and physiologic response during bacterial and fungal infections. Clin Transpl 1999;13(3):260–5.

[8] Chang FY, Singh N, Gayowski T, et al. Fever in liver transplant recipients: changing spectrum of etiologic agents. Clin Infect Dis 1998;26(1):59–65.

[9] Montoya JG, Giraldo LF, Efron B, et al. Infectious complications among 620 consecutive heart transplant patients at Stanford University Medical Center. Clin Infect Dis 2001;33(5): 629–40 [Epub 2001 Aug 6].

[10] Zorio Grima E, Blanes Julia M, Martinez Ortiz de Urbina L, et al. [Persistent fever, pancytopenia and spleen enlargement in a heart transplant carrier as presentation of visceral leishmaniasis]. Rev Clin Esp 2003;203(3):164–5 [in Spanish].

[11] Zedtwitz-Liebenstein K, Podesser B, Peck-Radosavljevic M, et al. Intestinal tuberculosis presenting as fever of unknown origin in a heart transplant patient. Infection 1999; 27(4–5):289–90.

[12] Berbari N, Johnson DH, Cunha BA. Respiratory syncytial virus pneumonia in a heart transplant recipient presenting as fever of unknown origin diagnosed by gallium scan. Heart Lung 1995;24(3):257–9.

[13] Dorschner L, Speich R, Ruschitzka F, et al. Everolimus-induced drug fever after heart transplantation. Transplantation 2004;78(2):303–4.

[14] Gelman R, Khankin E, Ben-Itzhak A, et al. Herpes simplex viral infection presenting as fever of unknown origin and esophagitis in a renal transplant patient. Isr Med Assoc J 2002;4(11 Suppl):970–1.

[15] Katafuchi R, Saito S, Yanase T, et al. A case of fever of unknown origin with severe stomatitis in renal transplant recipient resulting in graft loss. Clin Transpl 2000;14(Suppl 3):42–7.

[16] Lee CJ, Lian JD, Chang SW, et al. Lethal cytomegalovirus ischemic colitis presenting with fever of unknown origin. Transpl Infect Dis 2004;6(3):124–8.

[17] Kaaroud H, Beji S, Jebali A, et al. A rare cause of fever associated with leukopenia in a renal transplant patient. Nephrol Dial Transplant 2004;19(8):2140–1.

[18] Juskevicius R, Vnencak-Jones C. Pathologic quiz case: a 17-year-old renal transplant patient with persistent fever, pancytopenia, and axillary lymphadenopathy. Bacillary

angiomatosis of the lymph node in the renal transplant recipient. Arch Pathol Lab Med 2004;128(1):e12–4.

[19] Case records of the Massachusetts General Hospital. Weekly clinicopathological exercises. Case 29-2000. A 69-year-old renal transplant recipient with low grade fever and multiple pulmonary nodules. N Engl J Med 2000;343(12):870–7.

[20] Yilmaz E, Balci A, Sal S, et al. Tuberculous ileitis in a renal transplant recipient with familial Mediterranean fever: gray-scale and power Doppler sonographic findings. J Clin Ultrasound 2003;31(1):51–4.

[21] Parry RG, Playford EG, Looke DF, et al. Soft-tissue abscess as the initial manifestation of miliary tuberculosis in a renal transplant recipient with prolonged fever. Nephrol Dial Transplant 1998;13(7):1860–3.

[22] Muñoz P, Rodriguez C, Bouza E. *Mycobacterium tuberculosis* infection in recipients of solid organ transplants. Clin Infect Dis 2005;40(4):581–7, Epub 2005 Jan 25.

[23] Muñoz P, Palomo J, Muñoz R, et al. Tuberculosis in heart transplant recipients. Clin Infect Dis 1995;21(2):398–402.

[24] Sipsas NV, Boletis J. Fever, hepatosplenomegaly, and pancytopenia in a renal transplant recipient. Transpl Infect Dis 2003;5(1):47–52.

[25] Rajaram KG, Sud K, Kohli HS, et al. Visceral leishmaniasis: a rare cause of post-transplant fever and pancytopenia. J Assoc Physicians India 2002;50:979–80.

[26] Apaydin S, Ataman R, Serdengect K, et al. Visceral leishmaniasis without fever in a kidney transplant recipient. Nephron 1997;75(2):241–2.

[27] Moulin B, Ollier J, Bouchouareb D, et al. Leishmaniasis: a rare cause of unexplained fever in a renal graft recipient. Nephron 1992;60(3):360–2.

[28] Kher V, Ghosh AK, Gupta A, et al. Visceral leishmaniasis: an unusual case of fever in a renal transplant recipient. Nephrol Dial Transplant 1991;6(10):736–8.

[29] Fernandez-Guerrero ML, Aguado JM, Buzon L, et al. Visceral leishmaniasis in immuno-compromised hosts. Am J Med 1987;83(6):1098–102.

[30] Mahmood MN, Keohane ME, Burd EM. Pathologic quiz case: a 45-year-old renal transplant recipient with persistent fever. Arch Pathol Lab Med 2003;127(4):e224–6.

[31] Guetgemann A, Brandenburg VM, Ketteler M, et al. Unclear fever 7 weeks after renal transplantation in a 56-year-old patient. Nephrol Dial Transplant 2006;21(8):2325–7.

[32] Soman R, Vaideeswar P, Shah H, et al. A 34-year-old renal transplant recipient with high-grade fever and progressive shortness of breath. J Postgrad Med 2002;48(3):191–6.

[33] Chueh SC, Hong JC, Huang CY, et al. Drug fever caused by mycophenolate mofetil in a renal transplant recipient–a case report. Transplant Proc 2000;32(7):1925–6.

[34] Bauer C, Lidove O, Lamotte C, et al. [Sirolimus-associated interstitial pneumonitis in a renal transplant patient]. Rev Med Interne 2006;27(3):248–52, Epub 2005 Dec 27 [in French].

[35] Gurkan A, Yakupoglu U, Yavuz A, et al. Hemophagocytic syndrome in kidney transplant recipients: report of four cases from a single center. Acta Haematol 2006;116(2):108–13.

[36] Papanicolaou GA, Meyers BR, Meyers J, et al. Nosocomial infections with vancomycin-resistant *Enterococcus faecium* in liver transplant recipients: risk factors for acquisition and mortality. Clin Infect Dis 1996;23(4):760–6.

[37] Duchini A, Goss JA, Karpen S, et al. Vaccinations for adult solid-organ transplant recipients: current recommendations and protocols. Clin Microbiol Rev 2003;16(3):357–64.

[38] Braddy CM, Heilman RL, Blair JE. Coccidioidomycosis after renal transplantation in an endemic area. Am J Transplant 2006;6(2):340–5.

[39] Renaud CJ, Manjit K, Pary S. Dengue has a benign presentation in renal transplant patients: a case series. Nephrology (Carlton) 2007;12(3):305–7.

[40] Garcia JH, Rocha TD, Viana CF, et al. Dengue shock syndrome in a liver transplant recipient. Transplantation 2006;82(6):850–1.

[41] Martín-Rabadán P, Muñoz P, Palomo J, et al. Strongyloidiasis: the Harada-Mori test revisited. Clin Microbiol Infect 1999;5:374–6.

[42] Tan HP, Stephen Dumler J, Maley WR, et al. Human monocytic ehrlichiosis: an emerging pathogen in transplantation. Transplantation 2001;71(11):1678–80.

[43] Paterson DL, Dominguez EA, Chang FY, et al. Infective endocarditis in solid organ transplant recipients. Clin Infect Dis 1998;26(3):689–94.

[44] Mugnani G, Bergami M, Lazzarotto T, et al. [Intestinal infection by cytomegalovirus in kidney transplantation: diagnostic difficulty in the course of mycophenolate mofetil therapy]. G Ital Nefrol 2002;19(4):483–4 [in Italian].

[45] Bouza E, Merino P, Muñoz P, et al. Ocular tuberculosis: a prospective study in a general hospital. Medicine (Baltimore) 1997;76:53–61.

[46] Bouza E, Cobo-Soriano R, Rodriguez-Creixems M, et al. A prospective search for ocular lesions in hospitalized patients with significant bacteremia. Clin Infect Dis 2000;30(2): 306–12.

[47] Singh N, Gayowski T, Wagener MM, et al. Pulmonary infiltrates in liver transplant recipients in the intensive care unit. Transplantation 1999;67(8):1138–44.

[48] Mermel LA, Maki DG. Bacterial pneumonia in solid organ transplantation. Semin Respir Infect 1990;5(1):10–29.

[49] Jimenez-Jambrina M, Hernandez A, Cordero E, et al. Pneumonia after heart transplantation in the XXI century: a multicenter prospective study. Presented at the 45th Interscience Conference on Antimicrobial Agents and Chemoterapy. Washington, DC, December 2005.

[50] Fraser TG, Zembower TR, Lynch P, et al. Cavitary *Legionella pneumonia* in a liver transplant recipient. Transpl Infect Dis 2004;6(2):77–80.

[51] Singh N, Gayowski T, Wagener M, et al. Pulmonary infections in liver transplant recipients receiving tacrolimus. Changing pattern of microbial etiologies. Transplantation 1996;61(3): 396–401.

[52] Nichols L, Strollo DC, Kusne S. Legionellosis in a lung transplant recipient obscured by cytomegalovirus infection and *Clostridium difficile* colitis. Transpl Infect Dis 2002;4(1): 41–5.

[53] Horbach I, Fehrenbach FJ. Legionellosis in heart transplant recipients. Infection 1990; 18(6):361–3.

[54] Gupta RK, Jain M, Garg R. *Pneumocystis carinii* pneumonia after renal transplantation. Indian J Pathol Microbiol 2004;47(4):474–6.

[55] Renoult E, Georges E, Biava MF, et al. Toxoplasmosis in kidney transplant recipients: report of six cases and review. Clin Infect Dis 1997;24(4):625–34.

[56] Renoult E, Georges E, Biava MF, et al. Toxoplasmosis in kidney transplant recipients: a life-threatening but treatable disease. Transplant Proc 1997;29(1–2):821–2.

[57] Chang GC, Wu CL, Pan SH, et al. The diagnosis of pneumonia in renal transplant recipients using invasive and noninvasive procedures. Chest 2004;125(2):541–7.

[58] Stange BJ, Glanemann M, Nuessler NC, et al. Hepatic artery thrombosis after adult liver transplantation. Liver Transpl 2003;9(6):612–20.

[59] Caliskan Y, Demirturk M, Cagatay AA, et al. Isolated hepatic tuberculous abscess in a renal transplant recipient. Transplant Proc 2006;38(5):1341–3.

[60] Muñoz P, Menasalvas A, Bernaldo de Quiros JC, et al. Postsurgical mediastinitis: a case-control study. Clin Infect Dis 1997;25(5):1060–4.

[61] Thaler F, Gotainer B, Teodori G, et al. Mediastinitis due to *Nocardia asteroides* after cardiac transplantation. Intensive Care Med 1992;18(2):127–8.

[62] Levin T, Suh B, Beltramo D, et al. *Aspergillus* mediastinitis following orthotopic heart transplantation: case report and review of the literature. Transpl Infect Dis 2004;6(3): 129–31.

[63] Muñoz P. Management of urinary tract infections and lymphocele in renal transplant recipients. Clin Infect Dis 2001;33(Suppl 1):S53–7.

[64] Tolkoff Rubin NE, Rubin RH. Urinary tract infection in the immunocompromised host. Lessons from kidney transplantation and the AIDS epidemic. Infect Dis Clin North Am 1997;11(3):707–17.

[65] Kahana L, Baxter J. OKT3 rescue in refractory renal rejection. Nephron 1987;46(Suppl 1): 34–40.

[66] Singh N, Chang FY, Gayowski T, et al. Fever in liver transplant recipients in the intensive care unit. Clin Transpl 1999;13(6):504–11.

[67] Singh G. The study of prolonged fevers. J Assoc Physicians India 2000;48(4):454–5.

[68] Singh N. Posttransplant fever in critically ill transplant recipients. In: Singh N, Aguado JM, editors. Infectious complications in transplant patients. Norwell (MA): Kluwer Academic publishers; 2000. p. 113–32.

[69] Keven K, Basu A, Re L, et al. *Clostridium difficile* colitis in patients after kidney and pancreas-kidney transplantation. Transpl Infect Dis 2004;6(1):10–4.

[70] Ginsburg PM, Thuluvath PJ. Diarrhea in liver transplant recipients: etiology and management. Liver Transpl 2005;11(8):881–90.

[71] Altiparmak MR, Trablus S, Pamuk ON, et al. Diarrhoea following renal transplantation. Clin Transpl 2002;16(3):212–6.

[72] Kottaridis PD, Peggs K, Devereux S, et al. Simultaneous occurrence of *Clostridium difficile* and Cytomegalovirus colitis in a recipient of autologous stem cell transplantation. Haematologica 2000;85(10):1116–7.

[73] Kaplan B, Meier-Kriesche HU, Jacobs MG, et al. Prevalence of cytomegalovirus in the gastrointestinal tract of renal transplant recipients with persistent abdominal pain. Am J Kidney Dis 1999;34(1):65–8.

[74] Ponticelli C, Passerini P. Gastrointestinal complications in renal transplant recipients. Transpl Int 2005;18(6):643–50.

[75] Bouza E, Burillo A, Muñoz P. Antimicrobial therapy of *Clostridium difficile*-associated diarrhea. Med Clin North Am 2006;90(6):1141–63.

[76] Muñoz P, Palomo J, Yanez J, et al. Clinical microbiological case: a heart transplant recipient with diarrhea and abdominal pain. Recurring *C. difficile* infection. Clin Microbiol Infect 2001;7(8):451–2.

[77] West M, Pirenne J, Chavers B, et al. Clostridium difficile colitis after kidney and kidney-pancreas transplantation. Clin Transpl 1999;13(4):318–23.

[78] Apaydin S, Altiparmak MR, Saribas S, et al. Prevalence of clostridium difficile toxin in kidney transplant recipients. Scand J Infect Dis 1998;30(5):542.

[79] Sarmiento E, Rodriguez-Molina J, Muñoz P, et al. Decreased levels of serum immunoglobulins as a risk factor for infection after heart transplantation. Transplant Proc 2005;37(9): 4046–9.

[80] Muñoz P, Giannella M, Alcalá L. *Clostridium difficile*-associated diarrhea in heart transplant recipients. Is hypogammaglobulinemia the answer? Journal of Heart and Lung Transplantation 2007;26(9):907–14.

[81] Singh N, Paterson DL. Encephalitis caused by human herpesvirus-6 in transplant recipients: relevance of a novel neurotropic virus. Transplantation 2000;69(12):2474–9.

[82] Singh N, Husain S. Infections of the central nervous system in transplant recipients. Transpl Infect Dis 2000;2(3):101–11.

[83] Ponticelli C, Campise MR. Neurological complications in kidney transplant recipients. J Nephrol 2005;18(5):521–8.

[84] Deborska-Materkowska D, Lewandowski Z, Sadowska A, et al. Fever, human herpesvirus-6 (HHV-6) seroconversion, and acute rejection episodes as a function of the initial seroprevalence for HHV-6 in renal transplant recipients. Transplant Proc 2006;38(1): 139–43.

[85] Cervera C, Marcos MA, Linares L, et al. A prospective survey of human herpesvirus-6 primary infection in solid organ transplant recipients. Transplantation 2006;82(7): 979–82.

[86]  Ward KN. Human herpesviruses-6 and -7 infections. Curr Opin Infect Dis 2005;18(3): 247–52.

[87]  Nash PJ, Avery RK, Tang WH, et al. Encephalitis owing to human herpesvirus-6 after cardiac transplant. Am J Transplant 2004;4(7):1200–3.

[88]  Benito N, Ricart MJ, Pumarola T, et al. Infection with human herpesvirus 6 after kidney-pancreas transplant. Am J Transplant 2004;4(7):1197–9.

[89]  Yoshikawa T, Yoshida J, Hamaguchi M, et al. Human herpesvirus 7-associated meningitis and optic neuritis in a patient after allogeneic stem cell transplantation. J Med Virol 2003; 70(3):440–3.

[90]  Yoshida H, Matsunaga K, Ueda T, et al. Human herpesvirus 6 meningoencephalitis successfully treated with ganciclovir in a patient who underwent allogeneic bone marrow transplantation from an HLA-identical sibling. Int J Hematol 2002;75(4):421–5.

[91]  Tokimasa S, Hara J, Osugi Y, et al. Ganciclovir is effective for prophylaxis and treatment of human herpesvirus-6 in allogeneic stem cell transplantation. Bone Marrow Transplant 2002;29(7):595–8.

[92]  Murtagh B, Wadia Y, Messner G, et al. West Nile virus infection after cardiac transplantation. J Heart Lung Transplant 2005;24(6):774–6.

[93]  Kusne S, Smilack J. Transmission of West Nile virus by organ transplantation. Liver Transpl 2005;11(2):239–41.

[94]  Kumar D, Humar A. Emerging viral infections in transplant recipients. Curr Opin Infect Dis 2005;18(4):337–41.

[95]  Hoekstra C. West Nile virus: a challenge for transplant programs. Prog Transplant 2005; 15(4):397–400.

[96]  Hayes EB, Komar N, Nasci RS, et al. Epidemiology and transmission dynamics of West Nile virus disease. Emerg Infect Dis 2005;11(8):1167–73.

[97]  Cairoli O. The West Nile virus and the dialysis/transplant patient. Nephrol News Issues 2005;19(12):73–5.

[98]  Bragin-Sanchez D, Chang PP. West Nile virus encephalitis infection in a heart transplant recipient: a case report. J Heart Lung Transplant 2005;24(5):621–3.

[99]  Weiskittel PD. West Nile virus infection in a renal transplant recipient. Nephrol Nurs J 2004;31(3):327–9.

[100]  Shepherd JC, Subramanian A, Montgomery RA, et al. West Nile virus encephalitis in a kidney transplant recipient. Am J Transplant 2004;4(5):830–3.

[101]  Rosenberg RN. West Nile virus encephalomyelitis in transplant recipients. Arch Neurol 2004;61(8):1181.

[102]  Roos KL. West Nile encephalitis and myelitis. Curr Opin Neurol 2004;17(3):343–6.

[103]  Wiesmayr S, Tabarelli W, Stelzmueller I, et al. *Listeria meningitis* in transplant recipients. Wien Klin Wochenschr 2005;117(5–6):229–33.

[104]  Rettally CA, Speeg KV. Infection with *Listeria monocytogenes* following orthotopic liver transplantation: case report and review of the literature. Transplant Proc 2003;35(4):1485–7.

[105]  Hofer CB, Melles CE, Hofer E. Listeria monocytogenes in renal transplant recipients. Rev Inst Med Trop Sao Paulo 1999;41(6):375–7.

[106]  Limaye AP, Perkins JD, Kowdley KV. *Listeria* infection after liver transplantation: report of a case and review of the literature. Am J Gastroenterol 1998;93(10):1942–4.

[107]  Stamm AM, Smith SH, Kirklin JK, et al. Listerial myocarditis in cardiac transplantation. Rev Infect Dis 1990;12(5):820–3.

[108]  Ascher NL, Simmons RL, Marker S, et al. *Listeria* infection in transplant patients. Five cases and a review of the literature. Arch Surg 1978;113(1):90–4.

[109]  Summers SA, Dorling A, Boyle JJ, et al. Cure of disseminated cryptococcal infection in a renal allograft recipient after addition of gamma-interferon to anti-fungal therapy. Am J Transplant 2005;5(8):2067–9.

[110]  Rakvit A, Meyerrose G, Vidal AM, et al. Cellulitis caused by *Cryptococcus neoformans* in a lung transplant recipient. J Heart Lung Transplant 2005;24(5):642.

[111] Geusau A, Sandor N, Messeritsch E, et al. Cryptococcal cellulitis in a lung-transplant recipient. Br J Dermatol 2005;153(5):1068–70.

[112] Akamatsu N, Sugawara Y, Nakajima J, et al. Cryptococcosis after living donor liver transplantation: report of three cases. Transpl Infect Dis 2005;7(1):26–9.

[113] Utili R, Tripodi MF, Ragone E, et al. Hepatic cryptococcosis in a heart transplant recipient. Transpl Infect Dis 2004;6(1):33–6.

[114] Singh N, Husain S, De Vera M, et al. *Cryptococcus neoformans* infection in patients with cirrhosis, including liver transplant candidates. Medicine (Baltimore) 2004;83(3): 188–92.

[115] Lee YA, Kim HJ, Lee TW, et al. First report of *Cryptococcus albidus*–induced disseminated cryptococcosis in a renal transplant recipient. Korean J Intern Med 2004;19(1):53–7.

[116] Vilchez R, Shapiro R, McCurry K, et al. Longitudinal study of cryptococcosis in adult solid-organ transplant recipients. Transpl Int 2003;16(5):336–40.

[117] Bag R. Fungal pneumonias in transplant recipients. Curr Opin Pulm Med 2003;9(3):193–8.

[118] Singh N, Gayowski T, Marino IR. Successful treatment of disseminated cryptococcosis in a liver transplant recipient with fluconazole and flucytosine, an all oral regimen. Transpl Int 1998;11(1):63–5.

[119] Singh N, Gayowski T, Wagener MM, et al. Clinical spectrum of invasive cryptococcosis in liver transplant recipients receiving tacrolimus. Clin Transpl 1997;11(1):66–70.

[120] Wiesmayr S, Stelzmueller I, Tabarelli W, et al. Nocardiosis following solid organ transplantation: a single-centre experience. Transpl Int 2005;18(9):1048–53.

[121] Peraira JR, Segovia J, Fuentes R, et al. Pulmonary nocardiosis in heart transplant recipients: treatment and outcome. Transplant Proc 2003;35(5):2006–8.

[122] John GT, Shankar V, Abraham AM, et al. Nocardiosis in tropical renal transplant recipients. Clin Transpl 2002;16(4):285–9.

[123] Tripodi MF, Adinolfi LE, Andreana A, et al. Treatment of pulmonary nocardiosis in heart-transplant patients: importance of susceptibility studies. Clin Transpl 2001;15(6):415–20.

[124] Tan SY, Tan LH, Teo SM, et al. Disseminated nocardiosis with bilateral intraocular involvement in a renal allograft patient. Transplant Proc 2000;32(7):1965–6.

[125] Reddy SS, Holley JL. Nocardiosis in a recently transplanted renal patient. Clin Nephrol 1998;50(2):123–7.

[126] Kursat S, Ok E, Zeytinoglu A, et al. Nocardiosis in renal transplant patients. Nephron 1997;75(3):370–1.

[127] Bonatti H, Mendez J, Guerrero I, et al. Disseminated *Bartonella* infection following liver transplantation. Transpl Int 2006;19(8):683–7.

[128] Muñoz P, Arencibia J, Rodriguez C, et al. Trimethoprim-sulfamethoxazole as toxoplasmosis prophylaxis for heart transplant recipients. Clin Infect Dis 2003;36(7):932–3.

[129] Baden LR, Katz JT, Franck L, et al. Successful toxoplasmosis prophylaxis after orthotopic cardiac transplantation with trimethoprim-sulfamethoxazole. Transplantation 2003;75(3): 339–43.

[130] Wulf MW, van Crevel R, Portier R, et al. Toxoplasmosis after renal transplantation: implications of a missed diagnosis. J Clin Microbiol 2005;43(7):3544–7.

[131] Conrath J, Mouly-Bandini A, Collart F, et al. *Toxoplasma gondii* retinochoroiditis after cardiac transplantation. Graefes Arch Clin Exp Ophthalmol 2003;241(4):334–8, Epub 2003 Mar 22.

[132] Aboul-Hassan S, el-Shazly AM, Farag MK, et al. Epidemiological, clinical and laboratory studies on parasitic infections as a cause of fever of undetermined origin in Dakahlia Governorate. *Egypt.* J Egypt Soc Parasitol 1997;27(1):47–57.

[133] Ionescu DN, Dacic S. Persistent fever in a lung transplant patient. Arch Pathol Lab Med 2005;129(6):e153–4.

[134] Ortonne N, Ribaud P, Meignin V, et al. Toxoplasmic pneumonitis leading to fatal acute respiratory distress syndrome after engraftment in three bone marrow transplant recipients. Transplantation 2001;72(11):1838–40.

[135] Scherer M, Fieguth HG, Aybek T, et al. Disseminated *Aspergillus fumigatus* infection with consecutive mitral valve endocarditis in a lung transplant recipient. J Heart Lung Transplant 2005;24(12):2297–300.

[136] Ruttmann E, Bonatti H, Legit C, et al. Severe endocarditis in transplant recipients–an epidemiologic study. Transpl Int 2005;18(6):690–6.

[137] Sherman-Weber S, Axelrod P, Suh B, et al. Infective endocarditis following orthotopic heart transplantation: 10 cases and a review of the literature. Transpl Infect Dis 2004; 6(4):165–70.

[138] Bishara J, Robenshtok E, Weinberger M, et al. Infective endocarditis in renal transplant recipients. Transpl Infect Dis 1999;1(2):138–43.

[139] Chim CS, Ho PL, Yuen ST, et al. Fungal endocarditis in bone marrow transplantation: case report and review of literature. J Infect 1998;37(3):287–91.

[140] Sarkio S, Halme L, Arola J, et al. Gastroduodenal cytomegalovirus infection is common in kidney transplantation patients. Scand J Gastroenterol 2005;40(5):508–14.

[141] Huang HP, Chien YH, Huang LM, et al. Viral infections and prolonged fever after liver transplantation in young children with inborn errors of metabolism. J Formos Med Assoc 2005;104(9):623–9.

[142] Razeghi E, Hadadi A, Mansor-Kiaei M, et al. Clinical manifestation, laboratory findings, and the response of treatment in kidney transplant recipients with CMV infection. Transplant Proc 2007;39(4):993–6.

[143] Liebau P, Kuse E, Winkler M, et al. Management of herpes simplex virus type 1 pneumonia following liver transplantation. Infection 1996;24(2):130–5.

[144] Weiss RL, Colby TV, Spruance SL, et al. Simultaneous cytomegalovirus and herpes simplex virus pneumonia. Arch Pathol Lab Med 1987;111(3):242–5.

[145] Rodriguez-Moreno A, Sanchez-Fructuoso AI, Calvo N, et al. Varicella infection in adult renal allograft recipients: experience at one center. Transplant Proc 2006;38(8): 2416–8.

[146] Razonable RR, Paya CV. The impact of human herpesvirus-6 and -7 infection on the outcome of liver transplantation. Liver Transpl 2002;8(8):651–8.

[147] Thomasini RL, Sampaio AM, Bonon SH, et al. Detection and monitoring of human herpesvirus 7 in adult liver transplant patients: impact on clinical course and association with cytomegalovirus. Transplant Proc 2007;39(5):1537–9.

[148] Rogers J, Rohal S, Carrigan DR, et al. Human herpesvirus-6 in liver transplant recipients: role in pathogenesis of fungal infections, neurologic complications, and outcome. Transplantation 2000;69(12):2566–73.

[149] Persson L, Dahl H, Linde A, et al. Human cytomegalovirus, human herpesvirus-6 and human herpesvirus-7 in neutropenic patients with fever of unknown origin. Clin Microbiol Infect 2003;9(7):640–4.

[150] Friedrichs N, Eis-Hubinger AM, Heim A, et al. Acute adenoviral infection of a graft by serotype 35 following renal transplantation. Pathol Res Pract 2003;199(8):565–70.

[151] Wright JJ, O'Driscoll G. Treatment of parainfluenza virus 3 pneumonia in a cardiac transplant recipient with intravenous ribavirin and methylprednisolone. J Heart Lung Transplant 2005;24(3):343–6.

[152] Kumar J, Shaver MJ, Abul-Ezz S. Long-term remission of recurrent parvovirus-B associated anemia in a renal transplant recipient induced by treatment with immunoglobulin and positive seroconversion. Transpl Infect Dis 2005;7(1):30–3.

[153] Kumar D, Erdman D, Keshavjee S, et al. Clinical impact of community-acquired respiratory viruses on bronchiolitis obliterans after lung transplant. Am J Transplant 2005;5(8): 2031–6.

[154] Barton TD, Blumberg EA. Viral pneumonias other than cytomegalovirus in transplant recipients. Clin Chest Med 2005;26(4):707–20, viii.

[155] Slifkin M, Doron S, Snydman DR. Viral prophylaxis in organ transplant patients. Drugs 2004;64(24):2763–92.

[156] Mazzone PJ, Mossad SB, Mawhorter SD, et al. Cell-mediated immune response to influenza vaccination in lung transplant recipients. J Heart Lung Transplant 2004;23(10): 1175–81.

[157] Vilchez RA, McCurry K, Dauber J, et al. Influenza virus infection in adult solid organ transplant recipients. Am J Transplant 2002;2(3):287–91.

[158] Ison MG, Hayden FG. Viral infections in immunocompromised patients: what's new with respiratory viruses? Curr Opin Infect Dis 2002;15(4):355–67.

[159] Wadei H, Alangaden GJ, Sillix DH, et al. West Nile virus encephalitis: an emerging disease in renal transplant recipients. Clin Transpl 2004;18(6):753–8.

[160] Kleinschmidt-DeMasters BK, Marder BA, Levi ME, et al. Naturally acquired West Nile virus encephalomyelitis in transplant recipients: clinical, laboratory, diagnostic, and neuropathological features. Arch Neurol 2004;61(8):1210–20.

[161] DeSalvo D, Roy-Chaudhury P, Peddi R, et al. West Nile virus encephalitis in organ transplant recipients: another high-risk group for meningoencephalitis and death. Transplantation 2004;77(3):466–9.

[162] Khaled AS. Polyomavirus (BK virus) nephropathy in kidney transplant patients: a pathologic perspective. Yonsei Med J 2004;45(6):1065–75.

[163] Lipshutz GS, Flechner SM, Govani MV, et al. BK nephropathy in kidney transplant recipients treated with a calcineurin inhibitor-free immunosuppression regimen. Am J Transplant 2004;4(12):2132–4.

[164] de Bruyn G, Limaye AP. BK virus-associated nephropathy in kidney transplant recipients. Rev Med Virol 2004;14(3):193–205.

[165] Ramos E, Drachenberg CB, Portocarrero M, et al. BK virus nephropathy diagnosis and treatment: experience at the University of Maryland Renal Transplant Program. Clin Transpl 2002;16:143–53.

[166] Hirsch HH. [Polyomavirus associated nephropathy. A new opportunistic complication after kidney transplantation]. Internist (Berl) 2003;44(5):653–5 [in German].

[167] Lipshutz GS, Mahanty H, Feng S, et al. BKV in Simultaneous pancreas-kidney transplant recipients: a leading cause of renal graft loss in first 2 years post-transplant. Am J Transplant 2005;5(2):366–73.

[168] Arias LF, Alvarez T, Gonzalez L, et al. [BK virus in kidney allografts: a search for histologic evidence of the infection]. Nefrologia 2004;24(5):480–5, [in Spanish].

[169] Singh N, Paterson DL. *Mycobacterium tuberculosis* infection in solid-organ transplant recipients: impact and implications for management. Clin Infect Dis 1998;27(5):1266–77.

[170] Aguado JM, Herrero JA, Gavalda J, et al. Clinical presentation and outcome of tuberculosis in kidney, liver, and heart transplant recipients in Spain. Spanish Transplantation Infection Study Group. GESITRA. Transplantation 1997;63(9):1278–86.

[171] Muñoz P, de la Torre J, Bouza E, et al. Invasive Aspergillosis in transplant recipients. A large multicentric study. Presented at the 36th Interscience Conference of Antimicrobial Agents and Chemotherapy. American Society for Microbiology. New Orleans, September 1996.

[172] Paterson DL, Singh N. Invasive Aspergillosis in transplant recipients. Medicine 1999;78(2): 123–38.

[173] Muñoz P, Alcala L, Sanchez Conde M, et al. The isolation of *Aspergillus fumigatus* from respiratory tract specimens in heart transplant recipients is highly predictive of invasive aspergillosis. Transplantation 2003;75(3):326–9.

[174] Gavalda J, Len O, Rovira M, et al. Epidemiology of invasive fungal infections (IFI) in solid organ (SOT) and hematopoeitic stem cell (HSCT) transplant recipients: a prospective study from resitra. Presented at the 45th Interscience Conference on Antimicrobial Agents and Chemoterapy. Washington, DC, December 2005.

[175] Bonham CA, Dominguez EA, Fukui MB, et al. Central nervous system lesions in liver transplant recipients: prospective assessment of indications for biopsy and implications for management. Transplantation 1998;66(12):1596–604.

[176] Vagefi MR, Kim ET, Alvarado RG, et al. Bilateral endogenous *Scedosporium prolificans* endophthalmitis after lung transplantation. Am J Ophthalmol 2005;139(2):370–3.
[177] Husain S, Muñoz P, Forrest G, et al. Infections due to *Scedosporium apiospermum* and *Scedosporium prolificans* in transplant recipients: clinical characteristics and impact of antifungal agent therapy on outcome. Clin Infect Dis 2005;40(1):89–99, Epub 2004 Dec 08.
[178] Bouza E, Muñoz P. Invasive infections caused by *Blastoschizomyces capitatus* and Scedosporium spp. Clin Microbiol Infect 2004;10(Suppl 1):76–85.
[179] Muñoz P, Marin M, Tornero P, et al. Successful outcome of *Scedosporium apiospermum* disseminated infection treated with voriconazole in a patient receiving corticosteroid therapy. Clin Infect Dis 2000;31(6):1499–501.
[180] Bouza E, Muñoz P, Vega L, et al. Clinical resolution of *Scedosporium prolificans fungemia* associated with reversal of neutropenia following administration of granulocyte colony-stimulating factor. Clin Infect Dis 1996;23(1):192–3.
[181] Husain S, Alexander BD, Muñoz P, et al. Opportunistic mycelial fungal infections in organ transplant recipients: emerging importance of non-*Aspergillus* mycelial fungi. Clin Infect Dis 2003;37(2):221–9.
[182] Rodriguez M, Sifri CD, Fishman JA. Failure of low-dose atovaquone prophylaxis against *Pneumocystis jiroveci* infection in transplant recipients. Clin Infect Dis 2004;38(8):e76–8, Epub 2004 Mar 29.
[183] Radisic M, Lattes R, Chapman JF, et al. Risk factors for *Pneumocystis carinii* pneumonia in kidney transplant recipients: a case-control study. Transpl Infect Dis 2003;5(2):84–93.
[184] Muñoz P, Muñoz RM, Palomo J, et al. *Pneumocystis carinii* infections in heart transplant patients. Twice a week prophylaxis. Medicine (Baltimore) 1997;76:415–22.
[185] Husain S, Wagener MM, Singh N. *Cryptococcus neoformans* infection in organ transplant recipients: variables influencing clinical characteristics and outcome. Emerg Infect Dis 2001;7(3):375–81.
[186] Singh N, Lortholary O, Alexander BD, et al. Allograft loss in renal transplant recipients with *Cryptococcus neoformans* associated immune reconstitution syndrome. Transplantation 2005;80(8):1131–3.
[187] Singh N, Lortholary O, Alexander BD, et al. An immune reconstitution syndrome-like illness associated with *Cryptococcus neoformans* infection in organ transplant recipients. Clin Infect Dis 2005;40(12):1756–61, Epub 2005 Apr 29.
[188] Gupta RK, Khan ZU, Nampoory MR, et al. Cutaneous cryptococcosis in a diabetic renal transplant recipient. J Med Microbiol 2004;53(Pt 5):445–9.
[189] Singh N, Rihs JD, Gayowski T, et al. Cutaneous cryptococcosis mimicking bacterial cellulitis in a liver transplant recipient: case report and review in solid organ transplant recipients. Clin Transpl 1994;8(4):365–8.
[190] Basaran O, Emiroglu R, Arikan U, et al. Cryptococcal necrotizing fasciitis with multiple sites of involvement in the lower extremities. Dermatol Surg 2003;29(11):1158–60.
[191] Freifeld AG, Iwen PC, Lesiak BL, et al. Histoplasmosis in solid organ transplant recipients at a large Midwestern university transplant center. Transpl Infect Dis 2005;7(3–4):109–15.
[192] Nath DS, Kandaswamy R, Gruessner R, et al. Fungal infections in transplant recipients receiving alemtuzumab. Transplant Proc 2005;37(2):934–6.
[193] McGuinn ML, Lawrence ME, Proia L, et al. Progressive disseminated histoplasmosis presenting as cellulitis in a renal transplant recipient. Transplant Proc 2005;37(10):4313–4.
[194] Jha V, Sree Krishna V, Varma N, et al. Disseminated histoplasmosis 19 years after renal transplantation. Clin Nephrol 1999;51(6):373–8.
[195] Segall L, Moal MC, Doucet L, et al. Toxoplasmosis-associated hemophagocytic syndrome in renal transplantation. Transpl Int 2006;19(1):78–80.
[196] Walker M, Kublin JG, Zunt JR. Parasitic central nervous system infections in immunocompromised hosts: malaria, microsporidiosis, leishmaniasis, and African trypanosomiasis. Clin Infect Dis 2006;42(1):115–25.

[197] Toogood GJ, Roake JA, Morris PJ. The relationship between fever and acute rejection or infection following renal transplantation in the cyclosporin era. Clin Transpl 1994;8(4): 373–7.

[198] Singh N, Gayowski T, Marino IR, et al. Acute adrenal insufficiency in critically ill liver transplant recipients. Implications for diagnosis. Transplantation 1995;59(12):1744–5.

[199] Khan A, Ortiz J, Jacobson L, et al. Posttransplant lymphoproliferative disease presenting as adrenal insufficiency: case report. Exp Clin Transpl 2005;3(1):341–4.

[200] Heo JS, Park JW, Lee KW, et al. Posttransplantation lymphoproliferative disorder in pediatric liver transplantation. Transplant Proc 2004;36(8):2307–8.

[201] Carreno CA, Gadea M. Case report of a kidney transplant recipient converted to everolimus due to malignancy: resolution of bronchiolitis obliterans organizing pneumonia without everolimus discontinuation. Transplant Proc 2007;39(3):594–5.

[202] Mourad G, Rostaing L, Legendre C, et al. Sequential protocols using basiliximab versus antithymocyte globulins in renal-transplant patients receiving mycophenolate mofetil and steroids. Transplantation 2004;78(4):584–90.

[203] Khan SU, Salloum J, O'Donovan PB, et al. Acute pulmonary edema after lung transplantation: the pulmonary reimplantation response. Chest 1999;116(1):187–94.

[204] Singh N, Paterson DL, Gayowski T, et al. Predicting bacteremia and bacteremic mortality in liver transplant recipients. Liver Transpl 2000;6(1):54–61.

ELSEVIER
SAUNDERS

INFECTIOUS
DISEASE CLINICS
OF NORTH AMERICA

Infect Dis Clin N Am 21 (2007) 1055–1090

# Fever of Unknown Origin in Febrile Leukopenia

Anastasia Antoniadou, MD*,
Helen Giamarellou, MD, PhD

*University General Hospital ATTIKON, Fourth Department of Internal Medicine,
1 Rimini Street, 12462 Athens, Greece*

Febrile neutropenia (FN) is a syndrome commonly anticipated in patients receiving treatment for cancer. Its management for the last three decades includes the prompt administration of empiric antibacterial therapy, a tactic that resulted in a reduction in mortality. Challenges remain the administration of the most appropriate empiric treatment regimen adapted to evolving and changing epidemiology of infections in neutropenic patients and resistance rates; the development of markers of early diagnosis of severe bacterial or fungal infections; the risk stratification of patients; the establishment of targeted empiric (preemptive) antifungal therapy criteria; and the containment of antimicrobial resistance that compromises effective treatment efforts, through effective antibiotic policies and implementation of infection control measures, especially hand hygiene. The need for targeted antimicrobial or antifungal prophylaxis and supportive strategies like the use of growth factors awaits further clarification.

## Overview

*Definitions, epidemiologic features, risk factors*

As the first cellular component of the inflammatory response and a key component of innate immunity, neutrophils are the first line of defense against infection [1]. Nearly 40 years ago, Bodey and colleagues [2] reported that the risk of infection increases significantly when the absolute neutrophil count is reduced to less than 500 cells/mm$^3$. Neutropenia, defined as

* Corresponding author.
*E-mail address:* ananto@med.uoa.gr (A. Antoniadou).

0891-5520/07/$ - see front matter © 2007 Elsevier Inc. All rights reserved.
doi:10.1016/j.idc.2007.08.008
*id.theclinics.com*

neutrophils less than 500 cells/mm$^3$, remains the best characterized and most prominent form of immunocompromise in patients undergoing treatment for cancer, either solid tumors or hematologic malignancies. It is the leading cause of infectious complications in patients receiving antineoplastic chemotherapy, accounting for most chemotherapy-associated mortality and compromising treatment outcomes by causing dose reductions and treatment delays.

Neutropenia allows bacterial multiplication and invasion and compromises the mounting of clinically apparent inflammatory response, except from the presentation of fever [1]. Sickles and colleagues [3] demonstrated early the lack of typical manifestations of infections in neutropenic patients. In their study, 84% of patients with pneumonia and an adequate neutrophil count (> 1000 cells/mm$^3$) produced purulent sputum compared with only 8% of those with pneumonia and severe neutropenia (< 100 cells/mm$^3$). In a prospective study of 1001 cancer patients with FN, Pizzo [4] reported that only 45% of those with documented bacteremia had signs of infection other than fever. When neutrophils were less than 100 cells/mm$^3$, purulent exudates in patients with pharyngitis were present in 22%; dysuria, frequency, and pyuria was present in 44%, 33%, and 11%, respectively, of patients with urinary tract infections; and clinical signs of meningeal inflammation were absent in meningitis and fluctulence from perineal abscesses [3,4]. Fever can be the only sign of infection and 60% of febrile episodes in neutropenic patients are initially considered as fevers of unknown origin (FUO). Because 70% of these FUOs respond to empirical antimicrobial treatment, it is most likely that many of these episodes represent undetected infections, which if left untreated share a considerable mortality, especially if they represent an occult gram-negative bacteremia [5].

Febrile leucopenia, and most precisely FN, represents a syndrome comprising two components (fever and neutropenia), as defined by the Infectious Diseases Society of America (IDSA) [6] and the Immunocompromised Host Society [7]. Fever is defined as an oral temperature of greater than or equal to 38.3°C in a single measurement or a temperature of greater than or equal to 38°C lasting for greater than or equal to 1 hour. The Immunocompromised Host Society and other scientific societies [8] add also as a criterion of fever the presence of an oral temperature of greater than or equal to 38°C measured twice in 12 hours. Fever as a manifestation of infection or inflammation is not blunted in neutropenic patients because the proinflammatory cytokines necessary for its production are released from many types of cells (macrophages, lymphocytes, fibroblasts, epithelial, and endothelial cells) [9]. In the context of FN, every effort should be made to exclude fever related to noninfectious causes (drug fever, disease fever, transfusion related, and so forth). Rectal measurement of temperature should be avoided (along with other rectal-related procedures like rectal examination, enema, or endoscopy), because it may serve as a portal of entry for microorganisms, especially in patients with mucositis (diarrhea is the common presentation), hemorrhoids, or other topical lesions. Occasionally, the presence of fever can be blunted by immunosuppressive therapies (eg, corticosteroids); advanced age; or the presence of shock [10].

Neutropenia is defined as an absolute neutrophil count of either less than or equal to 500 cells/mm$^3$, or less than or equal to 1000 cells/mm$^3$ initially, predicted to decline to less than or equal to 500 cells/mm$^3$ in 24 to 48 hours. The incidence, severity, and recovery of infection are inversely proportional to the degree or depth of neutropenia [11,12]. The Common Toxicity Criteria of the National Cancer Institute delineates four grades of anticancer chemotherapy-related neutropenia: grade 0 is within normal limits ($\geq 2000$ cells/mm$^3$); and grades 1, 2, 3, and 4 are defined when the absolute neutrophil count is within the ranges of greater than or equal to 1500 to less than 2000 cells/mm$^3$, greater than or equal to 1000 to less than 1500 cells/mm$^3$, greater than or equal to 500 to less than 1000 cells/mm$^3$, and less than 500 cells/mm$^3$, respectively [13].

Duration of neutropenia is another variable that bears a direct relationship with the risk of infection [14]. It has been estimated [12] that all patients with grade 4 neutropenia that is prolonged for 3 weeks develop an infection. Duration of neutropenia after the onset of a febrile episode also affects response to antimicrobial treatment and the incidence of complications. Neutropenia lasting 7 days or less leads to 95% response rates compared with 32% in patients with neutropenia lasting more than 15 days [15].

Frequency of neutropenia is greatly influenced by the type and intensity of the chemotherapy regimen used; the type and stage of the underlying disease (high-dose chemotherapy, peripheral blood stem cell transplant and bone marrow transplantation [BMT] procedures, induction chemotherapy for acute myelogenous leukemia); the use of concomitant radiation therapy; the phase of therapy (greater risk in the earlier cycles, especially the first one); the degree of bone marrow involvement; and patient-specific factors, such as age, performance status, and comorbid conditions [16]. The risk of febrile episodes is increased if the neutrophil nadir at day 10 after cycle 1 of chemotherapy is less than 500 cells/mm$^3$ (Silber's model of prediction) [17].

Febrile episodes during neutropenic periods after antineoplastic chemotherapy, either FUO or documented infections, affect overall survival, probably because of substantial delays in treatment delivery, or the need for dose reductions. A study linking data from the National Cancer Institute with data from a survey in patients with aggressive non-Hodgkin's lymphoma found a significant association between the occurrence of FN, reduction in the number of cycles of CHOP delivered, and lower 5-year overall survival [18].

Neutropenic patients may present with other factors that further increase the risk and spectrum of potential complications: (1) the damage of mechanical barriers by chemotherapy-induced mucositis; bleeding disorders (low platelet count); or because of the presence of invasive devices like central venous catheters (implanted or not); (2) the alteration of patients' own flora by multiple hospitalizations and extensive use of antimicrobials and antifungals; (3) organ function alterations caused by the underlying disease (eg, kidney or liver failure); and (4) medications that affect other arms of the immune defense like the phagocytic function or the humoral response (monoclonal antibodies, fludarabine, corticosteroids) [16,19–23]. Recent studies point also to genetic factors that might influence the risk of infection and response to treatment in patients with neutropenia [24].

Patients with neutropenia not related to cancer, such as after a viral disease or because of drug toxicity, do not have the same risk of acute infection, probably because they retain mucosal integrity [25]. Lower risk characterizes also patients with congenital neutropenia or aplastic anemia. HIV-positive patients with FN have a possible infectious complication but with a lower relative risk compared with those who are neutropenic after cytotoxic chemotherapy [25].

FN for patients at high risk for infectious complications represents a medical emergency. In 50% of patients presenting with fever and neutropenia an occult infection may be present, whereas in 20% of those with grade 4 neutropenia, bacteremia is present [26]. Pseudomonal bacteremia, if untreated, bears a grave prognosis with a 33% to 75% mortality rate within the first 24 to 48 hours [27–29]. This is the reason why, since 1971, empiric use of intravenous broad-spectrum antibiotics has been introduced [30] and their initiation is immediately recommended (within the first hour after fever) in patients presenting with the syndrome of FN [6]. Schimppff and colleagues [30] showed that using this strategy mortality from FN could be dramatically decreased from 60% to 70% in the 1970s to 4% to 6% in adults and 0.4% to 1% in children nowadays [31–33]. During recent years and with the introduction of growth factors, it was realized that all FN patients were not the same. Patients with FN and a low risk for life-threatening infectious complications had a 70% chance to be treated as outpatients, with reduced costs and increased patient comfort, by orally administered broad-spectrum antimicrobial agents [16,34]. Validated prediction models have been developed to distinguish patients falling in different risk categories and they should be applied during the initial evaluation of the patient with FN and FUO.

*Patient risk assessment stratification*

Talcott and colleagues [35,36] were the first to develop a prospectively validated risk assessment tool. Before that only a variety of exclusion criteria for the prediction of patients in low risk for serious infectious complications had been used in studies, such as the presence of renal failure, shock, respiratory failure, HIV status, receipt of intravenous supportive therapy, allogeneic BMT, catheter-related infection, CNS infection, or risk of death within 48 hours postulated by Kern and colleagues [37]. The following factors were proposed by Freifeld and colleagues [38]: hemodynamic instability, abdominal pain, nausea or vomiting, diarrhea, neurologic or mental changes, new pulmonary infiltrates, catheter-related infection, and kidney or liver insufficiency. The clinical model by Talcott and colleagues [35,36] consisted of clinical factors assessable within 24 hours of admission and involved four categories of patients. Categories I, II, and III included patients at high risk: those being hospitalized at presentation of FN (category I); outpatients who presented with serious acute comorbidity, which could have been the reason for hospitalization independent of fever and leucopenia (category II); and patients without acute comorbidity but with uncontrolled cancer (leukemia not in complete remission and other cancers that progressed during the last assessable chemotherapy regimen). Complications in groups I to III were greater than 30% compared with 2% in group IV, which included patients not possessing risk factors present in the other groups [35,36]. Later, Klastersky and colleagues [39] postulated a scoring system based on the Multinational Association for Supportive Care in Cancer (MASCC) predictive model, which consisted of seven variables with a maximum score of 26:

1. Burden of illness with moderate (score 3) or mild (score 5) or absent symptoms (score 5)
2. Absence of hypotension (score 5)
3. Absence of chronic obstructive pulmonary disease (score 4)
4. Presence of solid tumor (4) or no history of previous fungal infection in case of hematologic malignancy (score 4)
5. Outpatient status (score 3)
6. Absence of dehydration (score 3)
7. Age less than 60 years for adults (score 2)

Compared with the Talcott model it offers increased sensitivity (71% versus 30%) and less miscalculations in the identification of low-risk patients at a cost of lower specificity (68% versus 90%) [39]. A score of greater than or equal to 21 predicts a less than 5% risk for severe complications during an episode of FN and a very low mortality (<1%). A prospective survey has validated the MASCC index in 611 episodes of FN in a mixed population of patients with solid tumors or leukemia [40–42]. The group with MASCC index of greater than or equal to 21 represents nearly 70% of an unselected population of patients with FN. A significant percentage (approximately 50%) of these patients are eligible for treatment with orally administered antibiotics and can be discharged early and safely from the hospital after a short (24–48 hours) observation period. The remaining 30% are at much higher risk for complications (25%) and death (14%) during the episode of FN and should be under close follow-up in the hospital while receiving intravenous antibiotics. It remains unclear if some of these patients could benefit from more aggressive therapies (eg, combination of antibiotics or the addition of growth factors) [42]. It is a challenge for the score validating systems to discriminate this group of patients among those with

MASCC index of less than 21, because patients in this high-risk category may not be identical: a score of 7 to 14 bears a mortality that is twice the mortality of patients with a score of 19 to 20 [40].

FUO seems to be a benign presentation, most commonly present in low-risk patients (49% versus 35% in high-risk patients). High-risk patients are more often bacteremic with gram-negatives (59% versus 31%), and less often with gram-positives (38% versus 62%). Bacteremic high-risk patients bear a higher complication (68% versus 24%) and mortality rate (28% versus 2%). A 45% mortality rate accompanies high-risk patients compared with no deaths in the low-risk group. Differences are less impressive between high- and low-risk groups in the subpopulation of patients with gram-positive bacteremia. High-risk febrile neutropenic patients have a significantly longer duration of neutropenia and an increased incidence of complications among patients not responding to the initial empiric therapy, whereas they lack differences in complications or mortality between patients with solid tumors and those with hematologic malignancies [40].

## Initial clinical evaluation

Despite the fact that FUO, as a term, entails the absence of signs of a localized infection, clinical evaluation of the FN patient should be thorough and repeated on a daily basis for the duration of the febrile episode. Although signs can be minimal, it should be mentioned that the commonest sites of infection noted in patients with FN, observed during the first consecutive EORTC trials, are the lungs (25%); mouth and pharynx (25%); soft tissue; skin and central venous catheters sites (15%); the perineum (10%); and less often the gastrointestinal and urinary tract (5%) and the nose sinuses (5%). All of these sites serve also as portals of entry for the offending pathogens [43].

During initial evaluation any piece of information leading to the probable occult infection must be gathered. From the patient's history, bits include the type and timing of antineoplastic chemotherapy; environmental exposures; contact with persons with viral diseases (common cold, chickenpox, measles, and so forth); administration of antibiotics or antifungals either as prophylaxis or treatment of previous infections; known allergies and drug interactions; and recent transfusion of blood or blood products.

Physical examination should include careful search for potential sites of infection, such as the oropharynx, skin and skin folds, the axilla, perineum, nails, eyes, sinuses, vascular access sites, and the lungs. If FN presents as FUO, physical examination initially is unrevealing but it must be repeated daily searching for skin nodules, ulcers, ecthyma gangrenosum, black eschars, pain in the perineum, facial or sinus pain, and swelling or eye redness, documenting clinical infection of microbial or fungal etiology. Vital signs, urine output, respiratory function parameters, and mental state should be evaluated and monitored because hemodynamic instability, hypoxemia, and confusion are signs of clinical deterioration and life-threatening infectious complications [19].

## Laboratory evaluation

Laboratory evaluation of all patients with FN should include complete blood count and biochemical tests and two sets of blood cultures. If a central venous catheter is present a set of cultures drawn one from a peripheral vein and the others from each central venous catheter lumen is obligatory to serve as a diagnostic criterion of catheter-related bloodstream infection, especially if differential time to positivity is used as a diagnostic method (ie, centrally drawn blood culture becomes positive $\geq 120$ minutes earlier compared with the peripherally drawn sample) [44]. Urine cultures are also recommended even if pyuria and dysuria are absent because neutropenia blunts these signs of urinary tract infection. Expectorated sputum samples are processed and cultured even in the absence of neutrophils in Gram stain for the previously mentioned reason. Cultures from other sites are sent if clinical suspicion of infection is present. Screening of normal flora is not indicated because it has not proved useful and cost effective in identifying early the causal pathogen. Screening for multidrug-resistant (MDR) pathogens, such as methicillin-resistant *Staphylococcus aureus* (MRSA), vancomycin-resistant enterococcus (VRE), or MDR gram-negative pathogens, is recommended only for infection control purposes (isolation or cohorting) [6].

A chest radiogram, although not expected to be abnormal even in the presence of pneumonia, should be initially done for later comparisons [45]. It should be repeated if FUO persists and accompanied by a high-resolution CT of the thorax, which can reveal early signs of fungal pneumonia (the "halo sign" in lung hyphomycoses) [46–48]. Right-sided abdominal pain and distention should prompt for a CT of the abdomen, which might reveal bowel wall thickening ($>4$ mm), indicative of typhlitis or neutropenic enterocolitis [49]. An ultrasound or CT examination of the abdomen can be useful in case of persisting FUO after neutrophil count recovery to normal levels, where multiple, hypodense lesions of liver and spleen are suggestive of chronic disseminated candidiasis in the form of hepatosplenic candidiasis (a condition with no other symptoms and signs except fever, increased serum alkaline phosphatase, and negative blood cultures, which necessitates administration of antifungal treatment for the duration of the chemotherapy cycles and for $\geq 6$ months afterward) [50].

Considering that acute bacterial infections and especially bacteremic infections have an increased rate of complications and mortality compared with FUO not representing an occult infection, it is useful for the successful management of the febrile episode in the neutropenic patient to have markers indicative, in case of FUO, of the infectious and bacterial origin of fever. Serum concentrations of several acute-phase proteins (eg, C-reactive protein), proinflammatory cytokines (tumor necrosis factor-α, interleukin-1, interferon-$\gamma$, interleukin-6, interleukin-8), and soluble adhesion molecules (soluble E-selectin, vascular cell adhesion molecule 1, intercellular adhesion molecule 1) have been investigated as to whether these may contribute to identifying infections as the cause of neutropenic fever. Unfortunately, the predictive values of all these parameters, based on the small and inconsistent amount of data available, are too low to influence the clinically based initial treatment decisions in patients with neutropenic fever [51]. More recently, procalcitonin (PCT), a precursor of calcitonin has been shown to increase in systemic bacterial infection especially if severe sepsis is present [52,53]. In healthy humans, PCT levels are almost undetectable ($<0.1$ ng/mL) [54]. PCT was measured on a daily basis and for the whole duration of the febrile episode in patients with neutropenia and cancer in several studies and it was found that it increases in serious systemic infections (values $>5$ ng/mL), with levels particularly elevated in patients with bacteremia and severe sepsis, whereas in viral or localized infections its levels remain much lower ($\leq0.1$ ng/mL) [55–58]. In one of the studies [55] blood samples were obtained from 115 patients with FN for determination of PCT levels before onset of fever and daily until the resolution of fever. The rise in PCT levels appeared early, with median values on the first day of fever of 8.23 ng/mL in patients with bacteremia, compared with 0.86 ng/mL in patients with localized bacterial infections ($P < .017$); 2.62 ng/mL in patients with severe sepsis; and 0.57 ng/mL in patients with clinically localized infections ($P < .001$). A dramatic decrease in PCT levels was documented after resolution of the infection, whereas elevations were noted when infections worsened, indicating that PCT may also serve as a marker useful for the follow-up of patients during the febrile episode. Pronounced PCT levels were also found in patients with FUO who were responding to antimicrobial chemotherapy (indicative of occult infection), compared with those not responding to treatment with antibiotics [59]. In other studies PCT levels were not found to rise during coagulase-negative staphylococci (CNS) bacteremia [59], whereas in only one study levels greater than 3 ng/mL were reported in BMT patients with invasive aspergillosis (IA) [60]. For the moment, because of low sensitivity and specificity, PCT adds little or no help to the diagnosis of invasive fungal infections (IFI) [61]. Accumulated data offer PCT a sensitivity range of 44% to 83% and a specificity range of 64% to 100% depending on the severity of the underlying infection and the cutoff value used. Most powerful is its negative prognostic value (NPV) for the presence of bacterial infection when levels are less than 0.5 ng/mL, which is greater than 85% [54]. PCT has probably lower values in neutropenic hosts necessitating lower cutoff values in the assessment of infectious risk. In a study with 95 FN patients, lowering PCT cutoff values to 0.2 ng/mL could strongly (97.1%–98.4%) predict for the infectious origin of fever [62]. If PCT evaluation is to be used, serial measurements are more helpful than an isolated determination. The value of PCT as a prognostic or treatment modification tool was studied prospectively in 101 episodes of fever- and chemotherapy-induced neutropenia in patients with hematologic malignancies. Values of less than or equal to 0.4 ng/mL 3 days after fever onset exhibited 91% to 100% NPV for the detection of complications, whereas daily values of less than or equal to 0.4 ng/mL for the first 8 days accurately predicted no subsequent complications [63].

A relevant issue studied recently is the prospective evaluation of PCT in the context of FN and the challenge to be able to discriminate early between patients at low or high risk of complications and how this compares and combines with the Talcott and MASCC criteria. The addition of PCT to clinical risk assessment scales, although not in a statistically significant way, seemed to augment sensitivity from 60% to 87% for the prediction of bacteremia and from 70% to 90% to predict treatment failure. More importantly, it incremented the NPV for the detection of bacteremia or treatment failure up to 98%, a determinant factor to decide whether a patient can be discharged safely and treated on an outpatient basis [54].

C-reactive protein is an acute-phase protein that is proved less useful in discriminating occult bacteria infection during an episode of FUO in FN patients, correlating more with the course of fever than with that of infection [64], and its value can be affected by the underlying disease or the presence of graft-versus-host disease. It increases late in the course of infection ($\geq 3$ days after the onset of fever) [65] and its normalization is also prolonged because of a long half-life. It is reported that serial measurements of C-reactive protein can be of help [65,66], with two consecutively low measurements bearing a good NPV for the presence of bacterial infection and stable, consecutively increasing values (levels $> 200$ mg/mL) in patients still febrile the fifth day of the febrile episode to be strongly predictive of mortality [67]. In a recent study levels of PCT and interleukin-6 varied significantly between bacteremic and not bacteremic episodes of FUO and neutropenia, whereas no differences were found in C-reactive protein concentrations indicating that PCT and interleukin-6 are more reliable markers than C-reactive protein for predicting bacteremia in patients with FN [63].

IFI, especially those caused by molds, have minimal signs and cultures are often negative (except for a 60% probability of positive blood cultures in fusariosis). The detection of specific antibodies or circulating fungal antigens or fungal metabolites is being investigated to lead to early or preemptive diagnosis of IFI. Among the most promising are the *Candida* antigens and antibodies in combination, the *Aspergillus* galactomannan (GM) (a major constituent of *Aspergillus* cell wall detected in bronchoalveolar lavage [BAL] and blood and recently in cerebrospinal fluid) and the polymerase chain reaction (PCR) for *Aspergillus*.

The recent advent of an improved commercial ELISA for the detection of circulating GM has contributed to the diagnosis of IA in many hematology and transplant centers [68,69]. GM is a cell wall polysaccharide released by *Aspergillus* sp during growth. Its kinetics in tissues is not completely understood. The optimal threshold for positivity remains a matter of debate and measurements must be repeated consecutively on a twice- or thrice-a-week basis in patients with neutropenia. Decreasing the index cutoff for positivity to 0.5 increases its sensitivity (with minimal loss of specificity) and the duration of test positivity before diagnosis by clinical means [70]. Sensitivity is highest in patients who did not receive antifungal prophylaxis with mold-active agents (87.5%) [71]. A rabbit model demonstrated that the level of circulating antigen correlated with the tissue fungus burden and a quantifiable response to antifungal therapy [72].

A series of allogeneic stem cell transplant recipients were monitored prospectively, and the relationship between antigenemia and other diagnostic triggers for initiation of antifungal therapy was analyzed. Antigenemia preceded diagnosis on the basis of radiologic examination or *Aspergillus* isolation by 8 and 9 days in 80% and 88.8% of patients, respectively, and initiation of therapy in 83.3% of patients. Detection of GM was especially useful when patients were receiving steroid treatment or when coexisting conditions masked the diagnosis of IA. Prospective screening for GM allows earlier diagnosis of aspergillosis than do conventional diagnostic criteria [68]. Studies have shown a sensitivity range of 75% to 100%, a specificity of 80% to 98%, and a high NPV of about 95% (with a sensitivity of 81% and a specificity of 89% in the studies leading to its clearance by the Food and Drug Administration) [73]. Physicians still must be aware of the potential for false-positive and false-negative results; the test does not replace careful microbiologic and clinical evaluation. The following have been identified as causes related to false-positive results (false-positive reactivity has been reported from 5% in adults to 83% in neonates) [72]: treatment with amoxicillin-clavulanate or piperacillin-tazompactam [74], early after lung transplantation (first week) [75] or BMT (first 15–30 days) [76]; in neonates (because of the heavy colonization of the neonatal gut by the cross-reacting *Bifidobacterium* spp) [77]; several cross-reacting food components, such as milk, rice, pasta, sogia, canned vegetables, or food supplements rich in proteins [78]; and technical factors, such as specimen transportation or airborne contamination with cross-reacting fungi (*Penicillium* sp, *Paecilomyces variotii*, *Alternaria* spp, and so forth) [79]. Although not validated methodologically, GM detection in other body fluids (urine, BAL, cerebrospinal fluid) has been studied. BAL testing seems more promising (sensitivity, 85%–100%; positive and negative predictive value of 100%), especially when combined with PCR for *Aspergillus* or high-resolution CT of the thorax. Airway colonization may produce false-positive results [80]. In a recent meta-analysis of 27 studies (1996–2005), which included 4230 patients among which 210 with proved IA GM detection presented moderate accuracy (sensitivity 71%, specificity 89%) to detect aspergillosis. There was significant heterogeneity and the test was more useful in patients with hematologic malignancies or BMT compared with solid-organ transplant recipients (sensitivity only 22%, specificity 84%) [81]. Further studies assessing the impact of false-positives and of antifungal therapy are needed.

GM in blood, BAL, or cerebrospinal fluid has been incorporated as a mycologic criterion in the new definitions for probable invasive fungal disease (www.doctorfungus.org). Accordingly, in a recent study Maertens and colleagues [82] investigated the clinical use of GM serial detection, incorporating its values in an algorithm for empiric antifungal treatment in 117 episodes of FN. As result, they noticed a 78% reduction in antifungal use without any effect on overall response or survival. One case of zygomycosis was missed.

Another test currently under investigation for the early diagnosis of invasive fungal disease is (1,3) β-D-glucan, which represents a panfungal test, as being a component of the cell wall of a variety of fungi (*Candida* sp, *Aspergillus* sp, *Acremonium* sp, *Fusarium* sp, *Trichosporon* sp, *P neumocystis jirovecii*) except *Cryptococcus* sp and *Zygomycetes*. In the commercially available test a cutoff of 60 pg/mL corresponds to 97% sensitivity and 93% specificity in candidemic patients [83]. False-positive results are correlated with hemodialysis and the use of cellulose membranes, with immunoglobulin and intravenous albumin products, with exposure to glucan-containing gauze, with gram-positive bacteremia and serum, and with hemolysis; questions exist about colonization, mucositis, and the use of polysaccharide antitumor agents [84]. Odabasi and colleagues [83] studied 283 patients with acute myelogenous leukemia or myelodysplasia by twice weekly sampling during neutropenia. Among 2070 specimens and using 60 pg/mL as a cutoff, they found a sensitivity of 38% to 65%, a specificity of 90% to 100%, and a NPV of 85% to 100% in the detection of 16 proved, 4 probable, and 33 possible invasive fungal diseases (aspergillosis, candidiasis, fusariosis, trichosporosis), according to the number of serial positive specimens and the strength of diagnosis. Compared with GM detection, (1,3) β-D-glucan exhibits a comparable high NPV (96.3%) and when combined to GM it can be useful in detecting false-positives [85]. When detected in blood, BAL, or cerebrospinal fluid, it is considered as a mycologic criterion in the new definitions of invasive fungal disease (www.doctorfungus.org).

Detection of *Aspergillus* sp DNA by PCR has been studied in blood and BAL samples with variable sensitivity (50%–100%), high specificity (93%–100%), and high NPV (96%–99%) in diagnosing aspergillosis [86]. Variable sensitivity is attributed to differences in assay characteristics (no standard platform assay, different DNA extraction methodologies); the type of patients evaluated (sensitivity rises at higher risk); the certainty of diagnosis (proved versus possible); and the presence of antimold therapy (lower sensitivity) [86].

In a prospective study including 205 treatment episodes in 165 patients, PCR for *Aspergillus* was validated compared with GM and was found superior to GM with respect to sensitivity rates. In patients at high risk for IA, positive results for *Aspergillus* by PCR of blood samples are highly suggestive for IA and contribute to the diagnosis [87]. The role of prospective blood screening for IA by PCR was studied in 95 febrile episodes in neutropenic patients with acute leukemia or BMT, among which 13 cases of IA were considered. Sensitivity and NPV noted were 100%. PCR positivity preceded clinical diagnosis by 14 days and if eligibility for empiric antifungal treatment relied on positive PCR, a 37% reduction in antifungal use would have been noted [88]. In 201 adult patients with hematologic malignancies where 55 cases of IA caused by *Aspergillus fumigatus* or *A flavus* were diagnosed, Florent and colleagues [89] found a 63.6% sensitivity and a NPV of 89.7% of PCR. Combination with GM detection increased sensitivity to 83.3% and NPV to 97.6%. Finally, White and colleagues using the most promising real-time PCR in 176 patients with hematologic malignancies at risk and having as controls 28 critical care patients with evidence of invasive candidiasis, with greater than or equal to two serial positive specimens as positivity criterion, reports a 92.3% sensitivity, a 94.6% specificity, a good correlation with high-resolution CT of the thorax, and a 76.7% agreement with GM [90]. High sensitivity and specificity is also reported in BAL, although false-positives may be an issue [91]. PCR is not included in the criteria for the new definitions for invasive fungal disease because of the lack of a PCR system externally validated for blood, tissue, or BAL (www.doctorfungus.org).

Detection of *Candida* antigens and antibodies is still under study in the evaluation of the FN patient at risk of candidiasis. In a study, circulating candidal antigens (mannan and [1-3] glucan) and IgG subclass antibodies to these cell wall antigens were analyzed in a limited number (14) of ICU or surgical patients with systemic candidiasis and cancer or diabetes. The (1-3) glucan antigen and the two subclass antibodies seemed to be early specific markers for the laboratory diagnosis of candidiasis, whereas the kinetics of (1-3) glucan appearance in serum were found to assist in evaluating the therapeutic efficacy of antifungal treatment. Combined, they offered a 92% sensitivity and a 100% specificity and positive predictive value [92]. In another study, the Platelia Candida-specific antigen and antibody assays were used to test serial serum samples from seven neutropenic adult patients with hematologic malignancies who had developed systemic *Candida tropicalis* infections. High and persistent mannanemias were detected in all patients during the neutropenic period, confirming the value of the combined detection of mannanemia and antimannan antibodies in individuals at risk of candidemia [93]. Further studies are needed to confirm these preliminary results.

In vitro fungal susceptibility testing still needs to be clinically interpreted and in vivo correlated with clinical outcomes. More solid and meaningful data exist about in vitro sensitivity of *Candida* sp against fluconazole, itraconazole, and flucytosine, using the Clinical and Laboratory Standards Institute standardized and clinically relevant methodology. Breakpoints were developed from data derived from patients with oropharyngeal or esophageal candidiasis (for fluconazole and itraconazole) and from nonneutropenic patients with candidemia (for fluconazole only) [94]. Application and clinical relevancy of data in the setting of febrile neutropenic patients with cancer is still under study and indications exist that in vitro susceptibility is a factor affecting outcome [95]. Reliable and convincing interpretative breakpoints are not available for amphotericin B and meaningful data do not exist yet for other compounds (echinocandins, newer azoles), although minimal inhibitory concentration data are available [96]. Epidemiologic studies have shown that *Candida* sp, such as *C albicans*, *C tropicalis*, and *C parapsilosis*, should be considered susceptible to fluconazole. Concern exists about the sensitivity of *C glabrata*, for which resistance rates of 15% against fluconazole are reported [97]. Identification of *Candida* to species level is of paramount importance for antifungal treatment selection and sensitivity testing is indicated in case of lack of clinical response after treatment initiation or when a change from a parenteral agent to oral fluconazole is considered.

## Therapeutic considerations

### The empirical approach

Prompt administration of empirical antibiotic therapy is essential in patients with FN and FUO because underlying infections may progress rapidly. Selection of proper empiric antimicrobial therapy should primarily be influenced by the local epidemiology and drug susceptibility patterns of bacterial pathogens at a certain institution and exposure of the patient to previous antimicrobial therapy [6]. Initial empiric therapy is primarily directed against bacterial pathogens, because fungal, viral, or protozoan etiology is rarely the cause of infection initially [10]. The local epidemiologic data are subject to dynamic changes and are influenced by resistance patterns in the community and the use of chemoprophylaxis, and the type of chemotherapy.

In environments where prophylaxis is not widely used gram-negative pathogens tend to predominate [98]. If prophylaxis is extensively used with agents active against gram-negatives, gram-positives consist of more 65% of pathogens [99]. In two large trials including more than 1000 patients, prophylaxis was given to less than 25% of patients and gram-negatives remained the most isolates [99,100]. In two recent studies, the one using chemoprophylaxis in more than 90% of patients and the second using nonabsorbable colistin for gut decontamination, gram-positives consisted of 66% and 67% of isolates, respectively, with CNS predominating in the first and *Streptococcus* sp in the latter [101,102].

Regarding the type of chemotherapy, regimens intensively cytotoxic and damaging to the mucosa increase the presence of viridans streptococci, enterococci, and gram-negative pathogens [10]. The type of pathogens that prevail during certain periods must not rely on data extracted only from blood isolates [103]. Bacteremias are documented only in 25% of patients with FUO and neutropenia [103]. Infections at other sites are commonly caused by gram-negative pathogens or are polymicrobial, a pattern that is currently emerging in 23% and 31% of documented bacterial infections in patients with hematologic malignancies or solid tumors, respectively. In these polymicrobial infections, 80% of pathogens are gram-negatives and in 33% of cases pathogens include only gram-negatives [104]. If data from all sites of infection are pooled together, gram-positives, which for the last 15 years are mentioned to predominate in bacteremias of FN patients, prove to have a prevalence of less than 50% [103]. *Pseudomonas aeruginosa* rates are stable, being the second most common gram-negative pathogen, at least at MD Anderson Cancer Center (18%), following *Escherichia coli* (29%) and followed by *Klebsiella* sp (16%) [105]. It seems to be more prevalent in warmer climates [106]. The initial empiric antimicrobial regimen should include coverage against gram-negatives including *P aeruginosa*, as traditionally is the practice since 1971, taking into consideration local resistance patterns at each institution.

Today, a challenging issue is the emergence of drug resistance among nosocomial pathogens, compromising the efficacy of the initial empiric antimicrobial regimen. Resistance to methicillin among CNS is 70% to 90% and among *S aureus* more than 50%. Rates of VRE are greater than or equal to 30%, whereas 50% to 60% of *Streptococcus viridans* and *Streptococcus pneumoniae* are resistant to penicillin [103,107]. *S viridans* can be the cause of fulminant bacteremia associated with acute respiratory distress syndrome, renal failure, and rapid death [108]. VRE is reported as the cause of outbreaks of bacteremias in leukemic patients, associated with high mortality [98]. Unusual gram-positive pathogens intrinsically resistant to vancomycin are emerging as pathogens causing catheter-related bloodstream infections or other systemic infections (*Leuconostoc* sp, *Pediococcus* sp, *Lactobacillus* sp, *C orynebacterium jeikeium*). *P aeruginosa* resistant to ciprofloxacin is a fact in many institutions and nonfermenting, intrinsically drug-resistant bacteria are rising in incidence (*Acinetobacter* sp, *S tenotrophomonas maltophilia*, *Alcaligenes* sp, *P* non-*aeruginosa*). Extended-spectrum β-lactamase (ESBL) producing *E coli* and *Klebsiella pneumoniae*, along with *Enterobacter* sp, renders problematic the use of cephalosporins. Extensive use of carbapenems led to 15% to 30% rates of MDR *P aeruginosa* reported from different parts of the world, sensitive only to colistin, which because of suboptimal efficacy cannot probably be used as a single agent [109,110]. Anaerobes are rarely isolated in blood cultures of patients with FN (<5%) for reasons that are not clearly defined [107,111], although their presence should be suspected in perineal abscesses, periodontal infections, or neutropenic enterocolitis.

Empiric antimicrobial therapy must be adapted to local epidemiology data, according to the previously mentioned factors. Usually it consists of an antipseudomonal cephalosporin (ceftazidime if ESBL do not prevail), piperacillin-tazobactam, cefepime, or an antipseudomonal carbapenem (imipenem, meropenem), combined with an aminoglycoside [6]. The combination is used for spectrum extension and rapid pathogen killing and not for synergy purposes, which could not be proved in meta-analysis studies [112]. Aminoglycosides, as drugs exhibiting a dose-dependent pattern of pharmacokinetics and pharmacodynamics, can be safely and effectively used in a once-daily dose regimen [113]. It is essential that if bacteremia or pseudomonas infection is not proved, the aminoglycoside must be (at 72–96 hours) discontinued early [6]. Otherwise, monitoring of kidney function and drug levels is recommended.

Monotherapy with ceftazidime, cefepime, meropenem, and imipenem or piperacillin-tazobactam was found in several studies to be equally effective with the conventional combination of a β-lactam and an aminoglycoside [101,114–116]. In a recent meta-analysis of monotherapy in FN that included 33 randomized controlled studies, cefepime was associated with higher all-cause mortality at 30 days. Carbapenems entailed fewer treatment modifications but increased rates of pseudomembranous colitis. Ceftazidime, piperacillin-tazobactam, and carbapenems seemed suitable agents for monotherapy [117]. When ESBL-producing pathogens prevail, cephalosporins may be problematic as empiric treatment and antipseudomonal carbapenems remain as first choice, probably followed by piperacillin-tazobactam as an alternative. Aminoglycosides clearly are not suitable as monotherapy [118] and the use of quinolones is discouraged in institutions where they are used as prophylaxis, although data are scarce and contradictory [119]. No universal guideline can be applied. Clinicians should be alert about the pathogen predominating in their institution.

Patients with intermediate or high risk must be hospitalized and must receive intravenous antibiotics. Patients falling in the low-risk category, after 24 to 48 hours evaluation at the hospital can be either sent home on oral regimen, or be hospitalized until defervescence and sent home to complete therapy with an oral regimen. Extensively used oral regimen is the combination of ciprofloxacin plus amoxicillin-clavulanate. The newer quinolones (moxifloxacin) are under study with limited data about their potential use as monotherapy in low-risk patients treated as out-patients [120]. The decision to treat a low-risk patient on an outpatient basis should rely on prerequisites like patient able to understand the risk, to receive oral medication, to have a telephone, to be able to reach a hospital within 1 hour, to have help at home, and the ability to offer a 24-hour service 7 days a week [121].

## Addition of vancomycin to the initial empirical regimen

The increased predominance of gram-positive microorganisms in bacteremias of patients with FN during the last 15 years led to the increased use of vancomycin as part of the initial empiric antimicrobial regimen. Study V of the EORTC in 1990 showed that the nonincorporation of vancomycin in the initial regimen and its use only when indicated by the isolation of a gram-positive microorganism did not lead to increased morbidity and mortality rates, except in patients with *S viridans* bacteremia not receiving a carbapenem, piperacillin-tazobactam, or cefepime [122]. In another study, the addition of vancomycin to imipenem did not affect efficacy [123]. A study by the National Cancer Institute confirmed that the gram-positive pathogens are not quickly lethal [124]. A recent meta-analysis of randomized controlled trials comparing antibiotics with anti–gram-positive spectrum with control or placebo, in addition to the same baseline antibiotic regimen in both arms (which included 13 studies with 2392 participants in total), concluded that the use of glycopeptides can be safely deferred until the documentation of a resistant gram-positive infection. Empirical anti–gram-positive antibiotics were assessed for the initial treatment in 11 studies, and for persistent fever in two states. Glycopeptides were assessed in nine trials. No significant difference in all-cause mortality and overall failure was observed, whereas adverse events were significantly more common with the additional antibiotic, and nephrotoxicity was significantly more common with additional glycopeptides [125,126]. The IDSA in its latest guidelines and taking into consideration the emergence of VRE under the selective pressure of vancomycin, recommends the addition of vancomycin to the initial regimen (1) in patients with hemodynamic instability (threat of septic shock); (2) when signs of or a documented gram-positive infection is present (tunnel infection, soft tissue infection); and (3) when high rates of S viridans or MRSA infections are prevalent in the institution, especially if the patient is known to be colonized with MRSA [6]. Considerations exist in some physicians for patients with chemotherapy-related substantial mucosal damage and history of quinolone prophylaxis during the period of FN. Sudden spikes of temperature greater than 40°C may be predicted of streptococcal sepsis [6]. Ceftazidime in this case should be avoided as empiric treatment because it lacks streptococcal activity.

Vancomycin remains the most widely used glycopeptide. Teicoplanin, widely used in Europe, is not approved in the United States. It is administrated once daily, rarely causes red-man syndrome, and is less nephrotoxic. Drug fever and thrombocytopenia, however, should be a consideration. In vitro studies have shown strains of Staphylococcus haemolyticus to be resistant to teicoplanin, whereas vancomycin retains its activity against them. The activity of teicoplanin in patients with cancer has been proved in several open and comparative trials [127,128].

Linezolid, an oxazolidinone active against MDR gram-positive pathogens (MRSA, VRE), has not been evaluated as empiric therapy in FN. It was compared with vancomycin in a randomized, double-blind study of 488 febrile neutropenic cancer patients with suspected or proved gram-positive infection. Linezolid demonstrated efficacy and safety outcomes equivalent to those of vancomycin [129].

Quinupristin-dalfopristin, also active against VRE, awaits further studies for evaluation in neutropenic patients [6]. Daptomycin, a new lipoglycopeptide also active against MDR gram-positive pathogens, has been used in small case-series of neutropenic patients and needs further evaluation

[130]. A major disadvantage is that the drug is not suitable for lung infections because of inactivation by the lung surfactant.

## Treatment options in the era of multiresistant bacteria

Mostly as a consequence of the extensive overuse and misuse of antibiotics, infections caused by MDR bacteria represent a daily challenge for the physician and patients worldwide, an event that is already influential to the immunocompromised host [131].

The current particularly problematic MDR pathogens are *Acinetobacter baumannii, Enterobacteriaceae* that produce ESBLs, *P aeruginosa*, MRSA, and vancomycin-resistant *Enterococcus faecium* [132]. The permanent, although decreasing, predominance of MRSA is not a real problem regarding therapeutic options, because newer antimicrobial agents with potent antistaphylococcal and anti–vancomycin-resistant *E faecium* activity, such as linezolid and daptomycin are already in the market, whereas such agents as oritavancin, dalbavancin, and telavancin are still waiting a license [132,133]. It should be pointed out, however, that clinical experience in FN or in the bacteriologically proved neutropenic host infections, does not exist. On the contrary, any newer antibiotic active against the gram-negatives is still an illusion.

It is characteristic that the number and spectrum of β-lactamases have increased dramatically in past years [134,135]. As of March 2007, more than 459 β-lactamases have been reported, among which ESBLs jumped to 354.The latter enzymes, which prevail among *E coli* and *Klebsiella* spp, and which have a broad substrate hydrolyzing all known β-lactams, including the inhibitors, were identified in 51.9% of *K pneumoniae* isolates in Latin America; in 16.7%, 24.4%, and 58.7% in northern, southern, and eastern Europe, respectively; and in 12.3% in Northern America. The problem is augmented by the cross-resistance of ESBL-producing organisms with the aminoglycosides, the fluoroquinolones, and trimethoprim-sulphamethoxazole [133]. It is of great importance that, in patients with ESBL-producing *K pneumoniae*, the failure to treat with an antibacterial with false in vitro activity resulted in a mortality rate of 64%, compared with 14% when an active antimicrobial agent was given [136].

Regarding in particular *P aeruginosa* the presence of metallo-β-lactamases, which number 32, is extremely harmful because they hydrolyze, with the exception of aztreonam, all β-lactams including carbapenems [137]. The increasing resistance rates of *P aeruginosa* strains are a worldwide problem. In the United States, according to the Nosocomial Infections Surveillance System, 33% of *P aeruginosa* isolates were found to be resistant to ciprofloxacin, 22% to imipenem, and 30% to ceftazidime for an increase from the period 1997 to 2001 of 37%, 32%, and 22%, respectively [138]. Relevant figures for ICU isolates derived from Europe are even worse, because from 1990 until 1999, resistance to aminoglycosides reached 37% to

70%, to ceftazidime 57%, to piperacillin-tazobactam 53%, to ciprofloxacin 56%, and to imipenem 52% [136].

The search for agents active against ESBL-positive Enterobacteriaceae led to tigecycline, which has been on the market in the United States for the last 2 years and recently in several European countries [137]. Tigecycline is a new semisynthetic glycylcycline representing a modified minocycline demonstrating antimicrobial activity against a wide range of bacteria including MRSA, penicillin-resistant *S pneumoniae*, VRE, MDR *A baumannii*, ESBL-producing Enterobacteriaceae, and *S maltophilia* strains, and against several anaerobic species including *Bacteroides* [139–141]. Tigecycline is not active against *P aeruginosa*, whereas its bacteriostatic activity renders its in vivo activity questionable in FN because experience even in established infections of the neutropenic host is lacking.

The emergence of MDR gram-negative bacilli, in parallel with the lack of new antibiotics, led to the revival of polymyxins, an old class of cyclic polypeptide antibiotic that was discovered in 1947. Colistin, which is identical to polymyxin E, exists commercially in two forms: colistin sulfate as tablets or syrup for bowel decontamination and as powder used topically for treating skin infections, and colistin methanesulfonate also under the names of colistimethate sodium, pentasodium colistimethanesulphate, or colistin sulfonylmethate [142].

Colistin is not active against gram-positive cocci and against *Proteus*, *Providencia* spp, *Morganella morganii*, *Serratia* spp, *Vibrios*, *Burkholderia cepacia* complex, *B pseudomallei* and *Edwardsiella* spp, and against anaerobes. On the contrary, colistin is very active in vitro against *P aeruginosa*, *Aeromonas* spp, *Acinetobacter* spp, *S maltophilia*, *E coli*, and *Klebsiella* spp, including ESBL producers *Enterobacter* and *Citrobacter* spp [143]. It should be pointed out that determination of susceptibilities to colistin should be performed with the E-test.

In vitro interaction of colistin methanesulfonate with rifampin has been evaluated against panresistant *P aeruginosa* strains, including colistin. Synergy was found in 11.8% to 41.7% of strains depending on exposure time [144].

Colistin methanesulfonate is administered intravenously, intramuscularly, intrathecally, or by inhalation. Parenterally and in patients with normal renal function, colistin methanesulfonate is given in the United States at a dose of 2.5 to 5 mg/kg (31.250–62.500 IU/kg) per day divided into two to four equal doses (1 mg of colistin equals 12.500 IU). The Greek experience has proved, however, that a higher dose of 3,000,000 IU (2.4 mg/kg) every 8 hours is safe [142]. Both the intrathecal and the intraventricular dose are equal to 125,000 to 500,000 IU per day [18]. Colistin methanesulfonate necessitates dosage modification in case of renal dysfunction because it is excreted mainly by the kidney.

The most common and important adverse effects of colistin reported in the old literature are nephrotoxicity and neurotoxicity. In contrast to older information, however, recent data indicate that nephrotoxicity in ICU patients after colistin methanesulfonate administration is lower, ranging from 8% to 18.6% [145].

Recently, the effectiveness of colistin at a dose of 5 mg/kg/d divided into two to four daily doses was studied retrospectively in 95 cancer patients diagnosed with infections caused by MDR *P aeruginosa* treated either with colistin or at least one active antipseudomonal agent (a β-lactam antibiotic or a quinolone) [146]. Thirty-one patients had been treated with colistin and 64 had been treated with an antipseudomonal non–colistin-containing regimen (control group). Compared with the control group, patients in the colistin group were more likely to have had nosocomial infections (87% and 64%, respectively; $P = .02$). Among patients, 45% and 37% were neutropenic, respectively, whereas *Pseudomonas* infection or colonization within the prior year was reported in 42% versus 48%. No difference in the incidence of nephrotoxicity (23% versus 22%); clinical and microbiologic response (52% versus 31% and 48% versus 41%); relapse rate (10% versus 11%); and infection-related mortality (26% versus 17%) or overall mortality (61% versus 47%) was observed. It is of interest, however, that multiple logistic regression analysis showed that those patients treated with colistin were 2.9 times more likely than those in the control group to experience a clinical response to therapy ($P = .026$). In particular, colistin-treated patients who were infected with a MDR *P aeruginosa* strain resistant to all available antipseudomonal drugs had also higher clinical and microbiologic responses than the control group rendering colistin a useful or a preferred alternative therapy for MDR infections in cancer-neutropenic patients.

In addition to the previously mentioned series, successful therapeutic results have also been described in two neutropenic patients with serious *P aeruginosa* soft tissue infections given polymyxin B (1 mg/kg intravenously every 12 hours) plus rifampin (10 mg/kg intravenously every 12 hours) [147]. In FN, while awaiting culture results, particularly in hospital settings with predominant MDR *P aeruginosa*, by extrapolating the limited but promising therapeutic results, colistin could serve for the empirical coverage either alone or in combination with an antipseudomonal β-lactam; de-escalation, however, applied after culture results.

Finally, a new carbapenem, doripenem, with enhanced antipseudomonal activity should be mentioned. It is a parenteral compound that is in Phase III clinical trials with an antimicrobial spectrum similar to that of imipenem and meropenem and with intrinsic activity against *P aeruginosa* superior to older carbapenems [27]. This compound has bactericidal action and is stable against a wide variety of β-lactamases and dehydropeptidase I; it is administered without an inhibitor. Doripenem is active against *P aeruginosa* and retains activity against some imipenem-resistant *P aeruginosa* isolates, with $MIC_{90}$ values reaching 8 μg/mL, but like the older carbapenems is not active in the presence of VIM and IMP metallo-β-lactamases [148]. Pharmacokinetic parameters of doripenem resemble those of meropenem with a half-life of approximately 1 hour. Because of weak inhibition of γ-aminobutyric acid receptors, low convulsive potential has been reported [149].

In October 2005 the Food and Drug Administration granted fast tract designation for doripenem for the treatment of nosocomial pneumonia. There are six Phase III clinical trials currently underway, including hospital-acquired pneumonia and complicated urinary tract and intra-abdominal infections. Despite doripenem's promising properties, no experience in neutropenic cancer patients has yet been reported.

## Empiric antifungal therapy

During the first week of neutropenia, efforts to evaluate fever primarily focus on the search for a bacterial pathogen, because at this time point bacteria account for most infections during FN. With the administration of antibiotics and the prolongation of neutropenia the risk of fungal infection emerges. *Candida* spp and *Aspergillus* spp are the most common fungal pathogens encountered. *Candida* infections occur during the second or subsequent week of neutropenia and *Aspergillus* infection later, during the third and subsequent weeks of neutropenia [150]. Therapies that cause short-term neutropenia lasting less than a week do not meet the risk of fungal infection. BMT patients are the patients at highest risk because of prolonged and deep neutropenia and the presence of other factors compromising immunity (graft-versus-host disease, corticosteroids) [150].

*Candida* may be the cause of fungemia, acute or chronic disseminated, or single-organ disease. Non-albicans strains are emerging. Aspergillosis initially is a lung or sinuses disease, to disseminate in 30% of patients, causing primarily CNS disease with 90% mortality rate. *Aspergillus* resistant to amphotericin B, such as *A terreus* and *A flavus*, has also emerged as a pathogen. Numerous others fungi are emerging as opportunistic pathogens: *Fusarium* spp (sinopulmonary infection, skin lesions, fungemia), *Muror* spp (sinopulmonary or disseminate disease), *Scedosporuim* spp, *Acremonium*, *Trichosporon*, and *Alternaria*, among others. They tend to present as breakthrough infections because of resistance against many antifungals [151].

Reasons necessitating the administration of empirical antifungal therapy include the high rates of morbidity and mortality associated with fungal infections, the difficulty of diagnosing IFI early during the course of infection, and the ineffectiveness of treatment when it is delayed.

Empiric antifungal therapy has been shown quite early [152,153] to improve the patient's outcome. In the recent IDSA guidelines the introduction of antifungal therapy is recommended in neutropenic patients with FUO not responding to greater than or equal to 5 days of appropriate antimicrobial treatment. Decisions could be individualized. For example, the appearance of lung infiltrates on chest radiograph, suspicious mucosal skin lesions, or eye-sinuses inflammation should prompt at any time point the initiation of antifungal treatment. History of a documented IFI is an indication for the administration of antifungal therapy, as secondary prophylaxis, as soon as the patient is rendered neutropenic (and for the whole duration of neutropenia) [150]. Amphotericin B, its lipid formulations, and caspofungin has been shown to be effective equally as empiric antifungal therapy in the management of neutropenic FUO [154,155]. Voriconazole has proved to cause fewer breakthrough fungal infections, but failed to reach the noninferiority end point compared with liposomal amphotericin B in the empiric antifungal treatment of neutropenic FUO [155]. Its extensive use as treatment or prophylaxis in patients with cancer is accompanied by reports of an increase in invasive zygomycosis incidence at the same centers [156,157]. Voriconazole should be the treatment of choice when the suspicion of IA is strong.

The optimal duration of empirical antifungal treatment has not been clearly established. If the patient is afebrile and the neutrophil count has recovered ($>500$ cells/mm$^3$), treatment can be discontinued. If the patient is afebrile and stable but neutropenia persists, treatment can be stopped after 2 weeks of administration. In an unstable, febrile, neutropenic patient treatment should continue until fever and neutropenia resolves [151].

In the future, empiric antifungal therapy may be transformed to preemptive antifungal therapy, based on nonculture methods (GM, PCR) and risk stratification efforts [150].

## Treatment strategy during the febrile episode

First time-point for the evaluation of the initial, empiric antimicrobial treatment is after 72 hours of treatment have been completed (Figs. 1–3). Elting and colleagues found that the median time to clinical response in hospitalized patients with cancer is 5 to 7 days, whereas in low-risk patients defervescence may be achieved in only 2 days [158,159]. If the patient is afebrile after 72 hours and the episode was a FUO, in a low-risk stable patient without mucositis, treatment continues until at least 7 days of treatment have been completed, or it can also be stepped down to an oral regimen and the patient sent home. For some clinicians, resolution of neutropenia before treatment discontinuation may be preferable [6]. If a pathogen has been identified treatment can be modified but its discontinuation or change of a broad-spectrum therapy is not recommended because of the risk of breakthrough infections [160]. For unstable patients with mucositis and profound neutropenia, treatment should be continued for at least 2 weeks and for as long as the patient is unstable or neutropenia profound ($<100$ cells/mm$^3$) [6].

If FUO persists after 5 days, patients need to be reassessed for occult fungal infection; a bacterial site of infection; atypical opportunistic infections (viruses, mycobacteria); resistant organisms; suboptimal dosing of antibiotics; or noninfectious causes of fever (drug fever, underlying disease,

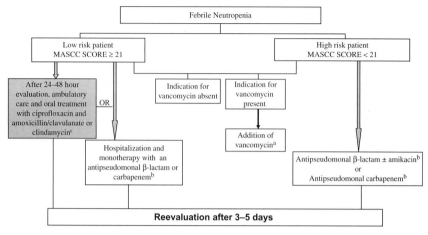

<sup>a</sup> Hemodynamic instability, MRSA carriage, clinical signs of gram-positive infection
<sup>b</sup> According to local epidemiology of resistance and previous antibiotic exposure
<sup>c</sup> Adequate home care is necessary, as is rapid access to the hospital

Fig. 1. Febrile neutropenia and initial empiric treatment. MRSA, methicillin-resistant *Staphylococcus aureus*.

graft-versus-host disease, phlebitis, transfusions, and so forth). Removal of central venous catheters without clear-cut evidence in case of FUO is not helpful [159]. If no other causes of persisting fever are revealed, the next step is the addition of empiric antifungal therapy, with or without

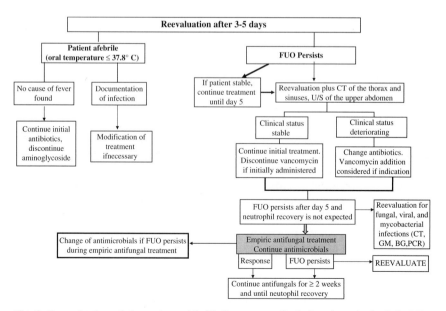

Fig. 2. Re-evaluation of the patient with febrile neutropenia during the episode. BG, β-D-glucan; CM, colistin methanesulfonate; PCR, polymerase chain reaction.

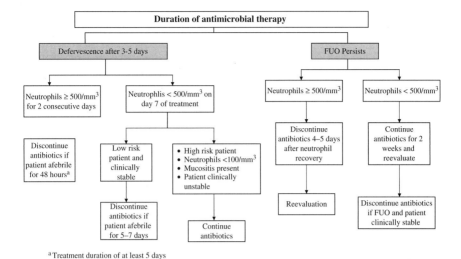

Fig. 3. Duration of antimicrobial treatment.

modification of the initial antimicrobial regimen [150]. Simultaneous continuation of the same antimicrobial regimen may be preferable for stable patients who are expected to have a rapid recovery of neutrophils. Modifying by changing from one broad-spectrum antibiotic to another (eg, from piperacillin-tazobactam to a carbapenem) may be done, epidemiology of resistance permitting, although is not supported by published evidence. Discontinuation of antimicrobials is not recommended [150]. Empirical addition of vancomycin is also not recommended because recent studies [126] have shown that the addition of a glycopeptide to persistently FN patients without evidence of a gram-positive infection is of no benefit. If a glycopeptide was a part of the initial regimen it should be discontinued in patients with persistent FUO or no isolation of a gram-positive pathogen [6]. If neutropenia and FUO persists, antimicrobial treatment should continue for at least 2 weeks [6]. If neutropenia resolves and FUO persists, the patient must be evaluated for chronic disseminated candidiasis or other fungal or viral diseases and antimicrobial treatment may be discontinued 5 days after neutrophil recovery [6].

Empirical antiviral therapy is not recommended at any time point [6]. It could be added in patients with oral lesions suggestive of herpes simplex virus infection (acyclovir); in patients with esophagitis (acyclovir or gancyclovir); or patients with viral respiratory disease indicative of respiratory syncytial virus (ribavirin), influenza, or parainfluenza infections (amantadine). Herpes simplex virus can cause serious morbidity in neutropenic patients after BMT, during the first month after transplantation, through systemic or CNS infection [161], although respiratory viruses can be the cause of serious pneumonias or interstitial pneumonitis leading to respiratory failure.

## Other considerations including prophylaxis

Colony-stimulating factors and granulocyte transfusions are not routinely recommended. They might be helpful in documented infections not responding to appropriate treatment; in severe uncontrolled fungal infections; and in specific life-threatening infections, such as pneumonia. They may be used as prophylaxis in high-risk patients with expected long duration of neutropenia ($\geq$ 10 days) and with a high risk of a febrile episode ($>$20%). The use of colony-stimulating factors in patients with FN caused by cancer chemotherapy does not affect overall mortality, but reduces the amount of time spent in hospital and the neutrophil recovery period, although it may permit the augmentation of the chemotherapy regimen. It is not clear whether colony-stimulating factors have an effect on infection-related mortality [162–165].

Routine use of antibacterial and antifungal prophylaxis for all patients with FN is not recommended in the latest versions of the IDSA's guidelines [6]. It may be beneficial in high-risk patients with expected prolonged neutropenia (eg, BMT patients) but it should be given for the shortest duration possible [6]. Two recent meta-analyses [166,167] published in 2005 come to doubt and reverse what during previous years was established as evidence-based knowledge by previous meta-analysis [168,169] and on which guidelines are based: that although oral antimicrobial prophylaxis reduces gram-negative and documented infections, the incidence of febrile episodes, and subsequently duration of hospitalization and days of antibiotics use, it does not decrease overall and infection-related mortality, contributing to emergence of resistance and accelerated toxicity. The first meta-analysis [166] (95 trials among which 52 were quinolone based) showed that in patients with hematologic malignancies, quinolone prophylaxis reduces overall and infectious-related mortality, whereas the second [167] (22 trials) confirmed also a reduction in infection-related mortality from bacterial causes in a mixed population of patients with solid tumors or hematologic malignancies receiving corimoxazole or a quinolone. Recently, two more trials explored the use of a newer quinolone, levofloxacin, as prophylaxis in afebrile neutropenic patients and in a setting of notable quinolone resistance. In the first randomized, double-blind, placebo-controlled trial levofloxacin prophylaxis was investigated in 1565 total afebrile neutropenic patients who received cytotoxic treatment for solid tumors and lymphomas. Febrile episodes and hospitalizations were reduced but the incidence of severe infections or mortality was not affected [170]. In the second study levofloxacin versus placebo was given in 760 cancer patients with neutropenia lasting more than 7 days. The risk for febrile episodes and the rate of microbiologically documented infections were lower but mortality was the same, whereas no differences were noted between patients with leukemia and solid tumors [171]. How this will affect future guidelines is not yet known, considering that studies have also shown that oral antimicrobials do not alter the protecting effect exhibited by growth factors in patients with chemotherapy-induced neutropenia.

Prophylaxis against *Pneumocystis carinii* pneumonia (cotrimoxazole) should be given to all patients at risk (BMT, lymphoma, or chronic lymphocytic leukemia patients, or patients treated with corticosteroids) [6]. Studies have shown the effective role of antifungal prophylaxis in the reduction of superficial infections and in the need for empirical antifungal treatment, in reduction of invasive fungal disease, and with a trend for reduced mortality [172]. The effective role of fluconazole against prevention of superficial infections and systemic candidiasis was shown in patients with BMT and for this population is recommended until engraftment in the dose of 400 mg/day [173]. Considerations exist today about the narrow spectrum of fluconazole and the increasing incidence of mold infections and infections caused by fluconazole-resistant *Candida* strains [174]. New data have been added by studies using intravenous itraconazole and liposomal amphotericin B as antifungal prophylaxis. New antifungal agents, such as the echinocandins and the new azoles, are available and may have a potential role in antifungal prophylaxis. Recently, two randomized, double-blind, placebo-controlled studies have been published, where posaconazole (a new broad-spectrum triazole) was used as antifungal prophylaxis. In the first study posaconazole was compared with oral fluconazole in 600 BMT patients with graft-versus-host disease [175]. Posaconazole was superior in preventing proved or probable IA. Overall mortality was the same but fungal-related mortality was lower in the posaconazole group [175]. In the second study in 304 patients with hematologic malignancies and neutropenia lasting more than 7 days, posaconazole prevented more effectively overall fungal infections and IA and improved survival [176]. A reappraisal of the issue of antifungal prophylaxis is pending. Future studies should also evaluate which strategy is more useful: prophylaxis or preemptive therapy [177].

High-efficiency particulate air filtration seems to be effective in reducing mold infections. It is recommended in BMT patients along with positive pressure rooms with more than 12 air exchanges per hour, especially in facilities undergoing construction and renovation. Debate exists about the effectiveness of laminal air flow systems, which are not generally recommended. All neutropenic patients require careful nursing including strict hygienic practices (gown, mask, sterile gloves); patient daily skin care and strict adherence to hand hygiene rules; avoidance of plants and flowers; and dietary restrictions that include raw vegetables and salads and everything that is not well cooked, boiled, or pasteurized. Visitors must be limited and without exposures to viral diseases. Adherence to such procedures is the first step toward effective prophylaxis [177,178].

Patients with FN, especially after BMT, who present with respiratory failure or hemodynamic instability may need the support of a medical ICU. Admission of cancer patients with serious medical complications to the ICU remains controversial primarily because of the high short-term mortality rates in these patients. A number of studies [179–183] have evaluated the risk factors for mortality and the differences between survivors and nonsurvivors among neutropenic patients admitted to the ICU. Admission to the ICU worsens the prognosis substantially but only the number of organ system failures at admission (expressed as number, SOFA or SAPS II score) and respiratory failure (requiring intubation and mechanical ventilation [19% survival rates in intubated patients versus 66% in nonintubated]), remains predictive of ICU mortality, which is comparable with severely ill noncancer patients (>47%). Septic shock among cancer patients admitted to the ICU has a mortality rate similar to that reported for mixed populations (>50%) and is particularly increased when hepatic or respiratory dysfunction develops. Neutropenia and its duration and underlying disease progression is not associated with a worse prognosis in terms of mortality, and general reluctance to admit cancer patients to an ICU does not seem to be justified. In the ICU, cerebrospinal fluid administration does not seem to alter the clinical outcome [184].

## Summary

FN is a syndrome commonly anticipated in patients receiving treatment for cancer. It presents with an incidence of 10% to 30% in patients treated for solid tumors and more than 80% in patients receiving aggressive treatment for hematologic malignancies. In 60% of cases and because of a blunted inflammatory reaction it presents as FUO and consists of a medical emergency because of the high mortality of occult gram-negative bacteremia that may be present. Its management for the last three decades includes the prompt administration of empiric antibacterial therapy, a tactic that resulted in a subsequent reduction in mortality. Challenges remain the administration of the most appropriate empiric treatment regimen adapted to evolving and changing epidemiology of infections in neutropenic patients and resistance rates; the development of markers of early diagnosis of severe bacterial or fungal infections; the risk stratification of patients; the establishment of targeted empiric (preemptive) antifungal therapy criteria; and the containment of antimicrobial resistance that compromises effective treatment efforts, through effective antibiotic policies and implementation of infection control measures, especially hand hygiene. The need for targeted antimicrobial or antifungal prophylaxis and supportive strategies, such as the use of growth factors, awaits further clarification.

## References

[1] Crawford J, Dale DC, Lyman GH. Chemotherapy-induced neutropenia: risks, consequences, and new directions for its management. Cancer 2004;100(2):228–37.
[2] Bodey GP, Buckley M, Sathe YS, et al. Quantitative relationships between circulating leukocytes and infection in patients with acute leukemia. Ann Intern Med 1966;64(2):328–40.

[3] Sickles EA, Greene WH, Wiernick PH. Clinical presentation of infection in granulocytopenic patients. Arch Intern Med 1975;135(5):715–9.

[4] Pizzo PA. Management of fever in patients with cancer and treatment induced neutropenia. N Engl J Med 1993;328(18):1323–32.

[5] Bodey GP. Unusual presentations of infection in neutropenic patients. Int J Antimicrob Agents 2000;16(2):93–5.

[6] Hughes WT, Armstrong D, Bodey GP, et al. 2002 guidelines for the use of antimicrobial agents in neutropenic patients with cancer. Clin Infect Dis 2002;34(6):730–51.

[7] Immunocompromized Host Society. The design, analysis and reporting of clinical trials on the empirical antibiotic management of the neutropenic patient. Report of a consensus panel. J Infect Dis 1990;161(3):397–401.

[8] Link H, Bohme A, Cornely OA, et al. Antimicrobial therapy of unexplained fever in neutropenic patients. Guidelines of the Infectious Diseases Working Party (AGIHO) of the German Society of Hematology and Oncology (DGHO) Study Group Interventional Therapy of Unexplained Fever. Ann Hematol 2003;82(Suppl 2):S105–17.

[9] Oude Nijhuis CS, Daenen SM, Vellenga E, et al. Fever and neutropenia in cancer patients: the diagnostic role of cytokines in risk assessment strategies. Crit Rev Oncol Hematol 2002; 44(2):163–74.

[10] Rolston KV. The Infectious Diseases Society of America 2002 guidelines for the use of antimicrobial agents in patients with cancer and neutropenia: salient features and comments. Clin Infect Dis 2004;39(Suppl 1):S44–8.

[11] Dompeling EC, Donnelly JP, Raemaekers JM, et al. Evolution of the clinical manifestations of infection during the course of febrile neutropenia in patients with malignancy. Infection 1998;26(6):349–54.

[12] Rolston KV. Prediction of neutropenia. Int J Antimicrob Agents 2000;16(2):113–5.

[13] National Cancer Institute. Common toxicity criteria, version 2.0. Available at: http://ctep. cancer.gov/forms/CTCv20_4-30-992.pdf. Accessed April 30, 1999.

[14] Dale DC, Guerry D IV, Wewerka JR, et al. Chronic neutropenia. Medicine (Baltimore) 1979;58(2):128–44.

[15] Rubin M, Hathorn JW, Pizzo PA. Controversies in the management of febrile neutropenic cancer patients. Cancer Invest 1988;6(2):167–84.

[16] Scott S. Identification of cancer patients at high risk of febrile neutropenia. Am J Health-Syst Pharm 2002;59(Suppl 4):S16–9.

[17] Silber JH, Fridman M, DiPaola RS, et al. First-cycle blood counts and subsequent neutropenia, dose reduction, or delay in early-stage breast cancer therapy. J Clin Oncol 1998; 16(7):2392–400.

[18] Chrischilles E, Link B, Scott S, et al. Factors associated with early termination of CHOP, and its association with overall survival among patients with intermediate-grade non-Hodgkin's lymphoma (NHL) [abstract 1539]. Proc Am Soc Clin Oncol 2002;21:385a.

[19] Giamarellou H, Antoniadou A. Infectious complications of febrile leukopenia. Infect Dis Clin North Am 2001;15(2):457–82.

[20] Viscoli C, Varnier O, Machetti M. Infections in patients with febrile neutropenia: epidemiology, microbiology, and risk stratification. Clin Infect Dis 2005;40(Suppl 4):S240–5.

[21] Dale DC, Crawford J, Lyman G. Chemotherapy-induced neutropenia and associated complications in randomized clinical trials: an evidence-based review [abstract 1638]. Proc Am Soc Clin Oncol 2001;20:410a.

[22] Gomez H, Hidalgo M, Casanova L, et al. Risk factors for treatment-related death in elderly patients with aggressive non-Hodgkin's lymphoma: results of a multivariate analysis. J Clin Oncol 1998;16(6):2065–9.

[23] Marty FM, Lee SJ, Fahey MM, et al. Infliximab use in patients with severe-graft- versus-host disease and other emerging risk factors of non-*Candida* invasive fungal infections in allogeneic hematopoietic stem cell transplant recipients: a cohort study. Blood 2003; 102(8):2768–76.

[24] Neth O, Turner MW, Klein NJ. Deficiency of mannose-binding lectin and burden of infection in children with malignancy: a prospective study. Lancet 2001;358(9282):614–8.

[25] Pizzo PA. Fever in immunocompromized patients. N Engl J Med 1999;341(12):893–900.

[26] Schimpff SC. Empiric antibiotic therapy for granulocytopenic cancer patients. Am J Med 1986;80(5c):13–20.

[27] Kreger BE, Craven DE, McCabe WR. Gram-negative bacteremia IV. Re-evaluation of clinical features and treatment in 612 patients. Am J Med 1980;68(3):344–55.

[28] Bodey GP, Jadeja L, Elting L. Pseudomonas bacteremia: retrospective analysis of 410 episodes. Arch Intern Med 1985;145(9):1621–9.

[29] Fergie JE, Schema SJ, Lott L, et al. *Pseudomonas aeruginosa* bacteremia in immunocompromised children: analysis of factors associated with a poor outcome. Clin Infect Dis 1994;18(3):390–4.

[30] Schimpff S, Satterlee W, Young V, et al. Empiric therapy with carbenicillin and gentamicin for febrile patients with cancer and granulocytopenia. N Engl J Med 1971;284(19):1061–5.

[31] Hann I, Viscoli C, Paesmans M, et al. A comparison of outcome from febrile neutropenic episodes in children compared with adults: results from four EORTC studies. International Antimicrobial Therapy Cooperative Group. (IATCG) of the European Organization for Research and Treatment of Cancer (EORTC). Br J Haematol 1997;99(3):580–8.

[32] Malik IA, Khan WA, Aziz Z, et al. Self-administered antibiotic therapy for chemotherapy-induced, low-risk febrile neutropenia in patients with nonhematologic neoplasms. Clin Infect Dis 1994;19(3):522–7.

[33] Klaassen RJ, Goodman TR, Pham B, et al. Low-risk prediction rule for pediatric oncology patients presenting with fever and neutropenia. J Clin Oncol 2000;18(5):1012–9.

[34] Vidal L, Paul M, Ben-Dor I, et al. Oral versus intravenous antibiotic treatment for febrile neutropenia in cancer patients. Cochrane Database Syst Rev 2004;18(4):CD003992.

[35] Talcott JA, Finberg R, Mayer RJ, et al. The medical course of cancer patients with fever and neutropenia: clinical identification of a low-risk subgroup at presentation. Arch Intern Med 1988;148(12):2561–8.

[36] Talcott JA, Siegel RD, Finberg R, et al. Risk assessment in cancer patients with fever and neutropenia: a prospective, two-center validation of a prediction rule. J Clin Oncol 1992;10(2):316–22.

[37] Kern WV, Cometta A, De Bock R, et al. Oral versus intravenous empirical antimicrobial therapy for fever in patients with granulocytopenia who are receiving cancer chemotherapy. International Antimicrobial Therapy Cooperative Group of the European Organization for Research and Treatment of Cancer. N Engl J Med 1999;341(5):312–8.

[38] Freifeld A, Marchigiani D, Walsh T, et al. A double-blind comparison of empirical oral and intravenous antibiotic therapy for low-risk febrile patients with neutropenia during cancer chemotherapy. N Engl J Med 1999;341(5):305–11.

[39] Klastersky J, Paesmans M, Rubenstein EB, et al. The multinational association for supportive care in cancer risk index: a multinational scoring system for identifying low-risk febrile neutropenic cancer patients. J Clin Oncol 2000;18(16):3038–51.

[40] Klastersky J. Management of fever in neutropenic patients with different risk of complications. Clin Infect Dis 2004;39(Suppl 1):S32–7.

[41] Uys A, Rapoport BL, Anderson R. Febrile neutropenia: a prospective study to validate the multinational association of supportive care of cancer (MASCC) risk-index score. Support Care Cancer 2004;12(8):555–60.

[42] Klastersky J, Paesmans M. Risk-adapted strategy for the management of febrile neutropenia in cancer patients. Support Care Cancer 2007;15:477–82.

[43] Meunier F. Infections in patients with acute leukemia and lymphoma. In: Mandel GL, Douglas JV, Bennett JE, editors. Principles and practice of infections diseases. 4th edition. Philadelphia: Churchill Livingstone Inc; 1995. p. 2675–86.

[44] Mermel LA, Farr BM, Sherertz RJ, et al. Guidelines for the management of intravascular catheter-related infection. Clin Infect Dis 2001;32(9):1249–72.

[45] Valdiviesco M, Gil-extremera B, Zornoza J, et al. Gram-negative bacillary pneumonia in the compromised host. Medicine (Baltimore) 1977;56(3):241–54.

[46] Heussel CP, Kauczor HU, Heussel GE, et al. Pneumonia in febrile neutropenic patients and in bone marrow and blood stem cell transplant recipients: use of high resolution computed tomography. J Clin Oncol 1999;17(3):796–805.

[47] Caillot D, Couaillier JF, Bernard A, et al. Increasing volume and changing characteristics of invasive pulmonary aspergillosis on sequential thoracic computed tomography scans in patients with neutropenia. J Clin Oncol 2001;19(1):253–9.

[48] Hauhhaard A, Ellis M, Ekelund L. Early chest radiography and CT in the diagnosis, management and outcome of invasive pulmonary aspergillosis. Acta Radiol 2002;43(3): 292–8.

[49] Gorschluter M, Mey U, Strehl J, et al. Neutropenic enterocolitis in adults: systematic analysis of evidence quality. Eur J Haematol 2005;75(1):1–13.

[50] Kontoyiannis DP, Luna MA, Samuels BI, et al. Hepatosplenic candidiasis. Infect Dis Clin North Am 2000;14(3):721–39.

[51] Sudhoff T, Giagonnidis A, Karthaus M. Evaluation of neutropenic fever: value of serum and plasma parameters in clinical practice. Chemotherapy 2000;46(2):77–85.

[52] Muller B, Becker KL, Schachinger H, et al. Calcitonin precursors are reliable markers of sepsis in a medical intensive care unit. Crit Care Med 2000;28(4):977–83.

[53] Tugrul S, Esen F, Celebi S, et al. Reliability of procalcitonin as a severity marker in critically ill patients with inflammatory response. Anaesth Intensive Care 2002;30(6):747–54.

[54] Jimeno A, Garia-Velasco A, del Val O, et al. Assessment of procalcitonin as a diagnostic and prognostic marker in patients with solid tumors and febrile neutropenia. Cancer 2004;100(11):2462–9.

[55] Giamarellos-Bourboulis EJ, Grecka P, Poulakou G, et al. Assessment of procalcitonin as a diagnostic marker of underlying infection in patients with febrile neutropenia. Clin Infect Dis 2001;32(12):1718–25.

[56] Ruokonen E, Nousiainen T, Pulkki K, et al. Procalcitonin concentrations in patients with neutropenic fever. Eur J Clin Microbiol Infect Dis 1999;18(4):283–5.

[57] Engel A, Steinbach G, Kern P, et al. Diagnostic value of procalcitonin serum levels in neutropenic patients with fever: comparison with interleukin-8. Scand J Infect Dis 1999;31(2): 185–9.

[58] Fleischhack G, Kambeck I, Cipic D, et al. Procalcitonin in paediatric cancer patients: its diagnostic relevance is superior to that of C-reactive protein, interleukin 6, interleukin 8, soluble interleukin 2 receptor and soluble tumour necrosis factor receptor II. Br J Haematol 2000;111(4):1093–102.

[59] Persson L, Engervall P, Magnuson A, et al. Use of inflammatory markers for early detection of bacteraemia in patients with febrile neutropenia. Scand J Infect Dis 2004;36(5):365–71.

[60] Ortega M, Rovira M, Filella X, et al. Prospective evaluation of procalcitonin in adults with febrile neutropenia after haematopoietic stem cell transplantation. Br J Haematol 2004; 126(3):372–6.

[61] Dornbusch HJ, Strenger V, Kerbl R, et al. Procalcitonin-a marker of invasive fungal infection? Support Care Cancer 2005;13(5):343–6.

[62] Schüttrumpf S, Binder L, Hagemann T, et al. Procalcitonin: a useful discriminator between febrile conditions of different origin in hemato-oncological patients? Ann Hematol 2003; 82(2):98–103.

[63] Persson L, Soderquist B, Engervall P. Assessment of systemic inflammation markers to differentiate a stable from a deteriorating clinical course in patients with febrile neutropenia. Eur J Haematol 2005;74(4):297–303.

[64] Arber C, Passweg JR, Fluckiger U, et al. C-reactive protein and fever in neutropenic patients. Scand J Infect Dis 2000;32(5):515–20.

[65] Yonemori K, Kanda Y, Yamamoto R, et al. Clinical value of serial measurement of serum C-reactive protein level in neutropenic patients. Leuk Lymphoma 2001;41(5-6):607–14.

[66] Manian FA. A prospective study of daily measurement of C-reactive protein in serum of adults with neutropenia. Clin Infect Dis 1995;21(1):114–21.

[67] Ortega M, Rovira M, Almela M, et al. Measurement of C-reactive protein in adults with febrile neutropenia after hematopoietic cell transplantation. Bone Marrow Transplant 2004;33(7):741–4.

[68] Maertens J, Van Eldere J, Verhaegen J, et al. Use of circulating galactomannan screening for early diagnosis of invasive aspergillosis in allogeneic stem cell transplant recipients. J Infect Dis 2002;186(9):1297–306.

[69] Viscoli C, Machetti M, Gazzola P. Aspergillus galactomannan antigen in the cerebrospinal fluid of bone marrow transplant recipients with probable cerebral aspergillosis. J Clin Microbiol 2002;40(4):1496–9.

[70] Maertens J, Theunissen K, Verbeken E, et al. Prospective clinical evaluation of lower cut-offs for galactomannan detection in adult neutropenic cancer patients and haematological stem cell transplant recipients. Br J Haematol 2004;126(6):852–60.

[71] Marr KA, Balajee SA, McLaughlin L, et al. Detection of galactomannan antigenemia by enzyme immunoassay for the diagnosis of invasive aspergillosis: variables that affect performance. J Infect Dis 2004;190(3):641–9.

[72] Mennink-Kersten MA, Donnelly JP, Verveij PE. Detection of circulating galactomannan for the diagnosis and management of invasive aspergillosis. Lancet Infect Dis 2004;4(6): 349–57.

[73] Wheat LJ. Rapid diagnosis of invasive aspergillosis by antigen detection. Transpl Infect Dis 2003;5(4):158–66.

[74] Mattei D, Rapezzi D, Mordini N, et al. False-positive *Aspergillus* galactomannan enzyme-linked immunosorbent assay results in vivo during amoxicillin-clavulanic acid treatment. J Clin Microbiol 2004;42(11):5362–3.

[75] Husain S, Kwak EJ, Obman A, et al. Prospective assessment of Platelia *Aspergillus* galactomannan antigen for the diagnosis of invasive aspergillosis in lung transplant recipients. Am J Transplant 2004 May;4(5):796–802.

[76] Blijlevens NM, Donnelly JP, Meis JF, et al. *Aspergillus* galactomannan antigen levels in allogeneic haematopoietic stem cell transplant recipients given total parenteral nutrition. Transpl Infect Dis 2002;4(2):64–5.

[77] Mennink-Kersten MA, Klont RR, Warris A, et al. Bifidobacterium lipoteichoic acid and false ELISA reactivity in *Aspergillus* antigen detection. Lancet 2004;363(9405):325–7.

[78] Pinel C, Fricker-Hidalgo H, Lebeau B, et al. Detection of circulating *Aspergillus fumigatus* galactomannan: value and limits of the Platelia test for diagnosing invasive aspergillosis. J Clin Microbiol 2003;41(5):2184–6.

[79] Swanink CM, Meis JF, Rijs AJ, et al. Specificity of a sandwich enzyme-linked immunosorbent assay for detecting *Aspergillus* galactomannan. J Clin Microbiol 1997;35(1):257–60.

[80] Klont RR, Mennink-Kersten MA, et al. Utility of *Aspergillus* antigen detection in specimens other than serum specimens. Clin Infect Dis 2004;39(10):1467–74.

[81] Pfeiffer CD, Fine JP, Safdar N. Diagnosis of invasive aspergillosis using a galactomannan assay: a meta-analysis. Clin Infect Dis 2006;42(10):1417–27.

[82] Maertens J, Theunissen K, Verhoef G, et al. Galactomannan and computed tomography-based preemptive antifungal therapy in neutropenic patients at high risk for invasive fungal infection: a prospective feasibility study. Clin Infect Dis 2005;41(9):1242–50.

[83] Odabasi Z, Mattiuzzi G, Estey E, et al. Beta-D-glucan as a diagnostic adjunct for invasive fungal infections: validation, cutoff development, and performance in patients with acute myelogenous leukemia and myelodysplastic syndrome. Clin Infect Dis 2004;39(2): 199–205.

[84] Pickering JW, Sant HW, Bowles CA, et al. Evaluation of a (1->3)-beta-D-glucan assay for diagnosis of invasive fungal infections. J Clin Microbiol 2005;43(12):5957–62.

[85] Pezos C, Pontoon J, Del Palacio A. Contribution of (1->3)-beta-D-glucan chromomeric assay to diagnosis and therapeutic monitoring of invasive aspergillosis in neutropenic adult

patients: a comparison with serial screening for circulating galactomannan. J Clin Microbiol 2005;43(1):299–305.

[86] Musher B, Fredrick's D, Leistering W, et al. *Aspergillus* galactomannan enzyme immunoassay and quantitative PCR for diagnosis of invasive aspergillosis with bronchoalveolar lavage fluid. J Clin Microbiol 2004;42(12):5517–22.

[87] Kapaau M, Kanda Y, Nanny Y, et al. Prospective comparison of the diagnostic potential of real-time PCR, double-sandwich enzyme-linked immunosorbent assay for galactomannan, and a (1–>3)-beta-D-glucan test in weekly screening for invasive aspergillosis in patients with hematological disorders. J Clin Microbiol 2004;42(6):2733–41.

[88] Holliday C, Hole R, Sorrell T, et al. Role of prospective screening of blood for invasive aspergillosis by polymerase chain reaction in febrile neutropenic recipients of haematopoietic stem cell transplants and patients with acute leukaemia. Br J Haematol 2005;132:478–86.

[89] Florent M, Katsahian S, Vekhoff A, et al. Prospective evaluation of a polymerase chain reaction-ELISA targeted to *Aspergillus fumigatus* and *Aspergillus flavus* for the early diagnosis of invasive aspergillosis in patients with hematological malignancies. J Infect Dis 2006; 193(5):741–7.

[90] White PL, Linton CJ, Perry MD, et al. The evolution and evaluation of a whole blood polymerase chain reaction assay for the detection of invasive aspergillosis in hematology patients in a routine clinical setting. Clin Infect Dis 2006;42(4):479–86.

[91] Buchheidt D, Baust C, Skladny H, et al. Clinical evaluation of a polymerase chain reaction assay to detect *Aspergillus* species in bronchoalveolar lavage samples of neutropenic patients. Br J Haematol 2002;116(4):803–11.

[92] Sendid B, Caillot D, Baccouch-Humbert B, et al. Contribution of the Platelia *Candida*-specific antibody and antigen tests to early diagnosis of systemic *Candida tropicalis* infection in neutropenic adults. J Clin Microbiol 2003;41(10):4551–8.

[93] Kondori N, Edebo L, Mattsby-Baltzer I. Circulating (1-3) glucan and immunoglobulin G subclass antibodies to *Candida albicans* cell wall antigens in patients with systemic candidiasis. Clin Diagn Lab Immunol 2004;11(2):344–50.

[94] Pappas PG, Rex JH, Sobel JD, et al. Guidelines for the treatment of candidiasis. Clin Infect Dis 2004;38(2):161–89.

[95] Antoniadou A, Torres HA, Lewis RE, et al. Candidemia in a tertiary care cancer center: in vitro susceptibility and its association with outcome of initial antifungal therapy. Medicine (Baltimore) 2003;82(5):309–21.

[96] Hospenthal DR, Murray CK, Rinaldi MG. The role of antifungal susceptibility testing in the therapy of candidiasis. Diagn Microbiol Infect Dis 2004;48(3):153–60.

[97] Pfaller MA, Diekema DJ. International Fungal Surveillance Participant Group. Twelve years of fluconazole in clinical practice: global trends in species distribution and fluconazole susceptibility of bloodstream isolates of *Candida*. Clin Microbiol Infect 2004;10(Suppl 1): 11–23.

[98] Ramphal R. Changes in the etiology of bacteremia in febrile neutropenic patients and the susceptibilities of the currently isolated pathogens. Clin Infect Dis 2004;39(Suppl 1):S25–31.

[99] Winston DJ, Lazarus HM, Beveridge RA, et al. Randomized, doubleblind, multicenter trial comparing clinafloxacin with imipenem as empirical monotherapy for febrile granulocytopenic patients. Clin Infect Dis 2001;32(3):381–90.

[100] Feld R, DePauw B, Berman S, et al. Meropenem versus ceftazidime in the treatment of cancer patients with febrile neutropenia: a randomized, double-blind trial. J Clin Oncol 2000; 18(21):3690–8.

[101] Del Favero A, Menichetti F, Martino P, et al. A multicenter, doubleblind, placebo-controlled trial comparing piperacillin-tazobactam with and without amikacin as empiric therapy for febrile neutropenia. Clin Infect Dis 2001;33(8):1295–301.

[102] Cordonnier C, Buzyn A, Leverger G, et al. Epidemiology and risk factors for gram-positive coccal infections in neutropenia: toward a more targeted antibiotic strategy. Clin Infect Dis 2003;36(2):149–58.

[103] Rolston KV. Challenges in the treatment of infections caused by gram-positive and gram-negative bacteria in patients with cancer and neutropenia. Clin Infect Dis 2005;40(Suppl 4): S246–52.

[104] Yadegarynia D, Tarrand J, Raad I, et al. Current spectrum of bacterial infections in patients with cancer. Clin Infect Dis 2003;37(8):1144–5.

[105] Rolston KV, Tarrand JJ. *Pseudomonas aeruginosa*: still a frequent pathogen in patients with cancer: 11-year experience at a comprehensive cancer center. Clin Infect Dis 1999;29(2): 463–4.

[106] Raje NS, Rao SR, Iyer RS, et al. Infection analysis in acute lymphoblastic leukaemia: a report of 499 consecutive episodes in India. Pediatr Hematol Oncol 1994;11(3): 271–80.

[107] Wisplinghoff H, Seifert H, Wenzel RP, et al. Current trends in the epidemiology of nosocomial blood stream infections in patients with haematological malignancies and sold neoplasms in hospitals in the United States. Clin Infect Dis 2003;36(9):1103–10.

[108] Tunkel AR, Sepkowitz KA. Infections caused by viridans streptococci in patients with neutropenia. Clin Infect Dis 2002;34(11):1524–9.

[109] Gales AC, Jones RN, Turnidge J, et al. Characterization of *Pseudomonas aeruginosa* isolates: occurrence rates, antimicrobial susceptibility patterns, and molecular typing in the global SENTRY Antimicrobial Surveillance Program, 1997–1999. Clin Infect Dis 2001; 32(Suppl 2):S146–55.

[110] Bell JM, Turnidge JD, Gales AC, et al. Prevalence of extended-spectrum beta-lactamase (ESBL)–producing clinical isolates in the Asia-Pacific region and South Africa: regional results from SENTRY Antimicrobial Surveillance Program (1998–99). Diagn Microbiol Infect Dis 2002;42(3):193–8.

[111] Fainstein V, Elting LS, Bodey GP. Bacteremia caused by non-sporulating anaerobes in cancer patients: a 12 year experience. Medicine (Baltimore) 1989;68(3):151–62.

[112] Paul M, Soares-weiser K, Leibovici L. β lactam monotherapy versus β lactam-aminoglycoside combination for fever with neutropenia: systematic review and meta-analysis. BMJ 2003;327(7399):1111–21.

[113] Aiken SK, Wetzstein GA. Once-daily aminoglycosides in patients with neutropenic fever. Oncol Pharm 2002;9(5):426–31.

[114] Pizzo PA, Hathorn JW, Himenez J, et al. A randomized trial comparing ceftazidime alone with combination antibiotic therapy in cancer patients with fever and neutropenia. N Engl J Med 1986;315(9):552–8.

[115] Yamamura D, Gucalp R, Carlisle P, et al. Open randomized study of cefepime versus piperacillin-gentamicin for treatment of febrile neutropenic cancer patients. Antimicrob Agents Chemother 1997;41(8):1704–8.

[116] Cometta A, Calandra T, Gaya H, et al. Monotherapy with meropenem versus combination therapy with ceftazidime plus amikacin as empiric therapy for fever in granulocytopenic patients with cancer. Antimicrob Agents Chemother 1996;40(5):1108–15.

[117] Paul M, Yahav D, Fraser A, et al. Empirical antibiotic monotherapy for febrile neutropenia: systematic review and meta-analysis of randomized controlled trials. J Antimicrob Chemother 2006;57(2):176–89.

[118] Bodey GP, Middleman E, Umsawadi T, et al. Infections in cancer patients: results with gentamycin sulfate therapy. Cancer 1972;29(6):1697–701.

[119] Giamarellou H, Bassaris HP, Petrikkos G, et al. Monotherapy with intravenous followed by oral high dose ciprofloxacin versus combination therapy with ceftazidime plus amikacin as initial empiric therapy for granulocytopenic patients with fever. Antimicrob Agents Chemother 2000;44(12):3264–71.

[120] Chamilos G, Bamias A, Efstathiou E, et al. Outpatient treatment of low-risk neutropenic fever in cancer patients using oral moxifloxacin. Cancer 2005;103(12):2629–35.

[121] Talcott JA. Out-patient management of febrile neutropenia. Int J Antimicrob Agents 2000; 16(2):169–71.

[122] European Organization for Research and Treatment of Cancer (EORTC) International Antimicrobial Therapy Cooperative Group, National Cancer Institute of Canada-Clinical Trials Group. Vancomycin added to empirical combination antibiotic therapy for fever in granulocytopenic cancer patients. J Infect Dis 1991;163(5):951–8.

[123] Raad II, Escalante C, Hachem RY, et al. Treatment of febrile neutropenic patients with cancer who require hospitalization: a prospective randomized study comparing imipenem and cefepime. Cancer 2003;98(5):1039–47.

[124] Rubin M, Hathorn JW, Marshall D, et al. Gram-positive infections and the use of vancomycin in 550 episodes of fever and neutropenia. Ann Intern Med 1988;108(1):30–5.

[125] Paul M, Borok S, Fraser A, et al. Empirical antibiotics against gram-positive infections for febrile neutropenia: systematic review and meta-analysis of randomized controlled trials. J Antimicrob Chemother 2005;55(4):436–44.

[126] Cometta A, Kern WV, De Bock R, et al. Vancomycin versus placebo for treating persistent fever in patients with neutropenic cancer receiving piperacillin-tazobactam monotherapy. Clin Infect Dis 2003;37(3):382–9.

[127] Erjavec Z, de Vries-Hospers HG, Laseur M, et al. A prospective, randomized, double-blinded, placebo-controlled trial of empirical teicoplanin in febrile neutropenia with persistent fever after imipenem monotherapy. J Antimicrob Chemother 2000;45(6):843–9.

[128] Menichetti F. The role of teicoplanin in the treatment of febrile neutropenia. J Chemother 2000;12(Suppl 5):S34–9.

[129] Jaksic B, Martinelli G, Perez-Oteyza J, et al. Efficacy and safety of linezolid compared with vancomycin in a randomized, double-blind study of febrile neutropenic patients with cancer. Clin Infect Dis 2006;42(5):597–607.

[130] Poutsiaka DD, Skiffington S, Miller KB, et al. Daptomycin in the treatment of vancomycin-resistant *Enterococcus faecium* bacteremia in neutropenic patients. J Infect 2007;54(6): 567–71.

[131] Badbugs, no drugs. Available at: www.idsociety.org. Accessed July 2004.

[132] Talbot GH, Bradley J, Edwards JE, et al. Bad bugs need drugs: an update on the development pipeline from the antimicrobial availability task force of the Infectious Diseases Society of America. Clin Infect Dis 2006;42(5):657–68.

[133] Giamarellou H. Multidrug resistance in gram-negative bacteria that produce extended-spectrum β-lactamases (ESBLs). Clin Microbiol Infect 2005;11(Suppl 4):1–16.

[134] Extended spectrum β-lactamases tables. Available at: www.lahey.org/studies/webt.htm. Accessed October 4, 2007.

[135] Turner PJ. Extended-spectrum β-lactamases. Clin Infect Dis 2005;41(Suppl 4):273–5.

[136] Paterson DL, Ko WC, Gottberg AV, et al. Antibiotic therapy for *Klebsiella pneumoniae* bacteremia: implications of production of extended spectrum β-lactamases. Clin Infect Dis 2004;39(1):31–7.

[137] Walsh TR, Toleman MA, Poirel L, et al. Metallo-β-lactamases: the quiet before the storm? Clin Microbiol Rev 2005;18(2):306–25.

[138] Nosocomial Infections Surveillance (NNIS) System report, data summary from January 1992 through June 2003, issued August 2003. Available at: www.cdc.gov/ncidod/dhqp/ pdf/nnis/2003NNISReport_AJIC.PDF.

[139] Souli M, Kontopidou FV, Koratzanis E, et al. In vitro activity of tigecycline against multiple-drug resistant, influencing pan-resistant, gram-negative and gram-positive clinical isolates from Greek hospitals. Antimicrob Agents Chemother 2006;50(9):3166–9.

[140] Ellis-Grosse EJ, Babinchak T, Dartois N, et al, for the Tigecycline 300 and 305 cSSSI Study Groups. The efficacy and safety of tigecycline in the treatment of skin and skin-structure infections: results of 2 double-blind phase 3 comparison studies with vancomycin/aztreonam. Clin Infect Dis 2005;41(Suppl 5):341–53.

[141] Bobinchak T, Ellis-Grosse E, Dartois N, et al, for the Tigecycline 301 and 306 Study Groups. The efficacy and safety of tigecycline for the treatment of complicated intra-abdominal infections: analysis of pooled clinical trial data. Clin Infect Dis 2005;41(Suppl 5):354–66.

[142] Falagas ME, Kasiakou SK. Colistin: the revival of polymyxins for the management of multi-drug resistant gram-negative bacterial infections. Clin Infect Dis 2005;40(9): 1333–41.

[143] Gales AC, Jones RN, Sader HS. Global assessment of the antimicrobial activity of polymyxin against 54731 clinical isolates of gram-negative bacilli: report from the SENTRY antimicrobial surveillance program(2001-2004). Clin Microbiol Infect 2006;12(4): 315–21.

[144] Giamarellos-Bourboulis EJ, Sambatakou H, Galani I, et al. In vitro interaction of colistin and rifampin on multidrug resistant *Pseudomonas aeruginosa*. J Chemother 2003;15(3): 235–8.

[145] Falagas ME, Fragoulis KN, Kasiakou SK, et al. Nephrotoxicity of intravenous colistin: a prospective evaluation. Int J Antimicrob Agents 2005;26(6):504–7.

[146] Hachem RY, Chemaly RF, Ahmar CA, et al. Colistin is effective in treatment of infections caused by multidrug-resistant *Pseudomonas aeruginosa* in cancer patients. Antimicrob Agents Chemother 2007;51(6):1905–11.

[147] Ostronoff M, Ostronoff F, Sucupira A, et al. Multidrug-resistant *Pseudomonas aeruginosa* infection in neutropenic patients successfully treated with a combination of polymyxin B and rifampin. Int J Infect Dis 2006;10:339–40.

[148] Jones RN, Sader HS, Fritsche T. Comparative activity of doripenem and three other carbapenems tested against gram-negative bacilli with various β-lactamase resistance mechanisms. Diagn Microbiol Infect Dis 2005;52(1):71–4.

[149] Horiuchi M, Kimura M, Tokumura M, et al. Absence of convulsive liability of doripenem, a new carbapenem antibiotic, in comparison with β-lactam antibiotics. Toxicology 2006; 222(1–2):114–24.

[150] Wingard JR. Empirical antifungal therapy in treating febrile neutropenic patients. Clin Infect Dis 2004;39(Suppl 1):S38–43.

[151] Sipsas NV, Bodey GP, Kontoyiannis DP, et al. Perspectives for the management of febrile neutropenic patients with cancer in the 21st century. Cancer 2005;103(6):1103–13.

[152] Pizzo PA, Robichaud KJ, Gill FA, et al. Empiric antibiotic and antifungal therapy for cancer patients with prolonged fever and granulocytopenia. Am J Med 1982;72(1):101–11.

[153] EORTC International Antimicrobial Therapy Cooperative Group. Empiric antifungal therapy in febrile granulocytopenic patients. Am J Med 1989;86(6 Pt 1):668–72.

[154] Walsh TJ, Finberg RW, Arndt C, et al. Liposomal amphotericin B for empirical therapy in patients with persistent fever and neutropenia. National Institute of Allergy and Infectious Diseases Mycoses Study Group. N Engl J Med 1999;340(10):764–71.

[155] Walsh TJ, Teppler H, Donowitz GR, et al. Caspofungin versus liposomal amphotericin B for empirical antifungal therapy in patients with persistent fever and neutropenia. N Engl J Med 2004;351(14):1391–402.

[156] Walsh TJ, Pappas P, Winston DJ, et al. Voriconazole compared with liposomal amphotericin B for empirical antifungal therapy in patients with neutropenia and persistent fever. N Engl J Med 2002;346(4):225–34.

[157] Vigourouz S, Morin O, Moreau P, et al. Zygomycosis after prolonged use of voriconazole in immunocompromised patients with hematologic disease: attention required. Clin Infect Dis 2005;40(4):e35–7.

[158] Chamilos G, Marom EM, Lewis RE, et al. Predictors of pulmonary zygomycosis versus invasive pulmonary aspergillosis in patients with cancer. Clin Infect Dis 2005;41(1):60–6.

[159] Elting LS, Rubenstein EB, Rolston K, et al. Time to clinical response: an outcome of antibiotic therapy of febrile neutropenia with implications for quality and cost of care. J Clin Oncol 2000;18(21):3699–706.

[160] Corey L, Boeckh M. Persistent fever in patients with neutropenia. N Engl J Med 2002; 346(4):222–4.

[161] Kern WV. Modifications of therapy. Int J Antimicrob Agents 2000;16(2):139–41.

[162] Leather HL, Wingard JR. Infections following hematopoietic stem cell transplantation. Infect Dis Clin North Am 2001;15(2):483–520.

[163] Clark OA, Lyman G, Castro AA, et al. Colony stimulating factors for chemotherapy induced febrile neutropenia. Cochrane Database Syst Rev 2003;(3):CD003039.

[164] Cheng AC, Stephens DP, Curie BJ. Granulocyte-colony stimulating factor (G-CSF) as an adjunct to antibiotics in the treatment of pneumonia in adults. Cochrane Database Syst Rev 2004;(3):CD004400.

[165] Smith TJ, Khatcharessian J, Lyman GH, et al. 2006 update of recommendations for the use of white blood cell growth factors: an evidence based clinical practice guideline. J Clin Oncol 2006;24(19):3187–205.

[166] Gafter-Gvilli A, Fraser A, Paul M, et al. Meta-analysis: antibiotic prophylaxis reduces mortality in neutropenic patients. Ann Intern Med 2005;142(12 Pt 1):979–95.

[167] van de Wetering MD, de Witte MA, Kremer LCM, et al. Efficacy of oral prophylactic antibiotics in neutropenic afebrile oncology patients: a systematic review of randomised controlled trials. Eur J Cancer 2005;41(10):1372–82.

[168] Engels EA, Lau J, Barza M, et al. Efficacy of quinolone prophylaxis in neutropenic cancer patients: a meta-analysis. J Clin Oncol 1998;16(3):1179–87.

[169] Cruciani M, Rampazzor R, Malena M, et al. Prophylaxis with fluoroquinolones for bacterial infections in neutropenic patients: a meta-analysis. Clin Infect Dis 1996;23(4): 795–805.

[170] Cullen M, Steven N, Billingham L, et al. Antibacterial prophylaxis after chemotherapy for solid tumors and lymphomas. N Engl J Med 2005;353:988–98.

[171] Bucaneve G, Micozzi A, Menichetti F, et al. Levofloxacin to prevent bacterial infection in patients with cancer and neutropenia. N Engl J Med 2005;353:977–87.

[172] Gotzsche PC, Johansen HK. Routine versus selective antifungal administration for control of fungal infections in patients with cancer. Cochrane Database Syst Rev 2002;(2):CD000026.

[173] Goodman JL, Winston DJ, Greenfield RA, et al. A controlled trial of fluconazole to prevent fungal infections in patients undergoing bone marrow transplantation. N Engl J Med 1992; 326(13):845–51.

[174] Kanda Y, Yamamoto R, Chizuka A, et al. Prophylactic action of oral fluconazole against fungal infection in neutropenic patients: a meta-analysis of 16 randomized, controlled trials. Cancer 2000;89(7):1611–25.

[175] Ullmann AJ, Lipton JH, Vesole DH, et al. Posaconazole or fluconazole for prophylaxis in severe graft-versus-host disease. N Engl J Med 2007;356:335–47.

[176] Cornely OA, Maertens J, Winston DJ, et al. Posaconazole vs. fluconazole or itraconazole prophylaxis in patients with neutropenia. N Engl J Med 2007;356:348–59.

[177] Ascioglou S, de Pauw BE, Meis J. Prophylaxis and treatment of fungal infections associated with haematological malignancies. Int J Antimicrob Agents 2000;15(3):159–68.

[178] Dykewicz CA. Hospital infection control in haematopoietic stem cell transplant recipients. Emerg Infect Dis 2001;7(2):263–7.

[179] Owczuk R, Wujtewicz MA, Sawicka W, et al. Patients with haematological malignancies requiring invasive mechanical ventilation: differences between survivors and non-survivors in intensive care unit. Support Care Cancer 2005;13(5):332–8.

[180] Blot F, Guiguet M, Nitenberg G, et al. Prognostic factors for neutropenic patients in an intensive care unit: respective roles of underlying malignancies and acute organ failures. Eur J Cancer 1997;33(7):1031–7.

[181] Staudinger T, Stoiser B, Mullner M. Outcome and prognostic factors in critically ill cancer patients admitted to the intensive care unit. Crit Care Med 2000;28(5):1322–8.

[182] Price KJ, Thall PF, Susannah KK, et al. Prognostic indicators for blood and marrow transplant patients admitted to an intensive care unit. Am J Respir Crit Care Med 1998;158(3): 876–84.

[183] Regazzoni CJ, Irrazabal C, Luna CM, et al. Cancer patients with septic shock: mortality predictors and neutropenia. Support Care Cancer 2004;12(12):833–9.
[184] Gruson D, Hilbert G, Vargas F. Impact of colony-stimulating factor therapy on clinical outcome and frequency rate of nosocomial infections in intensive care unit neutropenic patients. Crit Care Med 2000;28(9):3155–60.

ELSEVIER
SAUNDERS

INFECTIOUS
DISEASE CLINICS
OF NORTH AMERICA

Infect Dis Clin N Am 21 (2007) 1091–1113

# Fever of Unknown Origin in the Returning Traveler

Cristian Speil, MD, Adnan Mushtaq, MD,
Alys Adamski, BS, Nancy Khardori, MD, PhD*

*Division of Infectious Diseases, Department of Internal Medicine and Medical
Microbiology/Immunology, Southern Illinois School of Medicine, 701 North First Street,
PO Box 19636, Springfield, IL 62794–9636, USA*

Today's world has become a smaller place than it was even 10 years ago. With the larger availability of air travel to remote places, it has become possible for a person to go to virtually any place in the world in a matter of days. As the number of international travelers increases, so does the potential spread of infectious disease pathogens and their vectors [1]. The number of travelers with significant comorbidities and various degrees of immunosuppression is on the rise, thanks to the recent advances in biomedical sciences. HIV-infected individuals, for example, pose specific challenges both in terms of pretravel advice and management if and when they become ill returning travelers [2,3]. Other categories of immunosuppressed individuals, including solid organ transplant recipients, cancer patients, diabetics, and asplenic individuals, are at a higher risk of developing travel-related complications, both infectious and noninfectious [3,4].

The task of the physician caring for the ill returning traveler is not an easy one, because many of the diseases acquired during travel are not frequently encountered in the United States and diagnosing a tropical condition may be challenging for health care providers [5]. In this respect, however, the physician should be aware that in a febrile traveler, the chances for common diseases with a global distribution, like respiratory tract infections or urinary tract infections, are about as high as more exotic illnesses [6]. Noninfectious, travel-related diseases also should be considered. For example, air travelers on long flights are at risk for developing deep venous thrombosis of the lower extremities, which may present with fever [7].

---

* Corresponding author.
*E-mail address:* nkhardori@siumed.edu (N. Khardori).

0891-5520/07/$ - see front matter © 2007 Elsevier Inc. All rights reserved.
doi:10.1016/j.idc.2007.08.005
*id.theclinics.com*

Excellent books and reviews are available for the nonexpert physician who needs information on evaluating the febrile patient who has recently traveled overseas [5,8–13]. The World Health Organization and Centers for Disease Control and Prevention (CDC) Web sites are also useful and current sources of information. A list of some of the available resources on the World Wide Web is included in Box 1.

In evaluating the ill traveler, the highest priority should be given to diseases that are potentially fatal or are highly transmissible (and a potential public health risk) [5]. The threat of bioterrorism is on the rise with the current geopolitical situation and many of the potential bioterrorism class A and B agents cause natural diseases that may be acquired during travel (eg, viral hemorrhagic fevers or epidemic typhus) [14]. Common causes of fever in travelers, such as falciparum malaria, are potentially lethal unless treated early, and their diagnosis and presumptive management should be pursued aggressively if any suspicion exists. In a recent study from the Geo-Sentinel Surveillance Network, malaria was the leading cause of death among returning travelers with fever [15].

Travelers are a heterogeneous group from an epidemiologic standpoint, each category with its own specific risks [16]. For example, the extreme or adventure traveler or the immigrant visiting friends and relatives have different

---

**Box 1. International health references (free World Wide Web–based resources)**

- CDC Health Topics A-Z: www.cdc.gov
- CDC, general travel information: http://www.cdc.gov/travel/
- CDC, Health Information for International Travel 2008 (Yellow Book): http://wwwn.cdc.gov/travel/contentYellowBook.aspx
- CDC Morbidity and Mortality Weekly Report: http://www.cdc.gov/mmwr/about.html
- World Health Organization Health topics A-Z: http://www.who.int/topics/en/
- WHO Global Malaria Program, information about malaria: http://www.who.int/malaria/
- Global Monitoring Emerging Infectious Diseases (Promed): http://www.promedmail.org
- The International Society of Travel Medicine (ISTM) Web site, which includes a worldwide travel clinic directory: http://www.istm.org/
- GeoSentinel (the global surveillance network of the ISTM and CDC): http://www.istm.org/geosentinel/main.html
- European Network on Imported Infectious Disease Surveillance (TropNetEurop): http://www.tropnet.net/

risks and exposures, compared with the casual tourist or businessperson [17,18]. Fever in a United States–born tourist is unlikely to be caused by tuberculosis, but this is not the case in an immigrant from a country where the disease is endemic. Sometimes a puzzling situation may occur, where a non–United States traveler returning to his or her country of origin has fever as a result of an infection endemic in the United States. The authors recently managed a patient of Pakistani origin who returned to the United States with fever after spending a few weeks in her home country and was eventually diagnosed with disseminated histoplasmosis, which she likely acquired during her previous stay in central Illinois. Travel-related illnesses are largely associated with international travel. Domestic travel between various regions of the United States, however, may lead to acquisition of infectious agents endemic to that area; if they present at a later time, when the travel is already forgotten, the diagnosis may be delayed or not even considered.

## Causes of fever in travelers

One must keep in mind that the chances of fever being caused by a travel-related, tropical illness are not much higher than being caused by more mundane diseases that are an important worldwide cause of fever [6]. From a clinical and epidemiologic perspective, it is useful to group the patients presenting with fever in two broad categories: those presenting with a systemic febrile illness; and those with fever and focal symptoms, such as respiratory symptoms, diarrhea, or dermatologic conditions [15,19,20].

Large epidemiologic studies show that malaria is the leading cause of systemic febrile illness in travelers to the developing world and should be ruled out in any patient with fever returning from a tropical country [15,19]. Malaria was also the most common cause of hospital admissions in ill travelers in several studies from Europe, Australia, and Israel [21–25]. Dengue is the second most common cause of fever in travelers, being encountered more frequently than malaria in travelers to any developing region of the world except for sub-Saharan Africa and Central America [19]. Travelers to sub-Saharan and southern Africa are also at risk for tick-borne rickettsial infections, particularly African tick-bite fever [15,19]. Enteric fever caused by infection with *Salmonella enterica* serotype *typhi* or *paratyphi* is an important cause of fever in south central Asia, being as frequent as dengue and malaria in this region. Typhoid fever caused by *S typhi* is the most common cause of vaccine-preventable illness, with more than 70% occurring in south central and southeast Asia [15]. In the same study, the rare causes of systemic febrile illness were leptospirosis, amoebic liver abscess, viral meningitis, and relapsing fever.

Respiratory infections including influenza, diarrheal diseases, and urinary tract infections are, as a group, among the most common causes of fever in travelers [15,21,26]; the associated symptoms (cough, sore throat, diarrhea, urinary frequency, and so forth) should help in making the diagnosis.

## Approach to the patient

In evaluating the febrile traveler, the first priority is to exclude treatable diseases with high potential of causing severe disease and death, such as falciparum malaria and any infections that are a threat to public health, like tuberculosis and viral hemorrhagic fevers [9]. A differential list should be constructed based on history including travel history, physical examination, and pertinent laboratory data; as in the nontraveler, they should be viewed as interactive components, rather than treated sequentially. For example, signs and symptoms determine what laboratory test should be sought; reversely, physical findings or laboratory abnormalities may put the history in a different perspective and prompt further questioning [5].

### Travel history

Taking a good history is essential in trying to make a correct diagnosis in a traveler with fever. The travel history should include destination; type of activity and exposures; duration of travel; onset of symptoms in relation to travel; and immunization status, including pretravel vaccines and chemoprophylaxis.

### Destination

The travel history starts with areas visited, including such details as type of accommodation and urban versus rural environment. Destination is one of the strongest diagnostic predictors for tropical diseases [27]. Specific diseases are limited to or are more prevalent in certain locations, even within the same country. Tourists who stay in large cities are less exposed to insect and animal vectors or contaminated water than travelers to rural or remote areas. Malaria risk for a month of travel without chemoprophylaxis varies widely according to the destination; it is 1:5 in Oceania, 1:50 in Africa, 1:250 in south Asia, 1:2500 in southeast Asia, 1:5,000 in South America, and 1:10,000 in Mexico and Central America [28]. Malaria in sub-Saharan Africa is more likely to be caused by *Plasmodium falciparum* in contrast to the Pacific region, Central America, Mexico, and the Caribbean (with the exception of Haiti), where *Plasmodium vivax* is more prevalent [8,21].

Mosquito-borne diseases are usually not encountered at higher altitudes even in countries where they are endemic [26]. For example, in Peru, malaria is encountered in the low elevation jungle areas but not in the capital, Lima, or in the highland region [29].

### Activity and type of exposure

This includes purpose of travel and exposure history, including sexual encounters, eating and drinking places, recreational activities like spelunking, hobbies, and so forth. The usual tourist or the business traveler is less likely to be exposed to disease vectors or contaminated food or water; however, they still may engage in high-risk activities, such as unprotected sex [26]. Missionaries and health care personnel are at higher risk for contracting diseases that require prolonged or closer exposure, like tuberculosis [26]. The extreme or adventure traveler that goes to remote destinations and engages in high-risk activities is at higher risk for leptospirosis and rickettsial diseases [17].

People who are visiting friends or relatives are a heterogeneous category that deserves special consideration. They are immigrants from developing countries to the United States or they are Unites States–born children and they account for a significant proportion of international travelers [20,30]. They are at a higher risk for travel-related illnesses, because they are prone to stay for longer periods, in a rural environment, and have more exposure to the local population and contaminated food and water [10,20,30,31]. They are also less likely to seek pretravel advice and take prophylactic measures and more likely to have vaccine-preventable diseases than other categories of travelers [15]. A recent study that analyzed data from the GeoSentinel Surveillance Network found that immigrants going to their home countries to visit friends and relatives had higher risk of malaria and other significant infections and a higher rate of hospital admissions compared with tourist travelers [20].

Potential exposure to various pathogens or their vectors may offer important clues when correlated with the clinical presentation. Exposure to mosquitoes, ticks, animals, fresh water, raw or undercooked food, unpasteurized milk, or body fluids are all important in transmission of infectious agents and should be specifically addressed in the travel history. Unprotected sex puts the traveler at risk of acquiring various sexually transmitted diseases including HIV, depending on their prevalence in the region. Acute HIV syndrome, however, is a rare cause of fever in travelers [21]. Fresh water exposure is often seen in adventure travelers and may be associated with leptospirosis, schistosomiasis, and free-living amoebas [32,33]. Contact with contaminated food or water increases the risk for diseases with fecal-oral transmission, like viral hepatitis and typhoid fever. Exposure to ticks suggests rickettsial diseases, although often there is no recollection of a tick bite [34]. Brucellosis is the most common zoonosis worldwide and may be transmitted through ingestion of unpasteurized milk or cheese or undercooked meat from infected animals [35]. Animal bites or exposure to animals should arouse suspicion of rabies. Spelunking in bat-infested caves is associated with increased risk of histoplasmosis in endemic areas. An outbreak of pulmonary histoplasmosis was described in a group of Norwegian tourists who visited several caves in Guatemala and El Salvador [36].

## Duration of travel and time of onset

The length of travel and the time of onset are important in determining the risk of exposure and in approximating the incubation period. Although most infectious diseases have variable incubation periods, most are less than 30 days. Notable exceptions are vivax malaria, viral hepatitis, and tuberculosis [15]. Travelers with malaria caused by *P falciparum*, however, almost always become symptomatic within 1 month from their return [15,37]. Dengue has one of the shortest incubation periods, usually 4 to 8 days (range, 3–14 days), making it more likely to debut during travel [10,15,38].

*Pretravel immunization*

Pretravel immunizations are a major part of the travel history because it may help exclude certain diseases. The vaccines for hepatitis A and B and yellow fever are highly effective; if received, one can virtually rule them out [8,11]. In contrast, current vaccines against typhoid fever are only 50% to 80% effective [39]. Current malaria chemoprophylaxis drugs are 80% to 90% effective in preventing infection [40]. If infection occurs, however, they may alter the natural course of disease by prolonging the incubation period and decreasing symptoms severity and may prevent death from severe malaria [11,41].

*Host factors*

Associated factors that alter the immune response include comorbidities (diabetes mellitus, HIV infection, malignancies, asplenia, sickle cell disease); recent chemotherapy; immunosuppressive therapy in transplant recipients; and so forth. Travelers with HIV infection represent a particular challenge, especially those with a low CD4 count. In that case, not only are they at higher risk for more severe clinical infections, but the pretravel vaccines may not be as effective, especially if the CD4 count is less than 300 [42]. According to a recent study, less than half of HIV-infected travelers questioned received pretravel advice; they were also likely to be noncompliant with their antiretroviral medication and to have exposure to sharps and unprotected sexual encounters while traveling [2]. Travelers with HIV-AIDS are at particular risk for getting severe and persistent clinical infections with nontyphoidal *Salmonella* sp, which are a common cause of diarrhea and bacteremia in developing countries [3,43]. Malaria does not seem to be influenced or exacerbated by HIV infection, except for pregnant HIV patients, where there is increased risk for placental transfer and infant mortality [3,44]. *Penicillium marneffei* is a dimorphic fungus reported only from southeast Asia, where it has become a significant opportunistic infection in patients with AIDS [45]. In northern Thailand, penicilliosis is the third most common opportunistic infection, after tuberculosis, pneumocystis pneumonia, and cryptococcosis [45,46]. Visceral leishmaniasis, sometimes with atypical presentations, was also linked to advanced HIV disease and was considered an opportunistic infection in several studies from southern Europe [47,48].

## Presenting symptoms

Important symptoms include time of onset and characteristics of fever, and associated manifestations: diarrhea, rash, respiratory symptoms, localized pain, neurologic manifestations, or altered mentation.

Classical fever patterns have been described in the literature for many diseases but their use as a diagnostic tool is limited by errors of measurement; individual variations in normal body temperature; and intake of drugs that can interfere with fever, such as antipyretic, anti-inflammatory, or immunosuppressive agents [9,49]. For example, malaria can present as an intermittent or relapsing fever with daily or every 3 or 4 days temperature spike or as sustained fever (falciparum malaria) [49]. Dengue and yellow fever may be associated with a biphasic or saddle-back pattern, whereas mixed malaria infections and visceral leishmaniasis may cause the more specific pattern of double quotidian fever, with two temperature spikes in the same day [8,49–51].

Diarrhea is the most common travel-related symptom, but only 15% of patients with traveler's diarrhea have a fever [11]. Conversely, 15% of the patients with fever also had diarrhea in a recent study [15]. Invasive diarrhea caused by *Campylobacter jejuni*, *Shigella*, *Salmonella*, and *Yersinia* is more likely to be acute and cause fever [11].

## Physical examination

A thorough physical examination may offer important clues to the clinician. Key findings to consider are vital signs, including fever patterns; altered mentation; hemorrhagic manifestations; rash or other skin lesions; jaundice; organomegaly; and lymphadenopathy.

## Neurologic manifestations

Altered sensorium or neurologic manifestations associated with fever should be considered a medical emergency in any patient, with or without a history of travel. Specific considerations in travelers include meningococcal disease, malaria, rabies, tuberculosis, typhoid fever, and viral encephalidites [10].

Meningococcal disease presents as meningitis in 80% to 85% of the cases, with most cases occurring in epidemics in sub-Saharan Africa (meningitis belt) especially in the dry season [52]. The risk for the casual traveler is relatively low, although may increase with prolonged stay in confined spaces and close contact with the local population [52]. Invasive meningococcal disease has a high mortality even with early diagnosis and treatment.

## Organomegaly

Hepatomegaly is an important feature of visceral leishmaniasis (kala-azar) caused by *Leishmania donovani* and *Leishmania infantum-chagasi* in different parts of the world [53]. It is also seen in African sleeping sickness transmitted through the bite of infected tsetse fly, when it may be associated with a chancre at the site of inoculation [54]. Although rare in the United States, this disease should be considered in tourists returning with fever from trips to East Africa, particularly Tanzania [54,55].

Splenomegaly can be encountered in many diseases, including malaria, dengue, leptospirosis, typhus, viral hemorrhagic fevers, infectious mononucleosis syndromes, and HIV infection [8].

### Lymphadenopathy

Generalized lymphadenopathy is nonspecific but may be seen in acute HIV infection; mononucleosis-like syndromes; dengue fever; visceral leishmaniasis; and in disseminated histoplasmosis, blastomycosis, and coccidioidomycosis [8,11,56]. Regional lymphadenopathy close to the area of inoculation can be found in scrub typhus; tularemia; and plague (buboes) [8]. Local lymphadenopathy associated with an eschar at the site of inoculation was described in African tick-bite fever and other rickettsial infections [57]. Sexually transmitted diseases may present with tender inguinal adenopathy.

### Skin manifestations

Skin lesions and rash in travelers with and without associated fever are encountered in many tropical diseases and are well described in the literature [8,58]. Skin manifestations are often nonspecific; however, they are easily accessible and when associated with other signs and symptoms may provide important clues to the diagnosis and severity of illness.

Insect bites and cutaneous larva migrans are the most common causes of skin lesions overall in returning travelers, with cutaneous larva migrans being the most prevalent in the Caribbean region [19]. Bacterial skin infections and abscesses are the most common cause of skin lesions in travelers returning from sub-Saharan Africa [19].

Skin lesions can be maculopapular, petechial, nodular, or ulcerative. A black eschar may be seen in rickettsioses at the site of inoculation, usually accompanied by a generalized maculopapular, vesicular, or petechial rash [59,60].

A purpuric or petechial rash or other hemorrhagic manifestations could be the harbingers of a severe disease and deserve prompt and thorough evaluation. It may be encountered in invasive meningococcal disease and leptospirosis, in addition to dengue fever, viral hemorrhagic fevers, and some of the rickettsioses, most notably Rocky Mountain spotted fever, Mediterranean spotted fever, and epidemic typhus caused by *Rickettsia prowazeki* [11].

Multiple ulcerative lesions are typical for cutaneous leishmaniasis; a chancre at the site of inoculation can be seen in syphilis, chancroid, and African sleeping sickness [54].

A pink macular rash on the trunk ("rose spots") has been described in typhoid fever but it is rarely seen [61,62]. A diffuse maculopapular rash is mostly nonspecific and it may be encountered in many viral diseases, acute HIV syndrome, mononucleosis-like syndromes, most of the rickettsioses, secondary syphilis, drug reactions, and so forth. Schistosomal dermatitis appears shortly after exposure to contaminated fresh water and it manifests as a transient maculopapular and very pruritic eruption. A similar rash is caused by nonhuman, avian schistosomes with worldwide distribution, being commonly referred to as "swimmer or sea-bather's itch" [63–65]. Erythema limited to areas exposed to sun suggests a photosensitivity reaction, possibly related to medications including doxycycline.

Cutaneous larva migrans is the most common travel-related dermatologic illness in travelers to the Caribbean and it manifests as erythematous serpiginous pruritic lesions that reflect the migration of larvae. The infection is usually acquired by walking barefooted on contaminated sand and most lesions are seen on feet [63].

Jaundice associated with fever in a traveler is highly suggestive of viral hepatitis, more commonly type A or E [8]. Hepatitis A is still one of the most common vaccine- preventable diseases in travelers [66]. Other considerations are yellow fever, viral hemorrhagic fevers, dengue hemorrhagic fever, severe leptospirosis, and falciparum malaria [67,68].

*Laboratory evaluation*

All travelers presenting with fever should have a basic laboratory work-up that includes a complete blood count with differential, chemistry profile including liver function tests, urinalysis, and blood and urine cultures [69]. A chest radiograph should be done if respiratory symptoms are present. Thick and thin blood smears must be done in any febrile patient with a history of travel. One negative smear does not rule out malaria, however, and repeated smears should be performed 12 to 24 hours apart [70]. A stool specimen needs to be sent for fecal leukocytes, culture for enteric pathogens, ova, and parasites if diarrhea is present. Extra tubes of blood should be preserved in case paired serum samples are needed [11]. Laboratory abnormalities are often nonspecific, but corroborated with history and clinical data provide valuable tools in making a diagnosis.

Hematologic abnormalities are common in travel-related illnesses; leukocytosis with neutrophilia is usually seen in bacterial infections; leukopenia can be seen in typhoid fever, rickettsiae, and many viral diseases; atypical lymphocytes are a feature of infectious mononucleosis and have been described in malaria [71]; and thrombocytopenia is very frequent, seen in malaria, dengue fever, rickettsial diseases, viral hemorrhagic fevers, typhoid fever, and others [72]. Although anemia is also very common, hemoconcentration may suggest dengue fever [73]. Eosinophilia indicates a parasitic infection or a drug reaction rather than a bacterial infection [26]; significant eosinophilia increases the likelihood of a helminthic infection [74]. In a patient with headache, meningeal signs and paresthesias, and peripheral and cerebrospinal fluid eosinophilia is suggestive of eosinophilic meningitis most commonly caused by *Angiostrongylus cantonensis* [75]. Hypoglycemia is a feature of severe malaria [76,77]. Abnormal liver function tests are seen in various degrees and patterns in viral hepatitis, dengue fever, malaria, typhoid fever, many rickettsial and viral diseases, and in leptospirosis [77–81].

## Select specific diseases

### Malaria

Malaria is a major cause of morbidity and mortality worldwide and is the most common cause of fever and hospital admissions in the returning traveler [15,19,21–25]. It is estimated that 350 to 500 million cases occur annually, with 60% of all cases and 80% of all deaths in sub-Saharan Africa [82]. In the United States, about 1200 cases are seen every year [37,83].

Malaria is caused by intraerythrocytic protozoa of genus *Plasmodium* and transmitted to humans by the bite of infected female Anopheles mosquitoes. There are four species involved in human infections: *P falciparum*, *P vivax*, *P ovale*, and *P malariae*. *P falciparum* is the most common species in Africa, Haiti, and the Dominican Republic [84]. *P vivax* is rare in Africa and predominant in Central and South America. In Asia and Oceania, *P vivax* is more common, with *P falciparum* causing about one third of the cases [82]. *P malariae* is encountered in the same areas with *P falciparum* and *P ovale* is mostly seen in Africa, but their prevalence is lower [84].

Most cases of malaria imported in the United States involve *P falciparum*, seconded by *P vivax*, and most of cases of malaria in returning travelers are contracted in Africa, particularly West Africa [37,83]. *P falciparum* causes the most severe form of malaria and it was responsible for all the malaria deaths in the United States in 2005 [83]. Falciparum malaria has a shorter incubation period and most travelers become ill within 30 days after return or even during travel, whereas malaria caused by *P vivax* may have a later onset, with only 40% of the cases becoming symptomatic within 1 month from return [85]. Travelers without immunity resulting from previous exposures (eg, the United States–born children of immigrants) are at higher risk for severe disease [28]. Clinical manifestations are nonspecific, but fever with or without chills is present in most patients. Other symptoms at presentation may be nausea and vomiting, abdominal pain, diarrhea, chest pain, headaches, dizziness, myalgias, and arthralgias [86,87]. Physical findings vary with the severity of disease; a study at Grady Memorial hospital in Atlanta reviewed 126 cases of malaria and found tachycardia in 86%, hypotension in 14%, hepatomegaly in 21%, and splenomegaly in 15% of patients [77]. Another study looked at patients diagnosed with severe malaria caused by *P falciparum* and found jaundice in 62%; prostration (defined as confusion or behavioral changes with Glasgow Coma Score above 10) in 52%; coma in 7%; and seizures in 5% of patients [76]. Definition criteria for severe and complicated malaria according to the World Health Organization are available on their Web site (www.rbm.who.int/docs/hbsm.pdf).

Laboratory findings most common at presentation are anemia, thrombocytopenia, elevated L-lactate dehydrogenase, and abnormal liver enzymes [77]. Presence of atypical lymphocytes in the peripheral smear has also been described and it may be a clue to the diagnosis [71]. Complications associated with malaria caused by *P falciparum* are severe anemia; renal failure; acute respiratory distress syndrome; shock; hypoglycemia; disseminated intravascular coagulation; and neurologic manifestations (cerebral malaria [seizures, coma]) [76,77]. A large study from India that reviewed 3000 adult cases of falciparum malaria found that cerebral malaria occurred in 526 patients (18%), of which 175 (23%) died [68].

The diagnosis of malaria should be entertained in any febrile patient with a history of travel, even remote, and it should be on the differential list for fever of unknown origin, even without a history of travel [85,88]. Once considered, the laboratory diagnosis of malaria can be confirmed using Giemsa-stained thick and thin blood smears. The technique for preparing the smears is described on the CDC Web site [85]. Blood smears are the time-honored method for detection of malaria, but their accuracy is operator based and it decreases with low levels of parasitemia [89]. The smears should be read by a pathologist with experience in reading malaria smears, and if negative should be repeated every 12 to 24 hours for 48 to 72 hours [70]. Polymerase chain reaction–based methods are more sensitive but are available only in reference laboratories in the United States [85].

Current malaria prophylaxis is very effective in preventing clinical disease (although not completely) and in decreasing the severity of malaria caused by *P falciparum* [40,41]. Most patients with imported malaria in different case series did not take any prophylactic medication or took insufficient or inappropriate antimalarials [76,77,86,87]. In evaluating malaria prophylaxis one must consider possible drug resistance (eg, chloroquine-resistant *P falciparum* and *P vivax*), need for terminal prophylaxis with Primaquine to prevent recurrence caused by the exoerythrocytic phase of *P vivax*, and specific side effects of drugs, all weighted against risk of malaria in the area [90]. Guidelines and current issues in malaria prevention and chemoprophylaxis are widely available in the literature [40,90–93] and on the CDC Web site, at www.cdc.gov/malaria.

Malaria treatment in the United States has been recently reviewed [70]. Treatment should be directed at *P falciparum* if identification of species is in doubt. The widespread resistance of *P falciparum* to chloroquine needs to be taken into account, especially if area of exposure is not clearly determined. In such cases, oral quinine is the agent of choice for mild to moderate *P falciparum* malaria. Severe disease should be treated with intravenous quinidine (which is the only available parenteral option in the United States), combined with doxycycline or clindamycin, regardless of etiology [94].

Availability of quinidine is limited because there is less use for it as an antiarrhythmic agent and hospitals may not have it on formulary. If there is urgent need and the drug is not available locally, the manufacturer's (Eli Lilly Company) hotline should be contacted (800-821-0538) for a rapid shipment [95]. If oral therapy is feasible, quinine is an appropriate choice.

Artesunate, an artemisin derivative, was shown to decrease mortality in severe falciparum malaria when compared with intravenous quinine in several randomized trials and it may become available in the United States as an investigational drug in 2007 [70].

Exchange transfusion is recommended by the CDC for cerebral or complicated malaria or a high level of parasitemia (more than 10%) [94].

Key points for malaria include the following:

1. A travel history should be obtained from any patient with fever.
2. Malaria needs to be considered in any patient with fever and even a remote history of travel.
3. One negative blood smear does not rule out malaria.
4. History of chemoprophylaxis does not rule out malaria but it may alter the symptomatology.
5. Falciparum malaria is a medical emergency.
6. Most deaths from malaria are caused by a delay in seeking care, diagnosis, or treatment [85,96].
7. Treatment for malaria should be started immediately and be directed at *P falciparum* if species identification is not possible [70].

*Dengue fever*

Dengue fever is caused by four distinct serotypes (DEN-1, DEN-2, DEN-3, and DEN-4) of the dengue virus, a flavivirus transmitted to humans by *Aedes* mosquitoes, and is the most common cause of arboviral disease in the world [97]. Dengue is a major emerging infection worldwide and is second only to malaria as a cause of fever in travelers to the developing word [15,19]. In the United States there were 96 confirmed cases of travel-associated dengue, including one death reported in 2005, but that may be an underestimate because dengue is not a reportable disease [97]. Most of them were acquired from Mexico, Central America, and the Caribbean [97]. In contrast, of the 309 European travelers with dengue reported by the European network on imported infectious disease surveillance (Trop.Net.Europ), most acquired the infection in south and southeast Asia [98].

Dengue has a very short incubation period (range, 3–14 days) [73]. Clinical disease in most cases is self-limited and it manifests with fever; chills;

lymphadenopathy; headache and retro-orbital pain; myalgias; arthralgias; and back pain that can be incapacitating (hence the name "breakbone" fever) [99]. Hemorrhagic manifestations (petechiae, epistaxis, hematuria, hematemesis) can be absent or of variable severity [73].

A transient macular rash can be seen sometimes at onset, followed 3 to 4 days later by a maculopapular rash that spares palms and soles [5]. Bradycardia relative to the degree of fever and a "saddleback" fever pattern have also been described [51]. Neurologic manifestations are unusual but may be present and patients presenting with fever and diarrhea were also described [100,101]. Most prominent laboratory abnormalities are leukopenia with neutropenia and thrombocytopenia [102]. Dengue hemorrhagic fever and dengue shock syndrome are severe forms of disease that occur in a minority of infected travelers [98]. The main risk factor for dengue hemorrhagic fever seems to be previous infection with a different serotype, but viral virulence and other host factors may play a role [101]. A recent study showed that significant thrombocytopenia or elevated transaminases were also predictors of severe disease [78]. Dengue hemorrhagic fever, as defined by the World Health Organization, presents with fever; minor or major hemorrhagic manifestations; thrombocytopenia with a platelet count of less than 100,000; and evidence of plasma leakage (hemoconcentration, ascites or pleural effusions, and hypoalbuminemia) [73]. Some patients, however, may have severe manifestations without necessarily meeting all criteria for dengue hemorrhagic fever [78]. Diagnosis is confirmed by detection of viral DNA, viral culture, or serology. Elevated IgM or significant increases in IgG in paired serum samples are necessary for serologic diagnosis. Cross-reactivity with other flaviviruses may cause false-positive results and may be a problem in travelers that received yellow fever vaccination [99]. Treatment is largely supportive, and aspirin and other nonsteroidal anti-inflammatory agents should be avoided because of increased risk of bleeding and association with Reye's syndrome in children [73].

*Enteric fever*

Enteric fever is a potentially life-threatening illness caused by *S enterica* serotype *typhi* (typhoid fever) and *paratyphi* (paratyphoid fever). These pathogens are transmitted by fecal-oral route and infection is endemic in many regions around the globe. In the United States, there are about 400 cases reported every year to the CDC, most of them in returning travelers [103]. The highest risk is for travelers to south central and southeast Asia, particularly the Indian subcontinent, but there are other areas with high risk of transmission, including Mexico, the Caribbean, Central and South America, and parts of Africa [103,104]. Immigrants who live in the United States and are visiting friends and relatives in endemic areas are at particular risk because of longer stay, closer contact with the local population, and increased exposure to potentially contaminated food and water [20]. An incubation period of 7 to 14 days (range, 3–60 days) is followed by fever and flulike illness with headache, anorexia, nausea, and abdominal pain but with few physical findings [62,105]. Constipation has been described more often but some patients may present with diarrhea, particularly children and HIV-infected adults [106,107]. Hepatosplenomegaly and abdominal tenderness may be present and relative bradycardia is quite common [62,106,108]. Classically, a "stepladder" pattern of fever has been described but is not seen very often [61]. Regardless, the disease usually starts with low fever that becomes gradually higher over a few days, followed by a sustained high fever for 10 to 14 days. Most important complications are intestinal perforation, gastrointestinal bleeding, and encephalopathy, but they are usually seen with a prolonged course of untreated disease and are not commonly encountered in travelers [105,106]. Rose spots are pink blanching macules on abdomen and chest, classically associated with typhoid fever, but they may be difficult to detect [104]. Laboratory abnormalities include leukopenia, anemia, and thrombocytopenia, although leukocytosis may be seen in children or early disease [109]. Hepatic involvement with increased transaminases is common but they are less elevated than in viral hepatitis [79]. Definitive diagnosis is made by culturing the organism from urine, stool, blood, bone marrow, or from the rose spots. Studies have shown that bone marrow cultures have the highest sensitivity and should be performed in any patient with suspected enteric fever [110–112]. Additionally, bone marrow cultures are less likely to be influenced by prior antibiotic treatment [110]. Fluoroquinolones are the agents of choice for susceptible organisms; however, they are not routinely recommended in children and resistance is described in many areas of the world. Ceftriaxone or azithromycin are the first choice for presumptive therapy [104,113]. There are currently two available vaccines for typhoid fever: an oral live-attenuated vaccine and an injectable capsular polysaccharide Vi vaccine, both 50% to 80% effective [39]. Immunization should be considered for all travelers to high-risk areas, even if they are planning a short stay [39].

## Rickettsial diseases

Rickettsioses are febrile illnesses caused by intracellular pathogens that have a tropism for endothelial cells. Conventionally, they are divided into three main groups: (1) the spotted fever group (by far the largest, includes Rocky Mountain spotted fever, Mediterranean spotted fever, and African tick-bite fever); (2) the typhus group; and (3) the scrub typhus group (with only one member, the scrub typhus caused by *Orientia tsutsugamushi*) [114].

They usually present with nonspecific manifestations, such as fever and flulike illness, with headaches, myalgias, and arthralgias. A rash and an inoculation eschar with regional lymphadenopathy may be present [59,115,116].

Four rickettsioses are encountered most frequently in travelers: (1) African tick-bite fever, caused by *Rickesttsia africae*; (2) Mediterranean spotted fever, caused by *Ricketsia connorii*; (3) murine typhus, caused by *Ricketsia typhii*; and (4) scrub typhus, caused by *O tsutsugamushi* [117].

African tick-bite fever is by far the most common rickettsial disease diagnosed in the returning traveler [19]. *R africae* is the causative organism and it can be encountered in sub-Saharan and South Africa and the eastern Caribbean region [117]. The disease is transmitted to humans by cattle ticks of the genus *Amblyomma*, which also act as reservoirs [118]. Game hunting, travel between November and April, and travel to South Africa were identified as risk factors in a recent study [119]. After an incubation period of 5 to 10 days, the most common clinical manifestations are fever; a flulike illness; inoculation eschars (which may be multiple); regional lymphadenopathy; and a rash that is usually maculopapular or vesicular and rarely purpuric [118,120]. Most notable, an inoculation eschar was seen in 95% of patients in a study [120]. Mouth ulcerations may also be present [119]. The disease is usually mild and self limited. Serologic diagnosis can be made retrospectively by immunofluorescence assay, using paired serum samples taken 4 weeks apart; however, because no specific tests for *R africae* are available at the CDC, assays for *R conorii*, *R ricketsii*, or *R. akari* can be used [121]. *R africae* can be identified also in biopsy specimens from the eschar or from the rash using polymerase chain reaction or immunohistochemistry [121]. Doxycycline for 7 days is the recommended treatment, and it should be started based on clinical and epidemiologic diagnosis, because confirmation may be difficult [118].

Mediterranean spotted fevers are a group of diseases caused by serotypes of *R connorii* and are encountered along the Mediterranean basin in Europe and Africa (boutonneuse fever and Mediterranean tick fever); in South Asia (Indian tick typhus); in the Middle East (Israeli tick typhus); and in the north Caspian region of Russia (Astrakhan spotted fever) [122].

Mediterranean spotted fevers are transmitted by different species of dog ticks and usually cause mild disease, although complications are not uncommon and may include acute respiratory distress syndrome, peripheral gangrene, and neurologic manifestations, sometimes severe [117,123]. In a case series from Greece, a rash was present in 87% of patients and the classical inoculation eschar (tache noire) in more than half. Laboratory abnormalities included leukopenia and thrombocytopenia in about half of the patients and elevated transaminases in 80%. All patients were given doxycycline and recovered [34].

Murine typhus is caused by *R typhi* and is transmitted to humans by the bite of the rat flea. It has a worldwide distribution, especially in hot and humid regions [124]. Recently a new pathogen, *Rickettsia felis*, was identified that causes a murine typhus-like disease [124]. In a study from Texas, most common manifestations were fever, headache, gastrointestinal manifestations, myalgias, and a maculopapular rash [125]. Laboratory abnormalities include thrombocytopenia and elevated transaminases [125–127]. Complications including meningitis and renal involvement may occur [124,128]. Doxycycline is used for treatment [129].

Scrub typhus, caused by *O tsutsugamushi* and transmitted by the bite of infected trombiculid mites, is one of the most prevalent infectious diseases in rural areas of south and southeast Asia and Oceania [117]. It can be seen also in Japan; for example, in 1998 462 cases were reported from this country [130]. Most common findings in this study were fever in 98%, rash in 93%, and an inoculation eschar in 87%. Other symptoms were malaise, headache, and myalgias [130]. Complications include pneumonitis, acute respiratory distress syndrome, disseminated intravascular coagulation, renal failure, and meningoencephalitis [117,131,132]. Treatment of choice is doxycycline, given for a short course [133]. Azithromycin and telithromycin were also shown to be effective [134,135].

*Leptospirosis*

Leptospirosis is a zoonosis with worldwide distribution, caused by spirochetes of the genus *Leptospira* [136]. Human infection is caused by contact with the urine or tissues of carrier animals in endemic areas [137]. Leptospirosis is an uncommon cause of fever in travelers and it has been associated with recreational water exposure, such as swimming or rafting in contaminated lakes or rivers [32]. Clinical manifestations are variable, from subclinical or mild disease to a fulminant syndrome with jaundice, renal failure, and hemorrhagic manifestations (Weil's disease) [80,138]. Typically leptospirosis is described as a biphasic disease, with two distinct periods of fever and clinical symptoms, separated by a few days of remission. Most complications occur not in the initial, septicemic phase, but in the second, immune phase of the disease [139]. Although the absence of the classical biphasic illness does not rule out leptospirosis, this clinical scenario should raise suspicion for a point-source epidemic. In an outbreak among athletes participating in an Eco-challenge race in Borneo in 2000, the most commonly reported symptoms were fever, chills, headaches, myalgias, and diarrhea, whereas conjunctival suffusion, a classical finding in leptospirosis, was seen in 21% of patients; none had severe manifestations [33]. Complications include aseptic meningitis, pulmonary symptoms, renal failure, arrhythmias, jaundice, and hemorrhagic manifestations [33]. Laboratory diagnosis is most commonly made by serology, classically by the microscopic hemmaglutination test; newer and more reliable methods involve detection of leptospira-specific IgM by ELISA [33]. Culture from blood, cerebrospinal fluid, or urine may be done but it has a low sensitivity and may take several weeks to grow [136,138]. Doxycycline is used as short-term chemoprophylaxis for high-risk exposures. For the treatment of mild disease, either doxycycline or amoxicillin may be used. Severe disease is treated with intravenous penicillin G or ampicillin, although ceftriaxone and cefotaxime were shown to be as effective [138,140–142].

## Chikungunya fever

Chikungunya fever is a tropical arbovirosis present in areas of Africa and Asia, caused by the chikungunya virus, an alphavirus transmitted to humans by infected *Aedes* mosquitoes, also the vector of dengue fever [139]. The name of the disease comes from the language of the Makonde people in northern Mozambique and southeast Tanzania and means "that which bends up," a reference to the stooped posture that develops from severe arthritic pain [143]. The disease is not common in travelers, but it is probably underreported in the United States [139]. Major outbreaks where recently reported in the Indian Ocean islands, and a large epidemic is currently ongoing in India, where at least 1.4 million people have been affected [144]. Incubation period is short, on average 2 to 4 days (range, 1–12 days) [145]. In a study of imported Chikungunya fever in German travelers, fever and severe joint pain were encountered in all patients, a rash in 75%, and conjunctival injection in 20%. The small joints were more commonly involved; pain in wrists, ankles, and interphalangeal joints was seen in 90%. In the same study, laboratory abnormalities consisted of leukopenia, thrombocytopenia, and elevated transaminases [81]. Diagnosis can be confirmed by serology and paired serum samples (acute and convalescent) should be submitted to the CDC for testing [139]. Treatment is only symptomatic, with nonsteroidal anti-inflammatory drugs used for temporary relief of arthralgias [145].

## Summary

The returning traveler with fever presents a diagnostic challenge for the health care provider. When evaluating such a patient, the highest priority should be given to diseases that are potentially fatal or may represent public health threats. Common illnesses with a worldwide distribution, such as respiratory and urinary tract infections, are as likely to be the source of fever in travelers as they are in nontravelers. Malaria is the most common cause of fever in the international traveler and it should always be in the differential. A good history is paramount and needs to include destination, time and duration of travel, type of activity, onset of fever in relation to travel, associated comorbidities, and any associated symptoms. Pretravel immunizations and chemoprophylaxis may alter the natural course of disease and should be inquired about specifically. The fever pattern, presence of a rash or eschar, organomegaly, or neurologic findings are helpful physical findings. Laboratory abnormalities are nonspecific but when corroborated with clinical and epidemiologic data may offer a clue to diagnosis. Serial blood smears for malaria should be obtained in every patient with fever and a history of travel, even remote. The Web sites listed in Box 1 are excellent resources for the health care provider faced with a difficult to diagnose febrile illness in a returning traveler.

## References

[1] Tatem AJ, Rogers DJ, Hay SI. Global transport networks and infectious disease spread. Adv Parasitol 2006;62:293–343.

[2] Salit IE, Sano M, Boggild AK, et al. Travel patterns and risk behaviour of HIV-positive people travelling internationally. CMAJ 2005;172:884–8.

[3] Mileno MD, Bia FJ. The compromised traveler. Infect Dis Clin North Am 1998;12:369–412.

[4] Boggild AK, Sano M, Humar A, et al. Travel patterns and risk behavior in solid organ transplant recipients. J Travel Med 2004;11:37–43.

[5] Wilson ME. A world guide to infections: diseases, distribution, diagnosis. New York: Oxford University Press; 1991.

[6] Bottieau E, Clerinx J, Schrooten W, et al. Etiology and outcome of fever after a stay in the tropics. Arch Intern Med 2006;166:1642–8.

[7] Philbrick JT, Shumate R, Siadaty MS, et al. Air travel and venous thromboembolism: a systematic review. J Gen Intern Med 2007;22:107–14.

[8] Strickland GT. Fever in the returned traveler. Med Clin North Am 1992;76:1375–92.

[9] Magill AJ. Fever in the returned traveler. Infect Dis Clin North Am 1998;12:445–69.

[10] Ryan ET, Wilson ME, Kain KC. Illness after international travel. N Engl J Med 2002;347:505–16.

[11] Suh KN, Kozarsky PE, Keystone JS. Evaluation of fever in the returned traveler. Med Clin North Am 1999;83:997–1017.

[12] Strickland GT, editor. Hunter's tropical medicine and emerging infectious diseases. 8th edition. Philadelphia: W.B. Saunders Company; 2000.

[13] Mandell GL, Bennett JE, Dolin R, editors. Mandell, Bennett, Dolin's principles and practice of infectious diseases. 6th edition. Philadelphia: Elsevier; 2005.

[14] Borchardt SM, Ritger KA, Dworkin MS. Categorization, prioritization, and surveillance of potential bioterrorism agents. Infect Dis Clin North Am 2006;20:213–25.

[15] Wilson ME, Weld LH, Boggild A, et al. Fever in returned travelers: results from the GeoSentinel Surveillance Network. Clin Infect Dis 2007;44:1560–8.

[16] Bacaner N, Wilson ME. Evaluation of the ill returned traveler. Clinics in Family Practice 2005;7:805–34.

[17] Boulware DR. Travel medicine for the extreme traveler. Clinics in Family Practice 2005;7:745–59.

[18] Angell SY, Behrens RH. Risk assessment and disease prevention in travelers visiting friends and relatives. Infect Dis Clin North Am 2005;19:49–65.

[19] Freedman DO, Weld LH, Kozarsky PE, et al. Spectrum of disease and relation to place of exposure among ill returned travelers. N Engl J Med 2006;354:119–30.

[20] Leder K, Tong S, Weld L, et al. Illness in travelers visiting friends and relatives: a review of the GeoSentinel Surveillance Network. Clin Infect Dis 2006;43:1185–93.

[21] O'Brien D, Tobin S, Brown GV, et al. Fever in returned travelers: review of hospital admissions for a 3-year period. Clin Infect Dis 2001;33:603–9.

[22] Parola P, Soula G, Gazin P, et al. Fever in travelers returning from tropical areas: prospective observational study of 613 cases hospitalised in Marseilles, France, 1999–2003. Travel Med Infect Dis 2006;4:61–70.

[23] Stienlauf S, Segal G, Sidi Y, et al. Epidemiology of travel-related hospitalization. J Travel Med 2005;12:136–41.

[24] Antinori S, Galimberti L, Gianelli E, et al. Prospective observational study of fever in hospitalized returning travelers and migrants from tropical areas, 1997–2001. J Travel Med 2004;11:135–42.

[25] Doherty JF, Grant AD, Bryceson AD. Fever as the presenting complaint of travellers returning from the tropics. QJM 1995;88:277–81.

[26] McLellan SL. Evaluation of fever in the returned traveler. Prim Care 2002;29:947–69.

[27] Bottieau E, Clerinx J, Van den Enden E, et al. Fever after a stay in the tropics: diagnostic predictors of the leading tropical conditions. Medicine (Baltimore) 2007;86:18–25.

[28] Spira AM. Assessment of travellers who return home ill. Lancet 2003;361:1459–69.

[29] Malaria information for travelers to countries in Tropical South America. In: Travelers' health: regional malaria information. CDC; 2006 [vol. 2007].

[30] Bacaner N, Stauffer B, Boulware DR, et al. Travel medicine considerations for North American immigrants visiting friends and relatives. JAMA 2004;291:2856–64.

[31] Stauffer WM, Behrens RH. Providing travel medicine advice to visiting friends and relatives travelers: high risk and difficult to advise. Clinics in Family Practice 2005;7: 717–28.

[32] Outbreak of leptospirosis among white-water rafters—Costa Rica, 1996. MMWR Morb Mortal Wkly Rep 1997;46:577.

[33] Sejvar J, Bancroft E, Winthrop K, et al. Leptospirosis in "Eco-Challenge" athletes, Malaysian Borneo, 2000. Emerg Infect Dis 2003;9:702–7.

[34] Germanakis A, Psaroulaki A, Gikas A, et al. Mediterranean spotted fever in Crete, Greece: clinical and therapeutic data of 15 consecutive patients. Ann N Y Acad Sci 2006;1078: 263–9.

[35] Pappas G, Panagopoulou P, Christou L, et al. Category B potential bioterrorism agents: bacteria, viruses, toxins, and foodborne and waterborne pathogens. Infect Dis Clin North Am 2006;20:395–421.

[36] Nygard K, Brantsaeter A, Feruglio S, et al. [Histoplasmosis among travellers to Central America]. Tidsskr Nor Laegeforen 2006;126:2838–42 [in Norwegian].

[37] Thwing J, Skarbinski J, Newman RD, et al. Malaria surveillance—United States, 2005. MMWR Surveill Summ 2007;56:23–40.

[38] Wilder-Smith A, Schwartz E. Dengue in travelers. N Engl J Med 2005;353:924–32.

[39] Steinberg EB, Bishop R, Haber P, et al. Typhoid fever in travelers: who should be targeted for prevention? Clin Infect Dis 2004;39:186–91.

[40] Chen LH, Wilson ME, Schlagenhauf P. Controversies and misconceptions in malaria chemoprophylaxis for travelers. JAMA 2007;297:2251–63.

[41] Lewis SJ, Davidson RN, Ross EJ, et al. Severity of imported falciparum malaria: effect of taking antimalarial prophylaxis. BMJ 1992;305:741–3.

[42] Castelli F, Patroni A. The human immunodeficiency virus-infected traveler. Clin Infect Dis 2000;31:1403–8.

[43] Puthucheary SD, Ng KP, Hafeez A, et al. Salmonellosis in persons infected with human immunodeficiency virus: a report of seven cases from Malaysia. Southeast Asian J Trop Med Public Health 2004;35:361–5.

[44] Bloland PB, Wirima JJ, Steketee RW, et al. Maternal HIV infection and infant mortality in Malawi: evidence for increased mortality due to placental malaria infection. AIDS 1995;9: 721–6.

[45] Antinori S, Gianelli E, Bonaccorso C, et al. Disseminated Penicillium marneffei infection in an HIV-positive Italian patient and a review of cases reported outside endemic regions. J Travel Med 2006;13:181–8.

[46] Chariyalertsak S, Sirisanthana T, Saengwonloey O, et al. Clinical presentation and risk behaviors of patients with acquired immunodeficiency syndrome in Thailand, 1994–1998: regional variation and temporal trends. Clin Infect Dis 2001;32:955–62.

[47] Pasquau F, Ena J, Sanchez R, et al. Leishmaniasis as an opportunistic infection in HIV-infected patients: determinants of relapse and mortality in a collaborative study of 228 episodes in a Mediterranean region. Eur J Clin Microbiol Infect Dis 2005;24:411–8.

[48] Pintado V, Martin-Rabadan P, Rivera ML, et al. Visceral leishmaniasis in human immunodeficiency virus (HIV)-infected and non-HIV-infected patients: a comparative study. Medicine (Baltimore) 2001;80:54–73.

[49] Mackowiak PA, Bartlett JG, Borden EC, et al. Concepts of fever: recent advances and lingering dogma. Clin Infect Dis 1997;25:119–38.

[50] Cunha BA. The clinical significance of fever patterns. Infect Dis Clin North Am 1996;10: 33–44.

[51] Sideridis K, Canario D, Cunha BA. Dengue fever: diagnostic importance of a camelback fever pattern. Heart Lung 2003;32:414–8.

[52] Memish ZA. Meningococcal disease and travel. Clin Infect Dis 2002;34:84–90.

[53] Jeronimo SMB, Sousa ADQ, Pearson RD. Leishmania species: visceral (kala-azar), cutaneous, and mucocutaneous leishmaniasis. In: Mandell GL, Bennett JE, Dolin R, editors. Mandell, Bennett, Dolin's principles and practice of infectious diseases, vol. 2. 6th edition. Philadelphia: Elsevier; 2005. p. 3145–55.

[54] Moore AC, Ryan ET, Waldron MA. Case records of the Massachusetts General hospital. Weekly clinicopathological exercises. Case 20-2002. A 37-year-old man with fever, hepatosplenomegaly, and a cutaneous foot lesion after a trip to Africa. N Engl J Med 2002;346: 2069–76.

[55] Boonstra E. [Trypanosomiasis: a real risk for tourists visiting national parks in Tanzania]. Tidsskr Nor Laegeforen 2002;122:35–7 [in Norwegian].

[56] Saxe SE, Gardner P. The returning traveler with fever. Infect Dis Clin North Am 1992;6: 427–39.

[57] Jackson Y, Chappuis F, Loutan L. African tick-bite fever: four cases among Swiss travelers returning from South Africa. J Travel Med 2004;11:225–8.

[58] Wilson ME. Skin problems in the traveler. Infect Dis Clin North Am 1998;12:471–88.

[59] Walker DH. Rickettsial diseases in travelers. Travel Med Infect Dis 2003;1:35–40.

[60] Raoult D. Introduction to rickettsioses and ehrlichioses. In: Mandell GL, Bennett JE, Dolin R, editors. Mandell, Bennett, Dolin's principles and practice of infectious diseases, vol 2. 6th edition. Philadelphia: Elsevier; 2005. p. 2284–6.

[61] Gupta SP, Gupta MS, Bhardwaj S, et al. Current clinical patterns of typhoid fever: a prospective study. J Trop Med Hyg 1985;88:377–81.

[62] Mathura KC, Gurubacharya DL, Shrestha A, et al. Clinical profile of typhoid patients. Kathmandu Univ Med J (KUMJ) 2003;1:135–7.

[63] Jacobson CC, Abel EA. Parasitic infestations. J Am Acad Dermatol 2007;56:1026–43.

[64] Ross AG, Vickers D, Olds GR, et al. Katayama syndrome. Lancet Infect Dis 2007;7: 218–24.

[65] Burkhart CG, Burkhart CN. Swimmer's itch: an assessment proposing possible treatment with ivermectin. Int J Dermatol 2003;42:917–8.

[66] Mutsch M, Spicher VM, Gut C, et al. Hepatitis A virus infections in travelers, 1988–2004. Clin Infect Dis 2006;42:135–7.

[67] Anand AC, Puri P. Jaundice in malaria. J Gastroenterol Hepatol 2005;20:1322–32.

[68] Mishra SK, Mohanty S, Satpathy SK, et al. Cerebral malaria in adults: a description of 526 cases admitted to Ispat General Hospital in Rourkela, India. Ann Trop Med Parasitol 2007; 101:187–93.

[69] Pigott DC. Emergency department evaluation of the febrile traveler. J Infect 2007;54:1–5.

[70] Griffith KS, Lewis LS, Mali S, et al. Treatment of malaria in the United States: a systematic review. JAMA 2007;297:2264–77.

[71] Cunha BA. The diagnosis of imported malaria. Arch Intern Med 2001;161:1926–8.

[72] Cleri DJ, Ricketti AJ, Porwancher RB, et al. Viral hemorrhagic fevers: current status of endemic disease and strategies for control. Infect Dis Clin North Am 2006;20:359–93.

[73] van Zyl C, Abrahamian FM. Update on emerging infections: news from the Centers for Disease Control and Prevention. Travel-associated dengue infections—United States, 2001–2004. Ann Emerg Med 2005;46:420–3.

[74] Schulte C, Krebs B, Jelinek T, et al. Diagnostic significance of blood eosinophilia in returning travelers. Clin Infect Dis 2002;34:407–11.

[75] Slom TJ, Cortese MM, Gerber SI, et al. An outbreak of eosinophilic meningitis caused by Angiostrongylus cantonensis in travelers returning from the Caribbean. N Engl J Med 2002; 346:668–75.

[76] Badiaga S, Brouqui P, Carpentier JP, et al. Severe imported malaria: clinical presentation at the time of hospital admission and outcome in 42 cases diagnosed from 1996 to 2002. J Emerg Med 2005;29:375–82.

[77] Vicas AE, Albrecht H, Lennox JL, et al. Imported malaria at an inner-city hospital in the United States. Am J Med Sci 2005;329:6–12.

[78] Wichmann O, Gascon J, Schunk M, et al. Severe dengue virus infection in travelers: risk factors and laboratory indicators. J Infect Dis 2007;195:1089–96.

[79] El-Newihi HM, Alamy ME, Reynolds TB. Salmonella hepatitis: analysis of 27 cases and comparison with acute viral hepatitis. Hepatology 1996;24:516–9.

[80] Spichler A, Moock M, Chapola EG, et al. Weil's disease: an unusually fulminant presentation characterized by pulmonary hemorrhage and shock. Braz J Infect Dis 2005;9:336–40.

[81] Taubitz W, Cramer JP, Kapaun A, et al. Chikungunya fever in travelers: clinical presentation and course. Clin Infect Dis 2007;45:e1–4.

[82] World Malaria Report 2005. Geneva (Switzerland): World Health Organization; 2005.

[83] Skarbinski J, James EM, Causer LM, et al. Malaria surveillance—United States, 2004. MMWR Surveill Summ 2006;55:23–37.

[84] Taylor TE, Strickland GT. Malaria. In: Strickland GT, editor. Hunter's tropical medicine and emerging infectious diseases. 8th edition. Philadelphia: W.B. Saunders Company; 2000.

[85] Shah S, Filler S, Causer LM, et al. Malaria surveillance—United States, 2002. MMWR Surveill Summ 2004;53:21–34.

[86] Froude JR, Weiss LM, Tanowitz HB, et al. Imported malaria in the Bronx: review of 51 cases recorded from 1986 to 1991. Clin Infect Dis 1992;15:774–80.

[87] Kotwal RS, Wenzel RB, Sterling RA, et al. An outbreak of malaria in US army rangers returning from Afghanistan. JAMA 2005;293:212–6.

[88] Dorsey G, Gandhi M, Oyugi JH, et al. Difficulties in the prevention, diagnosis, and treatment of imported malaria. Arch Intern Med 2000;160:2505–10.

[89] Ndao M, Bandyayera E, Kokoskin E, et al. Comparison of blood smear, antigen detection, and nested-PCR methods for screening refugees from regions where malaria is endemic after a malaria outbreak in Quebec, Canada. J Clin Microbiol 2004;42:2694–700.

[90] Hill DR, Ericsson CD, Pearson RD, et al. The practice of travel medicine: guidelines by the Infectious Diseases Society of America. Clin Infect Dis 2006;43:1499–539.

[91] Franco-Paredes C, Santos-Preciado JI. Problem pathogens: prevention of malaria in travellers. Lancet Infect Dis 2006;6:139–49.

[92] Chen LH, Keystone JS. New strategies for the prevention of malaria in travelers. Infect Dis Clin North Am 2005;19:185–210.

[93] Guerin PJ, Olliaro P, Nosten F, et al. Malaria: current status of control, diagnosis, treatment, and a proposed agenda for research and development. Lancet Infect Dis 2002; 2:564–73.

[94] Part 3: alternatives for pregnant women § treatment: severe malaria. In: Malaria. CDC; 2007 [vol. 2007].

[95] Availability and use of parenteral quinidine gluconate for severe or complicated malaria. MMWR Morb Mortal Wkly Rep 2000;49:1138.

[96] Newman RD, Parise ME, Barber AM, et al. Malaria-related deaths among U.S. travelers, 1963–2001. Ann Intern Med 2004;141:547–55.

[97] Travel-associated dengue—United States, 2005. MMWR Morb Mortal Wkly Rep 2006;55: 700.

[98] Jelinek T, Muhlberger N, Harms G, et al. Epidemiology and clinical features of imported dengue fever in Europe: sentinel surveillance data from TropNetEurop. Clin Infect Dis 2002;35:1047–52.

[99] Jelinek T. Dengue fever in international travelers. Clin Infect Dis 2000;31:144–7.

[100] Helbok R, Dent W, Gattringer K, et al. Imported dengue fever presenting with febrile diarrhoea: report of two cases. Wien Klin Wochenschr 2004;116(Suppl 4):58–60.

[101] Guzman MG, Kouri G. Dengue: an update. Lancet Infect Dis 2002;2:33–42.

[102] Vaughn DW, Green S. Dengue and dengue hemorrhagic fever. In: Strickland GT, editor. Hunter's tropical medicine and emerging infectious diseases. 8th edition. Philadelphia: W.B. Saunders Company; 2000. p. 240–4.

[103] Chapter 4: prevention of specific infectious diseases. In: Travelers' health: Yellow book. CDC; 2007 [vol. 2007].

[104] Basnyat B, Maskey AP, Zimmerman MD, et al. Enteric (typhoid) fever in travelers. Clin Infect Dis 2005;41:1467–72.

[105] Connor BA, Schwartz E. Typhoid and paratyphoid fever in travellers. Lancet Infect Dis 2005;5:623–8.

[106] Parry CM, Hien TT, Dougan G, et al. Typhoid fever. N Engl J Med 2002;347:1770–82.

[107] Hoffner RJ, Slaven E, Perez J, et al. Emergency department presentations of typhoid fever. J Emerg Med 2000;19:317–21.

[108] Nasrallah SM, Nassar VH. Enteric fever: a clinicopathologic study of 104 cases. Am J Gastroenterol 1978;69:63–9.

[109] Pegues DA, Ohl ME, Miller SI. Salmonella species, including *Salmonella typhi*. In: Mandell GL, Bennett JE, Dolin R, editors. Mandell, Bennett, Dolin's principles and practice of infectious diseases, vol. 2. 6th edition. Philadelphia: Elsevier; 2005. p. 2636–54.

[110] Wain J, Pham VB, Ha V, et al. Quantitation of bacteria in bone marrow from patients with typhoid fever: relationship between counts and clinical features. J Clin Microbiol 2001;39: 1571–6.

[111] Vallenas C, Hernandez H, Kay B, et al. Efficacy of bone marrow, blood, stool and duodenal contents cultures for bacteriologic confirmation of typhoid fever in children. Pediatr Infect Dis 1985;4:496–8.

[112] Gilman RH, Terminel M, Levine MM, et al. Relative efficacy of blood, urine, rectal swab, bone-marrow, and rose-spot cultures for recovery of *Salmonella typhi* in typhoid fever. Lancet 1975;1:1211–3.

[113] Frenck RW Jr, Nakhla I, Sultan Y, et al. Azithromycin versus ceftriaxone for the treatment of uncomplicated typhoid fever in children. Clin Infect Dis 2000;31:1134–8.

[114] Raoult D. Scrub typhus. In: Mandell GL, Bennett JE, Dolin R, editors. Mandell, Bennett, Dolin's principles and practice of infectious diseases, vol. 2. 6th edition. Philadelphia: Elsevier; 2005. p. 2309–10.

[115] Jensenius M, Fournier PE, Raoult D. Tick-borne rickettsioses in international travellers. Int J Infect Dis 2004;8:139–46.

[116] Marschang A, Nothdurft HD, Kumlien S, et al. Imported rickettsioses in German travelers. Infection 1995;23:94–7.

[117] Jensenius M, Fournier PE, Raoult D. Rickettsioses and the international traveler. Clin Infect Dis 2004;39:1493–9.

[118] Jensenius M, Fournier PE, Kelly P, et al. African tick bite fever. Lancet Infect Dis 2003;3: 557–64.

[119] Jensenius M, Fournier PE, Vene S, et al. African tick bite fever in travelers to rural sub-equatorial Africa. Clin Infect Dis 2003;36:1411–7.

[120] Raoult D, Fournier PE, Fenollar F, et al. *Rickettsia africae*, a tick-borne pathogen in travelers to sub-Saharan Africa. N Engl J Med 2001;344:1504–10.

[121] McQuiston JH, Paddock CD, Singleton J Jr, et al. Imported spotted fever rickettsioses in United States travelers returning from Africa: a summary of cases confirmed by laboratory testing at the Centers for Disease Control and Prevention, 1999–2002. Am J Trop Med Hyg 2004;70:98–101.

[122] Chapter 4: prevention of specific infectious diseases. In: CDC; 2007 [vol. 2007].

[123] Caroleo S, Longo C, Pirritano D, et al. A case of acute quadriplegia complicating Mediterranean spotted fever. Clin Neurol Neurosurg 2007;109:463–5.

[124] Hernandez Cabrera M, Angel-Moreno A, Santana E, et al. Murine typhus with renal involvement in Canary islands, Spain. Emerg Infect Dis 2004;10:740–3.

[125] Whiteford SF, Taylor JP, Dumler JS. Clinical, laboratory, and epidemiologic features of murine typhus in 97 Texas children. Arch Pediatr Adolesc Med 2001;155:396–400.
[126] Suttor VP, Feller RB. Murine typhus mimicking acute cholecystitis in a traveller. Med J Aust 2006;184:475.
[127] Koliou M, Psaroulaki A, Georgiou C, et al. Murine typhus in Cyprus: 21 paediatric cases. Eur J Clin Microbiol Infect Dis 2007;26:491–3.
[128] Toumi A, Loussaief C, Ben Yahia S, et al. [Meningitis revealing *Rickettsia typhi* infection]. Rev Med Interne 2007;28:131–3 [in French].
[129] Dumler JS, Walker DH. *Rickettsia typhi* (murine typhus). In: Mandell GL, Bennett JE, Dolin R, editors. Mandell, Bennett, Dolin's principles and practice of infectious diseases, vol. 2. 6th editionPhiladelphia: Elsevier; 2005. p. 2306–8.
[130] Ogawa M, Hagiwara T, Kishimoto T, et al. Scrub typhus in Japan: epidemiology and clinical features of cases reported in 1998. Am J Trop Med Hyg 2002;67:162–5.
[131] Choi YH, Kim SJ, Lee JY, et al. Scrub typhus: radiological and clinical findings. Clin Radiol 2000;55:140–4.
[132] Pandey D, Sharma B, Chauhan V, et al. ARDS complicating scrub typhus in sub-Himalayan region. J Assoc Physicians India 2006;54:812–3.
[133] Song JH, Lee C, Chang WH, et al. Short-course doxycycline treatment versus conventional tetracycline therapy for scrub typhus: a multicenter randomized trial. Clin Infect Dis 1995; 21:506–10.
[134] Kim YS, Yun HJ, Shim SK, et al. A comparative trial of a single dose of azithromycin versus doxycycline for the treatment of mild scrub typhus. Clin Infect Dis 2004;39:1329–35.
[135] Kim DM, Yu KD, Lee JH, et al. Controlled trial of a 5-day course of telithromycin versus doxycycline for treatment of mild to moderate scrub typhus. Antimicrob Agents Chemother 2007;51:2011–5.
[136] Sellman J, Bender J. Zoonotic infections in travelers to the tropics. Prim Care 2002;29: 907–29.
[137] Levett PN. Leptospirosis. In: Mandell GL, Bennett JE, Dolin R, editors. Mandell, Bennett, Dolin's principles and practice of infectious diseases. vol. 2. 6th edition. Philadelphia: Elsevier; 2005. p. 2789–94.
[138] Bharti AR, Nally JE, Ricaldi JN, et al. Leptospirosis: a zoonotic disease of global importance. Lancet Infect Dis 2003;3:757–71.
[139] Chikungunya fever diagnosed among international travelers—United States, 2005–2006. MMWR Morb Mortal Wkly Rep 2006;55:955–62.
[140] Suputtamongkol Y, Niwattayakul K, Suttinont C, et al. An open, randomized, controlled trial of penicillin, doxycycline, and cefotaxime for patients with severe leptospirosis. Clin Infect Dis 2004;39:1417–24.
[141] Panaphut T, Domrongkitchaiporn S, Vibhagool A, et al. Ceftriaxone compared with sodium penicillin G for treatment of severe leptospirosis. Clin Infect Dis 2003;36:1507–13.
[142] Faucher JF, Hoen B, Estavoyer JM. The management of leptospirosis. Expert Opin Pharmacother 2004;5:819–27.
[143] Hochedez P, Jaureguiberry S, Debruyne M, et al. Chikungunya infection in travelers. Emerg Infect Dis 2006;12:1565–7.
[144] Mavalankar D, Shastri P, Raman P. Chikungunya epidemic in India: a major public-health disaster. Lancet Infect Dis 2007;7:306–7.
[145] Pialoux G, Gauzere BA, Jaureguiberry S, et al. Chikungunya, an epidemic arbovirosis. Lancet Infect Dis 2007;7:319–27.

ELSEVIER
SAUNDERS

INFECTIOUS
DISEASE CLINICS
OF NORTH AMERICA

Infect Dis Clin N Am 21 (2007) 1115–1135

# Fever of Unknown Origin in Rheumatic Diseases

## Thierry Zenone, MD

*Department of Medicine, Unit of Internal Medicine, Centre Hospitalier,
179 boulevard Marechal Juin, 26953 Valence cedex 9, France*

Despite advances in diagnostic techniques, fever of unknown origin (FUO) remains a great challenge [1]. In 1961, Petersdorf and Beeson [2] defined FUO as fever of at least 3 weeks duration, exceeding 38.3°C (101°F) on several occasions, with no established diagnosis after 1 week of evaluation in a hospital. Increasing costs of hospital care and changes in health systems (shift toward outpatient management, advances in diagnostic techniques, and accelerated pace of exploration), especially in Western countries, have motivated authors to revise the conventional definition. The most well-known revision, presented in 1991 by Durack and Street [3] and agreed by Petersdorf [4], limited the hospital stay to 3 days or more than two outpatient visits. To reduce selection bias, it has been proposed in recent years to change the quantitative criterion (diagnosis uncertain after 1 week, 3 days, or >2 outpatient visits) to a qualitative that requires the performance of certain investigations [1,4–6]. For future FUO studies, the use of a set of obligated investigations instead of time-related criterion is recommended [1].

Moreover, Durack and Street [3] proposed to divide FUO into four groups: (1) classic FUO, (2) nosocomial FUO, (3) neutropenic FUO, and (4) HIV-associated FUO. This article focuses on classic FUO; immunocompromised patients require an entirely specific approach.

The causes of classic FUO are usually classified into diagnostic categories: (1) infections; (2) malignancies; (3) noninfectious inflammatory diseases; (4) miscellaneous causes, including drug-related fever, habitual hyperthermia, and factitious fever; and (5) undiagnosed [6]. A noninfectious inflammatory disease is a category coined by De Kleijn and colleagues [5,7] that comprises connective tissue diseases, vasculitis syndromes, and

*E-mail address:* t.zenone@ch-valence.fr

granulomatous diseases. The group "noninfectious inflammatory diseases" can cause semantic problems, because it is designated by different investigators as rheumatic diseases, autoimmune diseases, systemic diseases, collagen vascular diseases, or vasculitides, and because several investigators use a separate category, namely granulomatous diseases, which are also inflammatory disorders that can be included in the noninfectious inflammatory diseases group [6].

This article focuses on noninfectious inflammatory diseases as a cause of classic FUO (mainly rheumatic diseases, such as vasculitis and connective tissue diseases).

## Distribution of the different disease categories

Historical series encompassing more than 100 patients satisfying the FUO definition are presented in Table 1 [8]. Cases are reclassified according to the previously mentioned diagnostic categories [5,6]. The noninfectious inflammatory diseases category gradually replaced the infectious category as the largest in Western countries. Authors who have presented an update of their previous FUO series also noted an increase in noninfectious inflammatory diseases [9].

Table 2 lists the diagnostic categories in a study of 144 nonimmunocompromised patients presenting to a single nonuniversity hospital in France between 1999 and 2005 (secondary level of the health care system) with a community-acquired FUO (corresponding to the so-called "classic FUO" of Durack and Street [3]) [10]. Among the 107 patients with a final diagnosis, noninfectious inflammatory diseases represented the most important cause of FUO in the study (38 cases, 35.5%). Giant cell arteritis and polymyalgia rheumatica were the most common etiology in this group (18 [47.4%] of 38) (Table 3) [10]. In the recent study conducted by Bleeker-Rovers and colleagues [1], 73 patients with FUO were recruited using qualitative criterion (instead of quantitative criterion). An infectious disease was the cause of the fever in 12 patients (16%); a neoplasm in five patients (7%); noninfectious inflammatory diseases in 16 patients (22%); and miscellaneous causes in three patients (4%). The cause of fever was not found in 51% of cases.

Table 4 lists the diagnosis of FUO in elderly patients (more than 65 years old) compared with the diagnosis in younger patients in the study [10]. Noninfectious inflammatory diseases, such as giant cell arteritis and polymyalgia rheumatica, account for 36.1% of causes in elderly patients. It is noteworthy that giant cell arteritis and polymyalgia rheumatica are, nowadays, one of the most common causes of FUO in the elderly. Other studies have shown a high prevalence of giant cell arteritis and polymyalgia rheumatica among patients with FUO [11–13]. In younger patients, adult-onset Still's disease is not an uncommon etiology.

Table 1
Comparison of the diagnostic categories in major series of FUO reported in the literature

| Author, publication date, study period, country | No. of patients | No diagnosis No. (%) | Diagnosis No. (%) | Diagnostic categories (% of diagnosed cases) | | | |
|---|---|---|---|---|---|---|---|
| | | | | Infections | Neoplasms | Inflammatory | Miscellaneous |
| *Fuo Criteria of Peterson and Beeson* | | | | | | | |
| Petersdof and Beeson [2] 1952–1957 United States | 100 | 9 (9) | 91 (91) | 39.6 | 20.9 | 18.7 | 20.9 |
| Larson et al [45] 1970–1980 United States | 105 | 17 (16.2) | 88 (83.8) | 36.4 | 37.5 | 14.8 | 11.4 |
| Barbado et al [46] 1968–1981 Spain | 133 | 29 (21.8) | 104 (78.2) | 39.4 | 25 | 19.2 | 16.3 |
| Knockaert et al [11] 1980–1989 Belgium | 199 | 51 (25.6) | 148 (74.4) | 30.4 | 9.5 | 31.1 | 29.1 |
| Likuni et al [47] 1982–1992 Japan | 153 | 18 (11.8) | 135 (88.2) | 32.6 | 16.3 | 34.8 | 16.3 |
| De Kleijn et al [5,7] 1992–1994 Netherlands | 167 | 52 (31.1) | 115 (68.9) | 37.4 | 18.3 | 33 | 11.3 |
| Tabak et al [8] 1984–2001 Turkey | 117 | 16 (13.7) | 101 (86.3) | 39.6 | 21.8 | 28.7 | 9.9 |
| *Fuo Criteria of Durack and Street* | | | | | | | |
| Vanderschueren et al [12] 1991–1999 Belgium | 223 | 98 (43.9) | 125 (56.1) | 25.6 | 19.2 | 36.8 | 18.4 |
| Zenone [10] 1999–2005 France | 144 | 37 (25.7) | 107 (74.3) | 30.8 | 13.1 | 35.5 | 20.6 |

*Adapted from* Zenone T. Fever of unknown origin in adults: evaluation of 144 cases in a non-university hospital. Scand J Infect Dis 2006;38:625–31; with permission.

Table 2
Diagnostic categories in a study of 144 patients with FUO

| Categories | No. of patients (%) | |
|---|---|---|
| Infections | 33 (22.9) | |
| Neoplasms | 14 (9.7) with diagnosis | 79.3% |
| Noninfectious inflammatory diseases (74.3%) | 38 (26.4) 107 | |
| Miscellaneous | 22 (15.3) | |
| Undiagnosed | 37 (25.7) | |

*Adapted from* Zenone T. Fever of unknown origin in adults: evaluation of 144 cases in a non-university hospital. Scand J Infect Dis 2006;38:625–31; with permission.

Although reported causes of FUO exceed 200 [14], a limited list of disorders accounted for most diagnoses. Petersdorf and Beeson [2] have already emphasized that most patients with FUO are not experiencing unusual diseases, but rather exhibit atypical manifestations of common illnesses.

## Vasculitis

### *Giant cell arteritis and polymyalgia rheumatica*

Giant cell arteritis and polymyalgia rheumatica are closely related conditions that affect individuals of middle age and older and frequently occur together [15–17]. Polymyalgia rheumatica is a common illness; giant cell arteritis is less frequent [16].

Polymyalgia rheumatica is an inflammatory condition of unknown cause characterized by aching and morning stiffness in the cervical region and

Table 3
Noninfectious inflammatory diseases as a cause of FUO in a study of 144 patients

| Diseases (Total no. of patients) | No. of patients |
|---|---|
| Connective tissue diseases (11) | |
| Adult-onset Still's disease | 4 |
| Rheumatoid arthritis | 4 |
| Systemic lupus erythematosus | 3 |
| Vasculitis syndromes (24) | |
| Giant cell arteritis and polymyalgia rheumatica | 18 |
| Polyarteritis nodosa | 3 |
| Behçet's disease | 1 |
| Henoch-Schönlein purpura | 1 |
| unclassified vasculitis | 1 |
| Granulomatous disorders (3) | |
| Sarcoidosis | 2 |
| Crohn's disease | 1 |
| Total (38) | |

*Adapted from* Zenone T. Fever of unknown origin in adults: evaluation of 144 cases in a non-university hospital. Scand J Infect Dis 2006;38:625–31; with permission.

Table 4
Diagnosis of FUO in elderly patients (more than 65 years old) compared with the diagnosis in younger patients in a study of 144 patients

| Diagnoses | Elderly (N = 61) | Young (N = 83) |
|---|---|---|
| Infections | 9 (14.8%) | 24 (28.9%) |
| Neoplasms | 9 (14.8%) | 5 (6%) |
| Noninfectious inflammatory diseases | 22 (36.1%) | 16 (19.3%) |
| Miscellaneous | 3 (4.9%) | 19 (22.9%) |
| Undiagnosed | 18 (29.5%) | 19 (22.9%) |

*Adapted from* Zenone T. Fever of unknown origin in adults: evaluation of 144 cases in a non-university hospital. Scand J Infect Dis 2006;38:625–31; with permission.

shoulder and pelvic girdles. Diagnostic criteria of Chuang and coworkers [18] and Healey [19] are presented in Box 1. The musculoskeletal pain worsens with the movements of the affected area and typically interferes with usual daily activities. Systemic symptoms and signs are present in approximately one third of patients and include fever, malaise or fatigue,

---

**Box 1. Sets of diagnostic criteria for polymyalgia rheumatica**

*Criteria of Chuang and coworkers[a]*
- Age of 50 years or older
- Bilateral aching and stiffness for 1 month or more and involving two of the following areas: neck or torso, shoulders or proximal regions of the arms, and hips or proximal aspects of the thighs
- Erythrocyte sedimentation rate greater than 40 mm/h
- Exclusion of all other diagnoses except giant cell arteritis

*Criteria of Healey[a]*
- Pain persisting for at least 1 month and involving two of the following areas: neck, shoulders, and pelvic girdle
- Morning stiffness lasting more than 1 hour
- Rapid response to prednisone (<20 mg/day)
- Absence of other diseases capable of causing the musculoskeletal symptoms
- Age of more than 50 years
- Erythrocyte sedimentation rate greater than 40 mm/h

---

[a] All the findings must be present for polymyalgia rheumatica to be diagnosed.
*Data from* Chuang TY, Hunder GG, Ilstrup DM, et al. Polymyalgia rheumatica: a 10-year epidemiologic and clinical study. Ann Intern Med 1982;97:672–80; and Healey LA. Long-term follow-up of polymyalgia rheumatica: evidence for synovitis. Semin Arthritis Rheum 1984;13:322–8.

anorexia, and weight loss [15,16,20]. Ultrasonography and MRI of the shoulders (subacromial and subdeltoid bursitis) are sometimes useful to confirm the diagnosis in patients with atypical symptoms [16]. Whereas the diagnosis of giant cell arteritis can be proved by temporal artery biopsy, however, no pathognomonic test is currently available for polymyalgia rheumatica [21]. It usually responds rapidly to low doses of corticosteroids and has a favorable prognosis [16].

Giant cell arteritis is a chronic vasculitis of large and medium-sized vessels. Although it may be widespread, symptomatic vessel inflammation usually involves the cranial branches of the arteries originating from the aortic arch [16]. Criteria for the classification of giant cell arteritis as formulated by the American College of Rheumatology are presented in Box 2 [22]. The most frequent symptoms are headache, scalp tenderness, and jaw claudication [16,21]. On physical examination, the superficial temporal arteries may be thickened, nodular, tender, or erythematous. Pulses may be decreased or absent [16]. Physicians need to be familiar with the typical manifestations of giant cell arteritis. The challenge, however, lies in recognizing atypical cases that lack the more specific manifestations or reflect vasculitis in less frequently involved territories [21]: peripheral neuropathy, transient ischemic attack and stroke, and dry cough [16,20,23,24]. Polymyalgia rheumatica occurs in 40% of patients with giant cell arteritis; peripheral arthritis and pitting edema of the hands and feet may occur [16]. Visual loss is the main complication caused by ischemia of the optic nerve [16,21].

Systemic symptoms are present in about half of patients. Although the fever is usually low grade, it can reach 39°C to 40°C and may be the

---

**Box 2. The American College of Rheumatology criteria for the classification of giant cell arteritis**

- Onset of disease at the age of 50 years or older
- New headache
- Temporal arteries abnormalities (tenderness to palpation or decreased pulsation)
- Erythrocyte sedimentation rate >50 mm/h
- Abnormal findings on temporal artery biopsy (vasculitis characterized by a predominance of mononuclear infiltrates or granulomas, usually with multinucleated giant cells)

---

A patient with vasculitis is said to have giant cell arteritis if at least three of these five criteria are met. These criteria are not useful for making the diagnosis in individual patients.

*Data from* Hunder GG, Bloch DA, Michel BA, et al. The American College of Rheumatology 1990 criteria for the classification of giant cell arteritis. Arthritis Rheum 1990;33:1122–8.

presenting clinical manifestation [16,25]. In the study conducted by Gonzales-Gay and colleagues [26], 10% of the 210 biopsy-proved giant cell arteritis patients had fever. Two of them fulfilled criteria of FUO. Sometimes, the systemic inflammatory syndrome (without manifestations of tissue ischemia) dominates clinical manifestations [21,27]. In these cases, FUO and a wasting syndrome with progressive weight loss, sweats, and anorexia are the presenting symptoms [21,25,27].

Acute-phase proteins are useful markers in giant cell arteritis and polymyalgia rheumatica [20,21]. Elevated erythrocyte sedimentation rate and C-reactive protein are seen in most patients [20,21]. The finding of a normal erythrocyte sedimentation rate, however, is not incompatible with the diagnosis of polymyalgia rheumatica and giant cell arteritis when other clinical findings suggest these diagnoses [15,16,21]. Most patients have anemia of chronic disease; thrombocytosis; and sometimes abnormal liver-function tests (particularly elevation of alkaline phosphatase levels) [21]. Tests for rheumatoid factor and antinuclear antibodies (ANA) are usually negative [15,16].

When giant cell arteritis is suspected, temporal artery biopsy is the diagnosis procedure of choice, even in the absence of arterial tenderness or nodularity [16,21,28]. The inflammatory involvement of arteries is intermittent rather than continuous, however, and 10% of patients with giant cell arteritis have negative findings on biopsy [16]. Because treatment involves prolonged courses of corticosteroid therapy, it is important to confirm the diagnosis with a biopsy [20]. Long biopsy specimens (> 2 cm) of the temporal artery, serial sectioning, and experienced pathologic assessment improve diagnostic yield [20,28].

Formerly considered an infrequent pattern of giant cell arteritis, large-vessel arteritis affecting the branches of the aortic arch, particularly the subclavian and axillary arteries, is increasingly recognized. Aortic involvement (aortitis) has been estimated to occur in 10% to 15% of patients [21]. These patients may have few of the usual symptoms of giant cell arteritis, so the diagnosis may be initially overlooked [16]. If a diagnosis of extracranial giant cell arteritis is suspected, ultrasonography, arteriography, CT, and MRI angiography are the required diagnostic tests [16]. The diagnosis of large-vessel arteritis is made by vascular imaging and not by biopsy [21]. 18 F-fluorodeoxyglucose positron emission tomography (FDG-PET) is not suitable for use in evaluation of the temporal arteries because of their small size, but it may be useful to demonstrate large-vessel inflammation, such as aortitis, in these patients [20].

Corticosteroids are the drug of choice to treat giant cell arteritis, and the response is rapid [17,20]. A lack of improvement should alert physicians to question the diagnosis [16]. The mortality rate in patients with giant cell arteritis is similar to that expected in general populations, although thoracic aortic aneurysms and dissection of the aorta are important late complications [16,17].

## Polyarteritis nodosa

Polyarteritis nodosa is a necrotizing vasculitis of the medium and small vessels. This commonly presents as a syndrome of multiorgan involvement (consequence of infarction and ischemia), on the background of constitutional upset (fever, malaise, weight loss). Peripheral neuropathy (mononeuritis multiplex) and symptoms from osteoarticular, renal artery, and gastrointestinal tract involvement are the most frequent manifestations [29]. Criteria for the classification of polyarteritis nodosa as formulated by the American College of Rheumatology are presented in Box 3 [30]. A clear distinction between limited versus systemic disease and idiopathic versus hepatitis B–related polyarteritis nodosa should be done because there are differences in treatment and prognosis [29]. Angiography of either the gastrointestinal tract or kidneys characteristically shows multiple aneurysms and irregular constrictions of vessels. A tissue biopsy of affected areas is the gold standard diagnostic test (necrotic inflammation of the medium-sized arteries). Polyarteritis nodosa can present initially as FUO [31]. In the author's study, it was the cause of FUO in three cases (see Table 3) [10].

## Behçet's disease

Behçet's disease can rarely cause FUO, mainly periodic fever [32]. This systemic vasculitis of unknown etiology is defined by the triad of oral

---

**Box 3. The American College of Rheumatology criteria for the classification of polyarteritis nodosa**

- Weight loss >4 kg
- Livedo reticularis
- Testicular pain or tenderness
- Myalgias, weakness, or leg tenderness
- Diastolic blood pressure >90 mm Hg
- Elevated blood urea nitrogen or creatinine levels
- Hepatitis B antigenemia
- Arteriography abnormality not resulting from atherosclerosis, fibromuscular dysplasia, or other noninflammatory causes
- Biopsy specimens of small or medium muscular artery showing granulocytes or mononuclear leukocytes in the artery wall

---

A patient with vasculitis is said to have polyarteritis nodosa if at least three of these criteria are met. These criteria are not useful for making the diagnosis in individual patients.

*Data from* Lightfoot RW, Michel BA, Bloch DA, et al. The American College of Rheumatology 1990 criteria for classification of polyarteritis nodosa. Arthritis Rheum 1990;33:1088–93.

ulceration, genital ulceration, and uveitis. Other manifestations include skin lesions, arthritis, venous thrombosis, artery aneurysm, and central nervous system involvement.

*Antineutrophil cytoplasmic antibody–associated vasculitis: Wegener's granulomatosis, microscopic polyangiitis, and Churg-Strauss syndrome*

Antineutrophil cytoplasmic antibody (ANCA)–associated vasculitis can be difficult to diagnose even for the most experienced of clinicians given the multifaceted and variable presentations, the overlap of signs and symptoms with much more common entities, and the low frequency of vasculitis in the general population [33]. Constitutional signs and symptoms, such as fever, myalgias, arthralgias, and malaise, often accompany small-vessel vasculitis. Many patients describe a flulike syndrome early in the course of their disease [34]. Main clinical scenarios suggestive of vasculitis in case of FUO are listed next.

Diffuse alveolar hemorrhage (diffuse alveolar infiltrates, hemoptysis, drop in hemoglobin level)
Acute glomerulonephritis (hematuria, proteinuria, renal insufficiency, edema, hypertension)
Deforming or ulcerating upper airway lesions (refractory chronic sinusitis)
Cavitary or nodular disease on chest imaging
Purpura (small-vessel leukocytoclastic cutaneous vasculitis)
Mononeuritis multiplex (sudden onset of a foot drop or wrist drop, paresthesias)

Wegener's granulomatosis, the most common ANCA-associated vasculitis, is clinically characterized by the triad of upper airway involvement (sinusitis, otitis, ulcerations); lower respiratory tract involvement (cough, chest pain, hemoptysis, shortness of breath); and glomerulonephritis [33]. Churg-Strauss syndrome is characterized by asthma and hypereosinophilia [33]; it is not a classic cause of FUO. Microscopic polyangiitis is often heralded by a long prodromal phase that is characterized by profound constitutional symptoms followed by the development of rapidly progressive glomerulonephritis [33,35].

ANCA has developed a prominent role in the diagnosis of small-vessel vasculitis. The following two distinct staining patterns have been described (indirect immunofluorescence): cytoplasmic ANCA, and perinuclear ANCA. Cytoplasmic ANCA has been shown primarily to recognize the enzyme proteinase 3, and the presence suggests a diagnosis of Wegener's granulomatosis. Perinuclear ANCA has been showed to interact most commonly with myeloperoxidase in case of microscopic polyangiitis or Churg-Strauss syndrome [33]. Anti-proteinase 3 and antimyeloperoxidase are demonstrated by ELISA.

## Takayasu's arteritis

Granulomatous arteritis can occur in individuals younger than 40 years of age (predominantly female). In contrast to giant cell arteritis, Takayasu's arteritis primarily targets the aorta and its proximal branches. The systemic, prepulseless, phase presents as fever, fatigue, weight loss, night sweats, arthralgias, and myalgias. It has been rarely described as a cause of FUO [36].

## Henoch-Schönlein purpura

Henoch-Schönlein purpura is most frequent in childhood. Purpura, arthralgias, and abdominal pain are the most frequent manifestations. Approximately half the patients have hematuria and proteinuria [34]. It has been rarely described as a cause of FUO [1,10].

## Cryoglobulinemic vasculitis

Cryoglobulinemic vasculitis is caused by the localization of mixed cryoglobulins in vessel walls, which incites acute inflammation. Patients have an average age of approximately 50 years. The most frequent manifestations are purpura, arthralgias, and nephritis. Mixed cryoglobulins and rheumatoid factor activity are typically detected in the serum. Most patients have an associated infection with hepatitis C virus [34]. Five cases of mixed cryoglobulinemia are reported in the study of 167 patients with FUO of De Kleijn and colleagues [5].

## Relapsing polychondritis

Relapsing polychondritis is a rare disease most commonly presenting as inflammation of the cartilage of the ears and nose. Auricular chondritis, with red ears resembling infectious cellulitis, is the most common initial finding; the earlobes are classically spared. It is frequently associated with fever; however, it is a rare cause of FUO. Chronic disease may result in a flabby, droopy ear; cauliflower ear; or saddle nose deformity. Acute involvement of the tracheal cartilage may cause collapse of the airway with obstruction and pulmonary infections. Arthritis may be oligoarticular or polyarticular, most often involving the costochondral junctions. Other manifestations include audiovestibular damage; heart valve disease; and neurologic or ocular involvement [37].

## Connective tissue diseases

### Adult-onset Still's disease

Adult-onset Still's disease is a systemic inflammatory disorder of unknown etiology, characterized by quotidian or double-quotidian high-spiking fevers with an evanescent rash, arthritis, and multiorgan involvement. It characteristically affects young people, with three quarters of the patients reporting disease onset between 16 and 35 years of age. Several cases, however, have been reported after the age of 60 [38].

Fever generally exceeds 39°C and is transient, typically lasting under 4 hours, with the highest temperatures seen in the late afternoon or the early evening. The typical rash is an evanescent, salmon-pink, maculopapular eruption, predominantly found on the proximal limbs and trunk [38]. The rash is seen during the fever spike and disappears when body temperature returns to normal [39]. Most patients have arthralgias or arthritis, typically symmetric. Joints affected most frequently are the knees, wrists, and ankles. Other common manifestations include sore throat, lymphadenopathy, splenomegaly, and myalgias. Liver abnormalities, predominantly hepato-megaly and abnormalities in liver biochemistry, are also frequent. Less common manifestations include pleuritis and pericarditis [38].

The erythrocyte sedimentation rate and C-reactive protein are raised. Common hematologic abnormalities include leukocytosis with neutrophilia, anemia of chronic disease, and reactive thrombocytosis. Pancytopenia should alert the physician to the presence of hemophagocytic syndrome [38]. Ferritin levels are usually high (> 1000 ng/mL) [40]. Very high levels ranging from 4000 to 30 000 ng/mL are not uncommon. A more specific di-agnostic marker than ferritin may be its glycosylated fraction. In adult-onset Still's disease, the glycosylated fraction of ferritin is often less than 20% [38]. The quantification of glycosylated ferritin is not available, however, in all centers [41]. Adult-onset Still's disease is not associated with rheumatoid factor or ANA [38]. The diagnosis of adult-onset Still's disease remains a clinical one. Seven sets of classification criteria have been proposed [41]. Yamaguchi criteria [42] and Fautrel criteria [43] are presented in Box 4.

Nonsteroidal anti-inflammatory drugs have limited efficacy; corticoste-roid therapy and disease-modifying antirheumatic drugs (mainly methotrex-ate) are usually required. Intravenous gamma globulin and anticytokine are also used in refractory cases [38,44].

Adult-onset Still's disease is a rare disease; however, according to major series of FUO published in the literature [2,5,10,11,45–48], it is not an un-common etiology among the connective tissue diseases category. Among the 130 patients with FUO, 20 had adult-onset Still's disease in the study of Mert and colleagues [39]. Rapid diagnosis of adult-onset Still's disease is frequently difficult because of nonspecific clinical and laboratory features. It is the most important noninfectious inflammatory disease closely to mimic infectious ones [39]. In the study of Mert and colleagues [39], most of the patients were given several antibiotics with presumed diagnoses of strepto-coccal pharyngitis, endocarditis, or sepsis. In a patient with FUO, an eva-nescent maculopapular rash observed with the fever spike, associated with arthralgia and sore throat, should raise the suspicion of adult-onset Still's disease [39]. In clinical practice, adult-onset Still's disease is usually

---

**Box 4. Sets of diagnostic criteria for adult-onset Still's disease**

*Criteria of Yamaguchi and colleagues[a]*
Major criteria
- Arthralgia >2 weeks
- Fever >39°C, intermittent, >1 week
- Typical rash
- Leucocytes >10,000 (>80% granulocytes)

Minor criteria
- Sore throat
- Lymphadenopathy or splenomegaly
- Liver function test abnormalities
- Negative rheumatoid factor and ANA

Exclusion criteria
- Infections
- Malignancies
- Rheumatic diseases

*Criteria of Fautrel and colleagues[b]*
Major criteria
- Spiking fever >39°C
- Arthralgia
- Transient erythema
- Pharyngitis
- Granulocytes >80%
- Glycosylated ferritin <20%

Minor criteria
- Maculopapular rash
- Leucocytes >10,000

---

[a] Diagnosis of adult-onset Still's disease: five criteria (at least two major).
[b] Diagnosis of adult-onset Still's disease: four major criteria or three major plus two minor.

*Data from* Yamaguchi M, Ohta A, Tsunematsu T, et al. Preliminary criteria for classification of adult Still's disease. J Rheumatol 1992;19:424–30; and Fautrel B, Zing E, Golmard JL, et al. Proposal for a new set of classification criteria for adult-onset Still disease. Medicine 2002;81:194–200.

---

considered a diagnosis of exclusion, particularly when it presents as FUO. Recently, Crispin and colleagues [41] designed a clinical scale that can be applied to patients with FUO to identify the subset of patients that can be diagnosed as having adult-onset Still's disease without further long and costly diagnostic work-up (Table 5). The clinical scale had a sensitivity of 76.9% and a specificity of 98%. The score can be calculated for a patient with FUO as soon as he or she is admitted [41].

Table 5
Clinical scale for the diagnosis of adult-onset Still's disease in the setting of FUO

| Criterion | Description | Points |
|---|---|---|
| Arthritis | Presence of synovitis | 10 |
| Pharyngitis | Present during the beginning of the disease | 7 |
| Rash | Macular or maculopapular pink-salmon nonpruriginous rash that accompanies the fever | 5 |
| Splenomegaly | Detected clinically or by imaging studies (> 11 cm) | 5 |
| Neutrophilia | Total neutrophil count > 9500 | 18 |

If a patient with FUO has 30 points or more, the diagnosis can be established without further diagnostic work-up, with a high specificity (98%).

*Data from* Crispin JC, Martinez-Banos D, Alcocer-Varela J. Adult-onset Still disease as the cause of fever of unknown origin. Medicine 2005;84:331–7.

## Systemic lupus erythematosus

Systemic lupus erythematosus is a multisystem, autoimmune, connective-tissue disorder with a broad range of clinical presentations. There is a peak age of onset in young women between their late teens and early 40s and a female/male ratio of 9:1 [49]. Polyarthritis and dermatitis (photosensitive skin rash) are the most common clinical manifestations of systemic lupus erythematosus, and the most common presenting symptoms. Any symptom or sign of the disease may be its first manifestation, however, and a single one, such as arthritis, thrombocytopenia, or pericarditis, may persist or recur for months or years before the diagnosis can be confirmed by the appearance of other features [50]. Chronic fatigue and low-grade fever are frequent in cases of lupus flare [51]. The American College of Rheumatology criteria for the classification of systemic lupus erythematosus are presented in Box 5 [52].

Common hematologic abnormalities include anemia, neutropenia, leucopenia, lymphopenia, and thrombocytopenia. Raised erythrocyte sedimentation rate with a normal C-reactive protein (or < 30 mg/L) is seen in most patients. C-reactive protein may be elevated, however, in patients with serositis or erosive arthritis. Because it is not very specific, a positive test for ANA is of limited value in support of an uncertain diagnosis, although strongly positive tests for antibody to Sm or native DNA carry more weight [50].

Antiphospholipid syndrome is defined as the occurrence of thrombosis, recurrent miscarriages, or both in association with laboratory evidence of persistent antiphospholipid antibodies (IgG or IgM anticardiolipin antibodies, lupus anticoagulant, false-positive serologic test for syphilis). Primary antiphospholipid syndrome occurs in patients without clinical evidence of another autoimmune disease, whereas secondary antiphospholipid syndrome occurs in association with autoimmune diseases, mainly systemic lupus erythematosus. Because symptoms of thrombosis are

---

**Box 5. The revised criteria of the American College of Rheumatology for the classification of systemic lupus erythematosus**

1. Malar rash
2. Discoid rash
3. Photosensitivity
4. Oral ulcers
5. Arthritis
6. Serositis
   a. Pleuritis
   b. Pericarditis
7. Renal disorder
   a. Proteinuria >0.5 g/24 h, or 3+, persistently
   b. Cellular casts
8. Neurologic disorder
   a. Seizures
   b. Psychosis
9. Hematologic disorders
   a. Hemolytic anemia
   b. Leucopenia
   c. Lymphopenia
   d. Thrombocytopenia
10. Immunologic disorders
    a. Raised anti-native DNA antibody binding
    b. Anti-Sm antibody
    c. Positive finding of antiphospholipid antibodies
11. ANA in raised titer

---

A patient is said to have systemic lupus erythematosus if at least 4 of the 11 criteria are met.

*Data from* Hochberg M. Updating the American College of Rheumatology revised criteria for classification of Systemic Lupus erythematosus. Arthritis Rheum 1997;40:1725–34.

---

predominant, prolonged fever is not usually the main clinical finding; antiphospholipid syndrome has been rarely described as a cause of FUO [53].

Kikuchi-Fujimoto disease is a necrotizing lymphadenitis. It usually affects the cervical lymph nodes in young women and has a self-limiting clinical course. This entity of uncertain etiology is sometimes associated with systemic lupus erythematosus. Kikuchi-Fujimoto disease can present as FUO [54].

## Rheumatoid arthritis

Rheumatoid arthritis is a chronic disorder whose main clinical manifestation is a symmetric polyarthritis. Fever is rare [51]. Fever is more frequently described in the case of rheumatoid vasculitis or Felty's syndrome (splenomegaly with lymphadenopathy, fever, and susceptibility to bacterial infections caused by neutropenia).

## Others

### Spondyloarthropathies

Ankylosing spondylitis and psoriatic arthritis are rarely described as a cause of FUO [1,51,55,56].

### Polymyositis

The idiopathic inflammatory myopathies (polymyositis and dermatomyositis) are characterized clinically by proximal muscle weakness and myalgias. General symptoms include fever, malaise, weight loss, and arthralgia [57]. Idiopathic inflammatory myopathies are a rare cause of FUO [51].

### Sjögren's syndrome

Sjögren's syndrome is a common inflammatory autoimmune disorder characterized by lymphocytic infiltration and destruction of exocrine glands, notably the lacrimal and salivary glands giving rise to dry eyes and dry mouth. The diagnosis is established by the characteristic signs with evidence of autoantibodies (anti-SSA/Ro and anti-SSB/La) and extensive lymphocytic infiltration on minor salivary gland biopsy. Fever is rare [51].

## Granulomatous disorders

### Sarcoidosis

Sarcoidosis is a multisystem disease of unknown etiology. Diagnosis is based on a compatible clinical presentation, supportive histologic evidence of noncaseating granulomas, and exclusion of other granulomatous diseases. The lungs are involved in over 90% of cases. Extrathoracic manifestations most commonly involve skin, eye, reticuloendothelial system, liver, and joints [58]. Occasionally, sarcoidosis can present as the diagnostically challenging patient with a FUO [59]. In the case of Löfgren's syndrome (arthralgia or arthritis, erythema nodosum, mediastinal lymphadenopathy) or Heerfordt's syndrome (uveitis, enlargement of the parotid glands, facial nerve palsy), fever is more frequent [51].

### Crohn's disease

Crohn's disease can cause FUO, mainly periodic fever [51].

## Miscellaneous

Habitual hyperthermia is sometimes associated with chronic fatigue syndrome or fibromyalgia [6,10]. Usually, it occurs in young women with low-grade fever (temperature usually does not rise >38.3°C; however, it can rise after physical or intellectual exertion) and without signs of inflammation [6]. In these women, progestogen component of oral contraceptive agents may induce a slight increase in body temperature, comparable with the minimal rise in body temperature during the second half of the menstrual cycle [10].

Another category of syndromes that may mimic the manifestations of rheumatic diseases in case of FUO are the hereditary periodic fever syndromes. Patients with familial Mediterranean fever often present with acute, self-limited episodes of fever accompanied by signs of peritonitis; pleuritis; or acute synovitis, mainly of the knee, ankle, wrist, or hip. Erysipelas-like erythema can accompany the fever, which usually lasts for 1 to 3 days. The disease often starts in childhood or early adolescence. A significant family history (including ethnic background) and response to colchicine can direct the clinician toward the correct diagnosis, which can be verified, in many cases, with genetic analysis for the *MEFV* gene [60]. Tumor necrosis factor receptor–associated periodic syndrome commonly starts in childhood and also has a strong familial distribution. Fever attacks last longer and are associated with ocular involvement, localized myalgia, and painful erythema. Arthralgia of large joints is common but arthritis is rare [60]. Hyper-IgD syndrome almost always develops in infancy. Cervical lymphadenopathy almost always accompanies the attack of fever. Arthralgias and arthritis of large joints are less common [60].

## Diagnostic work-up and diagnostic strategy

The differential diagnosis of FUO is the most extensive in medicine, and construction of algorithms covering all possible causes is difficult [1]. After a comprehensive history review, complete physical examination (including temporal arteries), a series of obligatory investigations are performed for each patient in a search for potentially diagnostic clues [1,5,10]. Initial diagnostic evaluation includes the following:

Erythrocyte sedimentation rate and C-reactive protein
Complete blood count including differential
Creatinine and electrolytes
Alkaline phosphatase, aspartate aminotransferase, alanine aminotransferase
Creatine phosphokinase, lactate dehydrogenase, ferritin
Protein electrophoresis
ANAs, rheumatoid factors
Microscopic urinalysis

Cultures of blood and urine (and other compartments if clinically indicated)
Chest radiography
Abdominal and pelvic ultrasonography

Potentially diagnostic clues are defined as all localizing signs, symptoms, and abnormalities potentially pointing toward a diagnosis [1,5]: weight loss, muscle weakness, skin changes, shortness of breath, chest or abdominal pain, arthralgia, morning stiffness, headache, abnormal urinalysis, abnormal chest radiograph, and so forth. With the help of the potentially diagnostic clues, a limited list of probable diagnoses is made and further diagnostic procedures are indicated, guided by this list [1]. It can also be used for rheumatic diseases: complements (C3, C4, CH50); cryoglobulins; ANCA; skin biopsy in case of skin changes; temporal artery biopsy in patients older than 55 years; chest and abdominal CT scan; renal biopsy in the setting of acute glomerulonephritis; and FDG-PET. Depending on the clinical scenario, additional rheumatologic serologies may also be useful, including the following: anticyclic citrullinated peptide for rheumatoid arthritis, anti-SSA/Ro and anti-SSB/La for systemic lupus erythematosus and Sjögren's syndrome, anti-native DNA for systemic lupus erythematosus, anti-JO1 for polymyositis, anticardiolipin antibody, and lupus anticoagulant for primary antiphospholipid syndrome.

In the study of FUO conducted by Bleeker-Rovers and colleagues [1], the presence of ANA was helpful in diagnosing systemic lupus erythematosus in all four patients diagnosed with this disease, but showed false-positive results in eight patients. In one patient with microscopic polyangiitis, the presence of ANCA was helpful, whereas ANCA was also present in five patients without vasculitis. The diagnostic yield of immunologic serology is relatively low in the case of FUO; ANA and ANCA are more often false-positive and are of little use without potentially diagnostic clues pointing to specific immunologic disorders [1]. As with any test, the predictive value of these assays depends on the prevalence of the disease in the patient population tested and the sensitivity and specificity of the test. False-positive testing may occur with infections.

Temporal artery biopsy is part of the routine approach in elderly patients with FUO [6,10,61]. In the study conducted by Bleeker-Rovers and colleagues [1], however, temporal artery biopsy was performed in 14 patients, but was useful to confirm the diagnosis of giant cell arteritis in only one patient, in whom FDG-PET already pointed large-vessel vasculitis. Temporal artery biopsy can be recommended for patients aged 55 years or older, however, because FDG-PET is not useful if the vasculitis is limited to the temporal arteries because of the small diameter of these vessels and high FDG uptake in the overlying brain. Sometimes, other types of vasculitis are found in the temporal artery. Fibrinoid necrosis, rarely encountered in giant cell arteritis, is a helpful clue to consider polyarteritis nodosa or an ANCA-related vasculitis [21,62].

In patients with FUO in relation with noninfectious inflammatory diseases, FDG-PET is of importance in the diagnosis of large-vessel vasculitis and seems to be useful in the visualization of other diseases, such as inflammatory bowel disease and sarcoidosis [63].

Diagnoses lacking persuasive confirmatory tests (eg, adult-onset Still's disease and polymyalgia rheumatica) are accepted only if sufficient standard criteria are met and follow-up allowed exclusion of other diseases.

## Empiric therapeutic

If the fever persists and the source remains elusive, supportive treatment with nonsteroidal anti-inflammatory drugs can be helpful in case of suspicion of rheumatic disease. Empirical therapeutic trials with steroids should be avoided, except in patients whose condition is deteriorating. The response to therapy is seldom proof of a single disease, because many undiagnosed FUO patients experience spontaneous resolution of fever [6]. A rapid response to corticosteroids is of high value in case of suspicion of giant cell arteritis or polymyalgia rheumatica.

## Summary

FUO remains one of the most difficult challenges facing the physician. The long list of more than 200 disorders encompasses both rare diseases and, more frequently, more common diseases that initially remain undiagnosed because of atypical presentation. In the future, the use of a qualitative criterion for FUO (the quality of the investigations counts, rather than an arbitrary number of investigational days or outpatient visits) will decrease the bias in series caused by individual experience of the investigators and the differences in diagnostic facilities between hospitals and countries.

Noninfectious inflammatory diseases emerged as the most frequent cause of FUO, particularly in the elderly. The number of patients eventually diagnosed with noninfectious inflammatory diseases will probably not decrease in the near future, because fever may precede more typical manifestations or serologic evidence by months in these diseases and many of noninfectious inflammatory diseases can only be diagnosed after prolonged observation and exclusion of other diseases. Among noninfectious inflammatory diseases, giant cell arteritis is the most frequent specific diagnosis in the elderly and adult-onset Still's disease the most frequent in younger patients.

## Acknowledgment

The author thanks Rawan Ghadban for her reviews and comments.

# References

[1] Bleeker-Rovers CP, Vos FJ, de Kleijn EMHA, et al. A prospective multicenter study on fever of unknown origin: the yield of a structured diagnostic protocol. Medicine 2007;86:26–38.

[2] Petersdorf RG, Beeson PB. Fever of unexplained origin: report on 100 cases. Medicine 1961; 40:1–30.

[3] Durack DT, Street AC. Fever of unknown origin: reexamined and redefined. Curr Clin Top Infect Dis 1991;11:35–51.

[4] Petersdorf RG. Fever of unknown origin: an old friend revisited. Arch Intern Med 1992;152: 21–2.

[5] De Kleijn EMH, Vandenbroucke JP, Van der Meer JWM. Fever of unknown origin (FUO) I: a prospective multicenter study of 167 patients with FUO, using fixed epidemiologic entry criteria. Medicine 1997;76:392–400.

[6] Knockaert DC, Vanderschueren S, Blockmans D. Fever of unknown origin in adults: 40 years on. J Intern Med 2003;253:263–75.

[7] De Kleijn EMH, Vandenbroucke JP, Van der Meer JWM. Fever of unknown origin (FUO) II: diagnostic procedures in a prospective multicenter study in 167 patients. Medicine 1997; 76:401–14.

[8] Tabak F, Mert A, Celik AD, et al. Fever of unknown origin in Turkey. Infection 2003;31: 417–20.

[9] Barbado FJ, Vasquez JJ, Pena JM, et al. Pyrexia of unknown origin: changing spectrum of diseases in two consecutive series. Postgrad Med J 1992;68:884–7.

[10] Zenone T. Fever of unknown origin in adults: evaluation of 144 cases in a non-university hospital. Scand J Infect Dis 2006;38:625–31.

[11] Knockaert DC, Vanneste LJ, Vanneste SB, et al. Fever of unknown origin in the 1980's: an update of the diagnostic spectrum. Arch Intern Med 1992;152:51–5.

[12] Vanderschueren S, Knockaert D, Adriaenssens T, et al. From prolonged febrile illness to fever of unknown origin: the challenge continues. Arch Intern Med 2003;163:1033–41.

[13] Knockaert DC, Vanneste LJ, Bobbaers HJ. Fever of unknown origin in elderly patients. J Am Geriatr Soc 1993;41:1187–92.

[14] Arnow PM, Flaherty JP. Fever of unknown origin. Lancet 1997;350:575–80.

[15] Salvarani C, Macchioni P, Boiardi L. Polymyalgia rheumatica. Lancet 1997;350:43–7.

[16] Salvarani C, Cantini F, Boiardi L, et al. Polymyalgia rheumatica and giant-cell arteritis. N Engl J Med 2002;24(4):261–71.

[17] Nordborg E, Nordborg C. Giant cell arteritis: epidemiological clues to its pathogenesis and an update on its treatment. Rheumatology 2003;42:413–21.

[18] Chuang TY, Hunder GG, Ilstrup DM, et al. Polymyalgia rheumatica: a 10-year epidemiologic and clinical study. Ann Intern Med 1982;97:672–80.

[19] Healey LA. Long-term follow-up of polymyalgia rheumatica: evidence for synovitis. Semin Arthritis Rheum 1984;13:322–8.

[20] Unwin B, Williams CM, Gillilland W. Polymyalgia rheumatica and giant cell arteritis. Am Fam Physician 2006;74:1547–54.

[21] Weyand CM, Goronzy JJ. Giant-cell arteritis and polymyalgia rheumatica. Ann Intern Med 2003;139:505–15.

[22] Hunder GG, Bloch DA, Michel BA, et al. The American College of Rheumatology 1990 criteria for the classification of giant cell arteritis. Arthritis Rheum 1990;33:1122–8.

[23] Zenone T, Souquet PJ, Bohas C, et al. Unusual manifestations of giant cell arteritis: pulmonary nodules, cough, conjunctivitis and otitis with deafness. Eur Respir J 1994;7: 2252–4.

[24] Cunha BA, Parchori S, Mohan S. Fever of unknown origin: temporal arteritis presenting with persistent cough and elevated serum ferritin levels. Heart Lung 2006;35:112–6.

[25] Calamia KT, Hunder GG. Giant cell arteritis (temporal arteritis) presenting as fever of undetermined origin. Arthritis Rheum 1981;24:1414–8.

[26] Gonzales-Gay MA, Garcia-Porrua C, Amor-Dorado JC, et al. Fever in biopsy-proven giant cell arteritis: clinical implications in a defined population. Arthritis Rheum 2004;51:652–5.

[27] Gonzales-Gay MA, Garcia-Porrua C, Amor-Dorado JC, et al. Giant cell arteritis without clinically evident vascular involvement in a defined population. Arthritis Rheum 2004;51: 274–7.

[28] Gonzales-Gay MA. The diagnosis and management of patients with giant cell arteritis. J Rheumatol 2005;32:1186–8.

[29] Colmegna I, Maldonado-Cocco JA. Polyarteritis nodosa revisited. Curr Rheumatol Rep 2005;7:288–96.

[30] Lightfoot RW, Michel BA, Bloch DA, et al. The American College of Rheumatology 1990 criteria for classification of polyarteritis nodosa. Arthritis Rheum 1990;33:1088–93.

[31] Henderson J, Cohen J, Jackson J, et al. Polyarteritis nodosa presenting as a pyrexia of unknown origin. Postgrad Med J 2002;78:685–6.

[32] Harmouche H, Maamar M, Sahnoune I, et al. Fever revealing Behcet's disease: two new cases. Eur J Intern Med 2007;18:146–7.

[33] Frankel SK, Cosgrove GP, Fischer A, et al. Update in the diagnosis and management of pulmonary vasculitis. Chest 2006;129:452–65.

[34] Jennette JC, Falk RJ. Small-vessel vasculitis. N Engl J Med 1997;337(21):512–23.

[35] Akar H, Ozbasli-Levi C, Senturk T, et al. MPO-ANCA-associated small vessel vasculitis presenting as fever of unknown origin. Report of one case. Nephron 2002;92:673–5.

[36] Erten N, Saka B, Karan MA, et al. Takayasu arteritis presenting with fever of unknown origin: two case reports. J Clin Rheumatol 2004;10:16–20.

[37] Rapini RP, Warner NB. Relapsing polychondritis. Clin Dermatol 2006;24:482–5.

[38] Efthimiou P, Paik PK, Bielory L. Diagnosis and management of adult onset Still's disease. Ann Rheum Dis 2006;65:564–72.

[39] Mert A, Ozaras R, Tabak F, et al. Fever of unknown origin: a review of 20 patients with adult-onset Still's disease. Clin Rheumatol 2003;22:89–93.

[40] Cunha BA. Fever of unknown origin caused by adult juvenile rheumatoid arthritis: the diagnostic significance of double quotidian fevers and elevated serum ferritin levels. Heart Lung 2004;33:417–21.

[41] Crispin JC, Martinez-Banos D, Alcocer-Varela J. Adult-onset Still disease as the cause of fever of unknown origin. Medicine 2005;84:331–7.

[42] Yamaguchi M, Ohta A, Tsunematsu T, et al. Preliminary criteria for classification of adult Still's disease. J Rheumatol 1992;19:424–30.

[43] Fautrel B, Zing E, Golmard JL, et al. Proposal for a new set of classification criteria for adult-onset Still disease. Medicine 2002;81:194–200.

[44] Efthimiou P, Georgy S. Pathogenesis and management of adult-onset Still's disease. Semin Arthritis Rheum 2006;36:144–52.

[45] Larson EB, Featherstone HJ, Petersdorf RG. Fever of undetermined origin: diagnosis and follow-up of 105 cases, 1970–1980. Medicine 1982;61:269–92.

[46] Barbado FJ, Vasquez JJ, Pena J, et al. Fever of unknown origin: a survey on 133 patients. J Med 1984;15:185–92.

[47] Likuni Y, Okada J, Kondo H, et al. Current fever of unknown origin 1982–1992. Intern Med 1994;33:67–73.

[48] Kazanjian PH. Fever of unknown origin: review of 86 patients treated in community hospitals. Clin Infect Dis 1992;15:968–73.

[49] D'Cruz DP, Khamashta MA, Hughes GRV. Systemic lupus erythematosus. Lancet 2007; 369:587–96.

[50] Mills JA. Systemic lupus erythematosus. N Engl J Med 1994;330:1871–9.

[51] Hachulla E. Fièvre intermittente symptomatique des maladies inflammatoires. Rev Prat 2002;52:160–6.

[52] Hochberg M. Updating the American College of Rheumatology revised criteria for classification of systemic lupus erythematosus. Arthritis Rheum 1997;40:1725–34.

[53] Ozaras R, Mete B, Hakko E, et al. Primary antiphospholipid syndrome: a cause of fever of unknown origin. Intern Med 2003;42:358–61.

[54] Parappil A, Rifaath AA, Doi SA, et al. Pyrexia of unknown origin: Kikuchi-Fujimoto disease. Clin Infect Dis 2004;39:138–43.

[55] Knockaert DC, Dujardin KS, Bobbaers HJ. Long-term follow-up of patients with undiagnosed fever of unknown origin. Arch Intern Med 1996;156:618–20.

[56] Knockaert DC, Vanneste LJ, Bobbaers HJ. Recurrent or episodic fever of unknown origin: review of 45 cases and survey of the literature. Medicine 1993;72:184–96.

[57] Dalakas MC, Hohlfeld R. Polymyositis and dermatopolymyositis. Lancet 2003;362:971–82.

[58] Johns CJ, Michele TM. The clinical management of sarcoidosis: a 50-year experience at the Johns Hopkins Hospital. Medicine 1999;78:65–111.

[59] Patel N, Krasnow A, Sebastian JL, et al. Isolated muscular sarcoidosis causing fever of unknown origin: the value of gallium-67 imaging. J Nucl Med 1991;32:319–21.

[60] Drenth JPH, Van der Meer JWM. Hereditary periodic fever. N Engl J Med 2001;345: 1748–57.

[61] Tal S, Guller V, Gurevich A, et al. Fever of unknown origin in the elderly. J Intern Med 2002; 252:295–304.

[62] Zenone T, Knefati Y, Sabatier JC. Polyarteritis nodosa presenting with jaw claudication and headache. Joint Bone Spine 2007;74:301–2.

[63] Meller J, Sahlmann CO, Scheel AK. 18F-FDG PET and PET/CT in fever of unknown origin. J Nucl Med 2007;48:35–45.

ELSEVIER
SAUNDERS

INFECTIOUS
DISEASE CLINICS
OF NORTH AMERICA

Infect Dis Clin N Am 21 (2007) 1137–1187

# Fever of Unknown Origin: Focused Diagnostic Approach Based on Clinical Clues from the History, Physical Examination, and Laboratory Tests

## Burke A. Cunha, MD, MACP[a,b,*]

[a]Infectious Disease Division, Winthrop-University Hospital, 259 First Street, Mineola, Long Island, NY 11501, USA
[b]State University of New York School of Medicine, Stony Brook, NY, USA

Few clinical problems are as challenging and difficult as that presented by the patient who has a febrile illness for more than 10 to 15 days, the origin of which remains obscure. No type of illness puts to a stronger test the physician's ability to approach a clinical problem effectively....

–Philip A. Tumulty, MD

Fever of unknown origin (FUO) was first and correctly termed "prolonged and perplexing fevers" by Kiefer and Leard [1]. Prolonged and perplexing fevers are difficult-to-diagnose febrile disorders aptly termed FUOs. FUOs may be conveniently divided into four general categories based on the etiology of the FUO: (1) infectious, (2) rheumatic-inflammatory, (3) neoplastic, or (4) miscellaneous disorders. Petersdorf and Beeson [2] in 1961 were the first to define FUO in terms of time-based diagnostic criteria. These have since been termed "classic" FUOs and may be defined as disorders with temperatures greater than or equal to 101°F that have persisted for at least 3 weeks that were not diagnosed after a week of intensive in-hospital testing. The classic and current causes of FUO have been modified, reflecting the changing spectrum of diseases and the availability of sophisticated diagnostic tests in the outpatient setting [3,4].

* Infectious Disease Division, Winthrop-University Hospital, 259 First Street, Mineola, Long Island, NY 11501.

0891-5520/07/$ - see front matter © 2007 Elsevier Inc. All rights reserved.
doi:10.1016/j.idc.2007.09.004

*id.theclinics.com*

The main diagnostic difficulty with FUOs is an efficient and effective diagnostic approach. Clinicians are advised that to diagnose FUOs effectively, they should be comprehensive. Unfortunately, often this has only resulted in excessive diagnostic testing to rule out every disorder causing FUOs. A nonfocused approach has the effect of incurring unnecessary expense, inconveniencing patients, and delaying or obscuring the FUO diagnostic work-up. The undesirable effect of the "shotgun approach" to diagnostic testing is that it underuses the FUO tests appropriate for the most likely diagnostic categories, and it overtests for unlikely diagnoses [5].

The diagnostic approach to the FUO patient should be focused and relevant to the clinical syndromic presentation. Because all patients with FUOs by definition have fevers, the clinician should identify the predominant features of the clinical presentation to determine the general category of FUO of the patient. With infectious FUOs, fevers are often accompanied by chills or night sweats. Weight loss without loss of appetite is another potential indicator of an infectious disease etiology. The clinical presentation of patients with FUOs caused by rheumatic-inflammatory disorders is dominated by arthralgias, myalgias, or migratory chest or abdominal pain. The predominant symptoms of patients with neoplastic FUOs are fatigue and weight loss with early or dramatic decrease in appetite. Night sweats may also be a feature of neoplastic disorders. Patients presenting with FUOs whose symptoms do not suggest an infectious, rheumatic-inflammatory, or neoplastic disorder should be considered as having an FUO of miscellaneous causes [6–8].

It makes little sense to get thyroiditis tests for every FUO patient if there is not an antecedent history of thyroid or autoimmune disease or physical findings referable to subacute thyroiditis. Similarly, just because subacute bacterial endocarditis (SBE) is a common cause of FUO, transthoracic echocardiography (TTE)–transesophageal echocardiography (TEE) should not be obtained on all FUO patients. In patients with FUOs, TTE-TEE should be obtained only in those with heart murmurs. In FUO patients with heart murmurs, vegetations seen on TTE-TEE can indicate SBE (culture positive and culture negative); systemic lupus erythematous (SLE; Libman-Sacks vegetations); or marantic (nonbacterial) endocarditis.

By using a focused approach the clinician can order tests that are more relevant to the presenting clinical syndrome; such tests more efficiently and effectively lead to a correct FUO diagnosis. The diagnostic approach to FUOs may be considered as consisting of three phases. The initial phase consists of the initial FUO history and physical examination and nonspecific laboratory tests. This phase provides the clinician with a general sense of whether the FUO is likely to be caused by an infection or by a rheumatic-inflammatory or neoplastic disorder. Phase II involves re-evaluating the patient using a focused FUO history and physical examination and additional nonspecific and specific laboratory tests. The focused FUO evaluation has the effect of narrowing diagnostic possibilities and eliminating possibilities from further diagnostic consideration [1,5].

Nonspecific laboratory tests included during the initial evaluation are helpful to increase the diagnostic probability of some entities, whereas decreasing or eliminating the diagnostic probability of others. Nonspecific laboratory tests, as with other clinical findings, are more significant when considered together rather than individually. For example, the combination of the following nonspecific laboratory tests, which alone are unhelpful diagnostically, should suggest a particular diagnosis (ie, increased lactate dehydrogenase, atypical lymphocytes in the peripheral smear, and thrombocytopenia should suggest the possibility of malaria in patients with an appropriate epidemiologic exposure). The patient exposed in malarious areas is also exposed to typhoid fever. Both typhoid fever and malaria have some clinical features in common and neither has localizing signs, making these infections difficult to diagnose if the epidemiologic history is not taken into account and the nonspecific laboratory clues are not appreciated for their diagnostic significance. The same three nonspecific laboratory tests argue strongly against typhoid fever and should point the clinician to the possibility of malaria as the cause of the patient's FUO [1,9].

## Fever of unknown origin: classic and current causes

FUOs fall into four general categories. The relative frequency of the causes of FUO in each category is the basis for a phased diagnostic approach. Phase I of an FUO evaluation consists of a FUO relevant history, physical examination, and nonspecific laboratory tests. The phase I evaluation provides the basis for determining the course of the FUO work-up. Features in the history, physical findings, and laboratory abnormalities in the initial FUO evaluation suggest which general category of disorder is responsible for the patient's FUO. Although all FUOs, by definition, are associated with fever, the predominant symptoms usually suggest a particular FUO category.

In general, infectious diseases may be associated with chills, night sweats, myalgias, or weight loss with an intact appetite. Arthralgias or myalgias are the predominant complaints of the patient presenting with rheumatic-inflammatory causes of FUO. These patients often have fatigue, but weight loss or night sweats are unusual findings. Even with some overlap in symptoms, the clinician can usually determine from the dominant clinical features whether the patient is likely to have an infectious, rheumatic-immunologic, or neoplastic cause of their FUO. Typically, in addition to fever and fatigue, neoplastic disorders have night sweats and weight loss accompanied by a dramatic and profound loss of appetite. Patients that do not fit in any of these categories have FUOs of a variety of miscellaneous causes. It is sometimes difficult to differentiate between infectious and neoplastic or infectious and rheumatic disorders. In such situations, the next phase of FUO investigation using a focused diagnostic approach provides additional information with a history and physical examination or additional laboratory tests, which clearly differentiate one group from another, and are able to narrow differential diagnostic possibilities within a category. Classic and current FUO causes have been reviewed (Table 1) [2,3,6,10–13].

## Fever of unknown origin: focused diagnostic approach

### Overview

After the initial FUO-relevant evaluation most of the common causes of FUOs in each category may be readily diagnosed. Combining the relevant FUO features on physical examination with selected nonspecific laboratory test abnormalities limits diagnostic possibilities and eliminates other causes from further diagnostic consideration. The diagnostic significance of selected nonspecific tests cannot be overemphasized. The clinical significance of nonspecific laboratory abnormalities is enhanced when they are considered together. As with FUO-relevant historical facts or physical findings, nonspecific laboratory abnormalities taken together increase diagnostic specificity and significance.

The function of the initial phase of FUO evaluation is to diagnose disorders, which are most easily diagnosed among the FUOs, and to limit differential diagnostic possibilities that direct the second phase of focused FUO evaluation. The focused FUO history of physical examination and laboratory tests has the purpose to refine further the differential diagnosis of disorders that have not been diagnosed during the initial evaluation [14,15].

### Fever of unknown origin: initial evaluation

Although the initial direction of the diagnostic work-up is suggested by FUO-relevant aspects of the history and physical examination, the basic battery of nonspecific laboratory tests helps to define further differential diagnostic possibilities. Many disorders in all categories of FUO are accompanied by some nonspecific laboratory abnormalities. The diagnostic significance of such findings alone and more critically taken together is often overlooked as having no importance because the abnormalities are not of sufficiently impressive magnitude or the abnormalities are associated with many potential disorders. The basic nonspecific laboratory test battery includes the complete blood count, erythrocyte sedimentation rate (ESR), C-reactive protein, and liver function tests. Imaging tests include a chest radiograph (if there are signs or symptoms referable to the chest) and CT and MRI scans of the abdomen and pelvis (as dictated by clinical clues suggesting an intra-abdominal or pelvic pathology. Blood cultures are also included as part of the initial diagnostic evaluation [1,16–19].

Blood cultures pick up common causes of SBE (bacteremia from an intra-abdominal or pelvic or renal-perinephric source), and intra-abdominal imaging provides important information for the focused phase of FUO evaluation. If the patient has a very highly elevated ESR ($\geq 100$ mm/h) it suggests possible FUO etiologies including abscesses, osteomyelitis, SBE, and adult Still's disease. Among the rheumatic inflammatory causes of FUO the ESR greater than or equal to 100 mm/h may point to adult Still's disease, polymyalgia rheumetica/temporal arteritis, late-onset rheumatoid arthritis, SLE, periarteritis nodosa, Takayasu's arteritis, Kikuchi's disease, or familial Mediterranean fever. Among neoplastic disorders an increased ESR rate may be present with any of them but an unelevated ESR has no differential diagnostic value and does not rule out neoplastic or other disorders. The high ESR rate may also point to drug fever and the miscellaneous category and elevated ESR rate may indicate drug fever, regional enteritis, subacute thyroiditis, deep vein thrombosis or small pulmonary emboli, and so forth.

Imaging tests (ie, CT and MRI scanning of the chest, abdomen, and pelvis) may show otherwise unsuspected adenopathy, hepatomegaly or splenomegaly, abscesses, or masses. The initial phase FUO evaluation provides the important diagnostic information that should guide the subsequent diagnostic process. The focused FUO diagnostic approach should be based on the initial FUO evaluation. Findings of the initial FUO evaluation should be based on this [5,10,16–20].

## Fever of unknown origin: focused FUO evaluation

The focused FUO evaluation builds on the initial FUO diagnostic impression. During the second phase of FUO evaluation focused diagnostic approach uses a more detailed history, physical examination, and additional nonspecific laboratory tests not obtained during the initial evaluation. The focused FUO evaluation confirms or eliminates any differential diagnostic difficulties encountered during the initial evaluation and is designed to identify less common causes of FUO in each category. The laboratory tests included in the focused test battery include antinuclear antibodies, rheumatoid factor, serum protein electrophoresis, serum ferritin, cold agglutinins, and so forth. Also included is serology for Epstein-Barr virus, cytomegalovirus, and *Bartonella*. If SLE is in the differential diagnosis, double-stranded DNA and anti–Smith antibodies are included. If malignancies are likely diagnostic possibilities, then additional nonspecific tests, such as uric acid, lactate dehydrogenase, and leukocyte alkaline phosphatase, are included. If diagnostic findings suggest the possibility of subacute thyroiditis, then tests for thyroid antibodies and thyroid function tests should be included. FUO patients with a heart murmur should have a TTE-TEE as part of the work-up for endocarditis. Patients with a heart murmur and a high-grade continuous bacteremia (with an organism associated with endocarditis) with or without peripheral manifestations are diagnosed with SBE. Patients with a heart murmur and negative blood cultures without peripheral manifestations of

Table 1
Classic causes of FUO

| Category | Most common | Common | Uncommon |
|---|---|---|---|
| Infectious diseases | Subacute bacterial endocarditis | Epstein-Barr virus mononucleosis (elderly) | Toxoplasmosis |
| | Intra-abdominal abscesses | Cytomegalovirus | Brucellosis |
| | Pelvic abscesses | Cat-scratch disease | Q fever |
| | Renal-perinephric abscesses | Visceral leishmaniasis (kala-azar) | Leptospirosis |
| | Typhoid-enteric fevers | | Histoplasmosis |
| | Miliary TB | | Coccidioidomycosis |
| | Renal TB | | Trichinosis |
| | TB meningitis | | Relapsing fever |
| | | | Rat-bite fever |
| | | | Lymphogranuloma venereum |
| | | | Chronic sinusitis |
| | | | Relapsing mastoiditis |
| | | | Subacute vertebral osteomyelitis |
| | | | Whipple's disease |
| Rheumatic-inflammatory disorders | Adult Still's disease (adult juvenile rheumatoid arthritis) | Late-onset rheumatoid arthritis | Takayasu's arteritis |
| | Polymyalgia rheumatica/ temporal arteritis | Systemic lupus erythematosus | Kikuchi's disease |
| | | Periarteritis nodosa/microscopic polyangiitis | Polyarticular gout |
| | | | Pseudogout |
| | | | Familial Mediterranean fever |
| | | | Sarcoidosis |

| Neoplastic disorders | Lymphomas (HL-NHL) | Hepatomas/liver metastases | Atrial myxomas |
|---|---|---|---|
| | Hypernephromas | Myeloproliferative disorders (CML-CLL) | Primary-metastatic CNS tumors |
| | | Preleukemias (AML) | Pancreatic carcinomas |
| | | Colon carcinomas | |
| Miscellaneous disorders | Drug fever | Crohn's disease (regional enteritis) | Cyclic neutropenia |
| | Alcoholic cirrhosis | Subacute thyroiditis | DVT/pulmonary emboli (small multiple/recurrent) |
| | | | Hypothalamic dysfunction |
| | | | Pseudolymphomas |
| | | | Schnitzler's syndrome |
| | | | Hyper-IgD syndrome |
| | | | Factitious fever |

*Abbreviations:* AML, acute myelogenous leukemia; CLL, chronic lymphatic leukemia; CML, chronic myelogenous leukemia; CNS, central nervous system; DVT, deep vein thrombosis; HL, Hodgkin's lymphoma; NHL, non-Hodgkin's lymphoma; TA, temporal arteritis; TB, tuberculosis.

SBE have marantic endocarditis. Patients with atrial myxomas have a heart murmur; vegetations on TTE-TEE with or without peripheral embolic phenomenon "culture-negative endocarditis" is a frequently misapplied diagnosis indicating heart murmur with negative blood cultures. True culture-negative endocarditis refers to patients with a heart murmur, vegetations on TTE-TEE (no evidence of an atrial myxoma), with peripheral manifestations of SBE [1,10,13].

Some tests obtained during the initial FUO evaluation may be of assistance with some disorders in this category (ie, regional enteritis [Crohn's disease]). Presenting as an FUO, Crohn's disease may be a difficult diagnosis when unaccompanied by abdominal complaints. If there are findings on the abdominal CT or MRI suggesting terminal ilial abnormalities then a gallium-indium scan may be obtained, which should also show increased uptake in the ileum. FUO patients with regional enteritis may present only with extraintestinal manifestations (eg, episcleritis). The diagnostic significance of episcleritis as an initial manifestation of Crohn's disease is easily overlooked in an FUO patient. The patient with regional enteritis may also have an increased ESR and monocytosis, which together with other findings suggests that Crohn's disease is indeed the cause of the patient's FUO (see the article by Cunha elsewhere in this issue for further exploration of this topic) [1,15–28].

## Diagnostic significance of fever patterns

### Morning temperature spikes

In obscure causes of FUO, fever curves are useful diagnostically and often provide the only clue to the diagnosis. The first step in evaluating fever patterns is to determine the time of the peak period during a 24-hour period. Most patients with fever have peak temperatures in the late afternoon or early evening. This means that there are relatively few disorders associated with morning temperature elevations. If not altered by antipyretic medications or devices, the periodicity of fever can be a useful diagnostic aid in obscure cases of FUO. The causes of FUO associated with morning temperature elevations are typhoid fever; tuberculosis; and among the noninfectious disorders, periarteritis nodosa [29,30].

### Relative bradycardia

A pulse-temperature deficit is termed "relative bradycardia" (Faget's sign). For a pulse temperature to be termed relative bradycardia there must be a significant pulse temperature deficit relative to the degree of fever. Relative bradycardia should not be applied to children or those with temperatures of less than 102°F or adults with temperatures of less than 102°F or those on β-blockers, diltiazem, verapamil, or who have pacemaker-induced rhythms or arrhythmias. The pulse rate for any given degree of temperature elevation is physiologic and predictable. For every degree of temperature elevation in degrees Fahrenheit there is a concomitant increase in pulse rate of 10 beats per minute. In the absence of the exclusion criteria mentioned, a temperature of 104°F should be accompanied by an appropriate pulse response of 130 beats per minute. This patient with relative bradycardia would have a pulse less than or equal to 120 beats per minute. Appropriate pulse-temperature relationships are shown in Table 2. Applied correctly in the appropriate clinical context in patients with FUO relative bradycardia is an important diagnostic sign. In FUO patients, relative bradycardia may occur in association with malaria, typhoid fever, any central nervous system disorder, some lymphomas, and drug fever. Simultaneous pulses should be obtained in all patients with FUOs to determine if relative bradycardia is present. Relative tachycardia refers to an inappropriately rapid pulse for a given degree of temperature, and is only associated with pulmonary emboli among the causes of FUO [29–31].

## Double quotidian fevers

Double quotidian fevers refer to two temperature spikes occurring within a 24-hour period. Although double quotidian fevers are not a common fever pattern, they are most helpful when present in febrile patients presenting with a differential diagnosis. Infectious causes of FUO associated with double quotidian fevers include miliary tuberculosis, visceral leishmaniasis, and mixed malarial infections. In returning travelers from India, malaria and typhoid fever are important differential diagnostic considerations. In such a patient with a double quotidian fever, typhoid fever is immediately eliminated from further diagnostic consideration. Although malaria caused by one *Plasmodium* species does not present with a double quotidian fever, a mixed malarial infection may be accompanied by a double quotidian fever pattern. For example, in a returning traveler from India, a double quotidian fever eliminates a mixed malarial infection and typhoid fever from diagnostic consideration, and the astute clinician should then consider the possibility of visceral leishmaniasis.

Table 2
Physiologic pulse-temperature relationships

| Appropriate temperature | Pulse rate (beats/min) | Pulse in relative bradycardia[a] |
|---|---|---|
| 106°F (41.1°C) | 150 | <140 |
| 105°F (40.6°C) | 140 | <130 |
| 104°F (40.7°C) | 130 | <120 |
| 103°F (39.4°C) | 120 | <110 |
| 102°F (38.9°C) | 110 | <100 |

[a] In adults with temperature > 102°F and not on β-blockers, verapamil, diltiazem, or with pacemaker pulses/second/third degree heart block.

*Data from* Cunha BA. Antibiotic essentials. 6th edition. Royal Oak (MI): Physicians Press; 2007.

Among noninfectious causes of FUO, a double quotidian fever pattern is a key diagnostic finding in adult Still's disease. Patients with adult Still's disease often present as an FUO without many multisystem symptoms or findings. If the clinical syndromic presentation includes adult Still's disease then a double quotidian fever pattern is a key diagnostic finding because no other rheumatic-inflammatory disorder is associated with a double quotidian fever.

In febrile patients, double quotidian fevers may be artificially induced by intermittent antipyretic medications; devices (eg, hypothermia blankets); or other body cooling mechanisms. Before using a double quotidian fever pattern as diagnostic sign the clinician must be sure that the patient has not been subjected to antifever medications or maneuvers [29,30].

*Camelback (dromedary) fevers*

A camelback or dromedary fever curve is one that has a few days with fever, separated by a decrease in fever between the febrile episodes over the period of a week. Graphed on temperature chart the two periods of temperature prominence are separated by a period of decreased temperatures, resembling a two-humped camel or dromedary silhouette. As with other unusual fever curves, camelback fever patterns are of most use when the differential diagnosis includes obscure otherwise difficult-to-diagnose infections presenting as FUOs. A camelback fever curve may occur in leptospirosis, brucellosis, and ehrlichiosis [29,30].

*Relapsing fevers*

Relapsing fevers refer to those that are recurring and separated by periods with low-grade fever or no fever. Rat-bite fever, relapsing fever, *Bartonella*, tuberculosis, and relapsing fever patterns are important in FUOs because, by definition, the fever in patients with FUOs is of long duration (ie, $\geq 3$ weeks). Inherent in the definition of a relapsing fever is the notion that the underlying disorder responsible for ongoing fever continues to be clinically active in terms of its febrile expression. In contrast, recurrent fevers recur periodically and are associated with fever flares, which is an expression of the flare of the underlying disorder (eg, SLE). A relapsing fever pattern may be difficult to appreciate in acute fevers where the duration of the fever may not permit an appreciation of the relapsing nature of the fever.

Among the infectious causes of FUO, relapsing fever pattern is classically associated with relapsing fever (*Borrelia recurrentis*) but has also been associated with typhoid fever, malaria, brucellosis, and rat-bite fever [29,30].

Nonrelapsing fevers may also be caused by a variety of noninfectious etiologies. In the FUO patient, noninfectious causes of relapsing fever include cyclic neutropenia, familial Mediterranean fever, SLE, vasculitis, hyperimmunoglobulinemia D syndrome, and Schnitzler's syndrome. Relapsing fevers may be mimicked by antipyretic interventions, and by inappropriately or partially treated infectious diseases in FUO patients (Tables 3–21) [29,30,32].

Table 3
Sequence of diagnostic approach to FUO

| Initial FUO assessment | Focused FUO assessment (after initial FUO evaluation) |
|---|---|
| I. Initial FUO history | I. ID etiology suspected based on focused ID history and physical examination |
| | A. See Tables 3–10 |
| A. Initial FUO infectious disease history | II. RD etiology suspected based on focused RD history and physical examination |
| PMH-FMH of infectious disease | A. See Tables 11–14 |
| Pet-animal contact | III. ND etiology suspected based on focused ND history and physical examination |
| STD history | |
| Travel | A. See Tables 15,16 |
| Heart murmur | IV. Miscellaneous disorders suspected based on a negative focused ID, RD, ND history and physical examination |
| Surgical-invasive procedures | |
| B. Initial FUO rheumatic history | |
| PMH-FMH of rheumatic disorder | A. See Table 17 |
| SLE | V. Definitive FUO laboratory tests |
| RA | A. ID suspected |
| Gout | TTE-TEE (if heart murmur) |
| Sarcoidosis | Naprosyn test (if DDx between ND and ID) |
| HA, mental confusion | Special blood culture-media incubation |
| Eye symptoms | Specific relevant serology |
| Neck or jaw pain | Tissue biopsy of appropriate nodes, liver, bone marrow, and so forth |
| Sore throat | |
| Mouth ulcers | B. Rheumatic disorder suspected |
| Acalculous cholecystitis | TTE-TEE (if heart murmur) |
| Abdominal pain (intermittent, recurrent) | Specific relevant serology |
| Heart murmur | Tissue biopsy of appropriate nodes, liver, bone marrow, and so forth |
| Myalgias, arthralgias | |
| Joint swelling, effusion | C. Neoplastic disorder suspected |
| C. Initial FUO neoplastic history | TTE-TEE (if heart murmur) |
| PMH-FMH of malignancy | Tissue biopsy of appropriate nodes, liver, bone marrow, and so forth |
| Night sweats | |
| Decrease in appetite with weight loss | Naprosyn test (if DDx between neoplastic and infectious disorders) |
| Fundi | |
| D. Initial FUO miscellaneous history | D. Miscellaneous disorder suspected |
| Drug, medication, fume or exposure | History, physical examination, and laboratory tests negative for infectious, rheumatic, or neoplastic disorders |
| Alcoholism | |
| Thyroid, autoimmune disorders | |
| IBD | Individualized tests for obscure causes |
| II. Initial FUO physical examination | |
| A. Infectious disease physical examination | |
| Fever pattern | |
| Fundi | |
| Nodes | |
| Liver tenderness, hepatomegaly | |
| Spleen tenderness, hepatomegaly | |
| B. Rheumatic disease physical examination | |

(*continued on next page*)

Table 3 (*continued*)

| Initial FUO assessment | Focused FUO assessment (after initial FUO evaluation) |
|---|---|
| Fever pattern | |
| Temporal artery tenderness | |
| Fundi | |
| Mouth ulcers | |
| Nodes | |
| Heart murmur | |
| Epididymitis | |
| Joint swelling, effusion | |
| C. Neoplastic physical examination | |
| Heart murmur | |
| Sternal bone tenderness | |
| D. Miscellaneous disease physical examination | |
| Fever pattern | |
| Adenopathy | |
| Splenomegaly | |
| Signs of alcoholic cirrhosis | |
| III. Initial infectious, rheumatic, and neoplastic disorders; FUO laboratory tests | |
| A. CBC (manual differential count) | |
| B. ANA | |
| C. RF | |
| D. SPEP | |
| E. Cold agglutinins | |
| F. ESR | |
| G. Ferritin levels | |
| H. CT or MRI of chest, abdomen, pelvis (if suggested by history and clinical findings) | |

*Abbreviations:* ANA, antinuclear antibodies; BCs, blood cultures; CBC, complete blood count; CT, computed tomography scan; CXR, chest radiograph; ESR, erythrocyte sedimentation rate; ID, infectious disease; KUB, kidney, ureter, bladder film; LDH, lactate dehydrogenase; LFTs, liver function tests; MRI, magnetic resonance imaging; ND, neoplastic disorder; PET, positron emission tomography; RD, rheumatic disorder; SPEP, serum protein electrophoresis; TTE-TEE, transthoracic-transesophageal echocardiogram; UA-UC, urinalysis and urine culture.

## Fever of unknown origin: diagnostic usefulness of the Naprosyn test

The Naprosyn test was first developed by Chang [32], an oncologist. Using Naprosyn (naproxen) over a 3-day period (375 mg orally twice daily) he was able to differentiate neoplastic from infectious FUOs. The Naprosyn test is considered positive when there is a rapid or sustained defervescence during the 3 days of the test period. Fever in patients with neoplastic disorders recurs after cessation of the Naprosyn test. Those with infectious diseases undergo little or no drop in their temperatures during the test

Table 4
Common infectious disease causes of FUO: focused infectious disease history*

| Historical clues | SBE | Abscess | CNS TB | Renal TB | Miliary TB | Typhoid | CMV | EBV | HIV | CSD | TOXO |
|---|---|---|---|---|---|---|---|---|---|---|---|
| Recent or close contact with similar illness | - | - | - | - | - | - | ± | + | + | - | - |
| Recent contaminated water or food exposure | - | - | - | - | - | + | - | - | - | - | - |
| History of blood transfusion | - | - | - | - | - | - | + | - | + | - | - |
| HIV exposure | - | - | - | - | - | - | + | - | + | - | - |
| Recent insect, rodent, animal exposure | - | - | - | - | - | - | - | - | - | + | - |
| Recent travel to Asia, Latin America, Africa | - | - | - | - | - | ± | - | - | ± | - | - |
| Consumption of contaminated or unpasteurized milk or cheese | - | - | - | - | - | - | - | - | - | - | - |
| History of TB or TB exposure | - | - | + | + | + | - | - | - | - | - | - |
| Eye pain, visual complaints | - | - | - | - | - | - | - | - | - | - | - |
| History of heart murmur | + | - | - | - | - | - | - | - | - | - | - |
| Night sweats | + | + | ± | ± | + | + | - | - | - | - | - |
| Weight loss | + | ± | - | ± | + | - | - | - | - | - | - |
| Headaches, mental status changes | + | - | + | - | - | + | - | - | ± | + | - |
| Arthralgias, arthritis | + | - | - | - | - | - | - | - | - | - | - |
| Prominent myalgias | - | - | - | - | - | - | - | - | - | - | - |
| New onset of back pain | ± | - | - | - | - | ± | - | - | - | - | - |

*Abbreviations:* Abscess, intra-abdominal, pelvic; CMV, cytomegalovirus; CSD, cat-scratch disease; EBV, Epstein-Barr virus; HIV, human immunodeficiency virus; KA, kala-azar (visceral leishmaniasis); SBE, subacute bacterial endocarditis; TB, tuberculosis; TOXO, toxoplasmosis; Typhoid, typhoid, enteric fever.

+, Usually present; ±, may be present; -, Usually not present.

* When presenting as an FUO.

Table 5
Uncommon and rare infectious disease causes of FUO: focused infectious disease history*

| Historical clues | EHR/ANA | LEPTO | BRU | Q Fever | TRICH | Malaria | HISTO | COCCI | KA | RBF | RF | LGV | WD |
|---|---|---|---|---|---|---|---|---|---|---|---|---|---|
| Recent or close contact with same illness | − | − | − | − | − | − | − | − | − | − | − | + | − |
| Recent contaminated water exposure | − | + | − | − | − | − | − | − | − | − | − | − | − |
| History of blood transfusion | − | − | − | − | − | ± | − | − | − | − | − | − | − |
| Recent insect, rodent, animal exposure | + | + | + | + | + | + | − | − | + | + | + | − | − |
| Recent travel to Asia, Latin America, Africa | − | + | ± | ± | − | + | − | − | + | ± | ± | − | − |
| Consumption of contaminated or unpasteurized milk or cheese | − | − | + | ± | − | − | − | − | − | − | −ᵃ | − | − |
| Sleep disturbances | − | + | + | − | − | − | − | − | − | − | + | − | − |
| Sore throat | − | + | + | − | − | − | − | − | − | + | − | − | − |
| Tongue tenderness | − | − | − | − | − | − | − | − | − | − | + | − | − |
| History of heart murmur | − | − | +ᵇ | + | − | − | +ᵇ | ±ᵇ | − | − | − | − | +ᵇ |
| Night sweats | − | − | ± | + | − | − | + | ± | ± | − | − | − | − |
| Weight loss | − | − | − | + | − | − | + | ±ᵇ | ± | − | − | − | + |
| Headaches, mental status changes | + | + | + | + | + | + | + | − | − | + | + | − | + |
| Arthralgias, arthritis | − | − | + | − | + | − | ± | + | − | + | + | + | + |
| Prominent myalgias, new-onset back pain | + | + | + | − | + | + | − | + | − | + | + | +ᶜ | − |
| Diarrhea | − | − | − | − | − | − | − | − | − | − | − | − | + |

*Abbreviations:* BRU, brucellosis; COCCI, coccidiomycosis; EHR/ANA, ehrlichosis-anaplasmosis; HISTO, histoplasmosis; KA, kala-azar (visceral leishmaniasis); LEPTO, leptospirosis; LGV, lymphogranuloma venereum; RBF, rat-bite fever (*Streptobacillus minus*, *S moniliformis*); RF, relapsing fever (*Borrelia recurrentis*); TRICH, trichinosis; WD, Whipple's disease.

+, Usually present; ±, may be present; −, usually not present.

* When presenting as an FUO.

ᵃ *Streptobacillus moniliformis.*

ᵇ If SBE, CNS coccidiomycosis may be only manifestation of disseminated coccidiomycosis.

ᶜ In females.

Table 6
Common infectious disease causes of FUO: focused infectious disease physical examination*

| Physical clues | SBE | Abscess | CNS TB | Renal TB | Miliary TB | Typhoid | CMV | EBV | HIV | CSD | TOXO |
|---|---|---|---|---|---|---|---|---|---|---|---|
| Morning temperature spikes | − | − | + | + | + | + | − | − | − | − | − |
| Relative bradycardia[a] | − | − | ± | − | + | + | − | − | − | − | − |
| Double quotidian fever | − | − | − | − | − | − | − | − | − | − | − |
| Vitritis[b] | − | − | − | − | − | − | + | − | − | − | + |
| Chorioretinitis | − | − | − | − | − | − | + | − | − | + | + |
| Lacrimal gland enlargement | − | − | − | − | ±[c] | − | − | − | − | − | − |
| Conjunctival suffusion | − | − | − | − | − | − | − | − | − | − | − |
| Roth's spots | + | − | − | − | + | − | − | − | − | + | + |
| Optic neuritis (with macular star) | − | − | + | − | − | − | + | − | + | + | + |
| Cytoid bodies (cotton wool spots) | − | − | − | − | − | − | + | − | + | − | − |
| Retinal hemorrhages | − | − | − | − | − | − | + | − | + | − | ± |
| Palatal petechiae | + | − | − | − | − | − | − | + | − | − | − |
| Tender fingertips | + | +[d] | − | − | − | − | − | − | − | − | − |
| Trapezoid (upper border) muscle tenderness | − | − | − | − | − | − | − | − | − | − | − |
| Spinal tenderness | ± | − | − | − | − | − | − | − | − | − | − |
| Heart murmur | + | − | − | − | − | − | − | − | − | +[e] | − |
| Regional or localized adenopathy | − | − | − | − | − | − | + | − | + | + | + |

(continued on next page)

Table 6 (continued)

| Physical clues | SBE | Abscess | CNS TB | Renal TB | Miliary TB | Typhoid | CMV | EBV | HIV | CSD | TOXO |
|---|---|---|---|---|---|---|---|---|---|---|---|
| Generalized adenopathy | − | − | − | − | + | − | ± | + | + | ± | ± |
| Splenomegaly | + | − | − | − | + | + | ± | + | − | ± | ± |
| Hepatomegaly | − | +[f] | − | − | ± | ± | − | − | − | − | − |
| Thigh tenderness | − | − | − | − | − | − | − | − | − | − | − |
| Epididymo-orchitis, epididymal nodule | − | − | − | + | − | − | − | + | − | − | − |
| Arthritis, joint effusion | ± | − | − | − | − | ± | − | − | − | − | − |
| Skin hyperpigmentation | − | − | − | − | +[g] | − | − | − | − | − | − |

*Abbreviations:* Abscess, intra-abdominal, pelvic; CMV, cytomegalovirus; CSD, cat-scratch disease; EBV, Epstein-Barr virus; HIV, human immunodeficiency virus; KA, kala-azar (visceral leishmaniasis); SBE, subacute bacterial endocarditis; TB, tuberculosis; TOXO, toxoplasmosis; Typhoid, typhoid, enteric fever.

+, Usually present; ±, may be present; −, usually not present.
* When presenting as an FUO.
[a] Pulse temperature deficit.
[b] Vitreitis ("headlight in the fog").
[c] Phlyctenular keratoid conjunctivitis.
[d] Subdiaphragmatic.
[e] If SBE.
[f] If liver abscess large.
[g] If Addison's disease.

Table 7
Uncommon and rare infectious disease causes of FUO: focused infectious disease physical examination*

| Physical clues | EHR-ANA | LEPTO | BRU | Q fever | TRICH | Malaria | HISTO | COCCI | KA | RBF | RF | LGV | WD |
|---|---|---|---|---|---|---|---|---|---|---|---|---|---|
| Relative bradycardia[a] | + | + | + | + | – | – | – | – | + | – | – | – | – |
| Double quotidian fever | – | – | – | – | – | +[b] | – | – | – | – | – | – | – |
| Long eyelashes | – | – | – | – | – | – | – | – | + | – | – | – | – |
| Epistaxis | – | – | – | – | – | – | – | – | – | – | – | – | – |
| Conjunctivitis | – | – | – | – | – | – | – | – | –[c] | – | – | – | – |
| Conjunctival suffusion | – | + | – | – | + | ± | – | – | – | ± | + | – | – |
| Uveitis | – | – | – | – | – | ± | +[d] | – | + | ± | – | + | + |
| Chorioretinitis | – | ± | – | – | – | – | + | ± | – | – | – | – | – |
| Roth's spots | – | – | – | – | – | +[e,f] | – | – | – | – | – | – | – |
| Tongue ulcer | – | – | – | – | – | – | + | – | – | – | – | – | – |
| Trapezoid (upper border) muscle tenderness | – | – | – | – | – | – | – | – | – | – | – | – | – |
| Spinal tenderness | – | – | + | – | + | – | – | ± | – | – | – | – | – |
| Abdominal wall tenderness | – | + | ±[g] | – | + | – | – | – | – | + | – | – | – |
| Heart murmur | – | – | ±[g] | +[g] | – | – | ±[g] | – | – | +[g] | +[h] | – | +[g] |
| Regional, localized adenopathy | – | – | – | – | – | – | – | – | + | + | – | ± | – |
| Generalized adenopathy | – | ±± | + | – | – | – | + | – | + | –[i] | + | + | + |
| Splenomegaly | ± | ±± | ± | + | – | + | + | – | + | +[i] | + | – | – |

(continued on next page)

Table 7 (continued)

| Physical clues | EHR-ANA | LEPTO | BRU | Q fever | TRICH | Malaria | HISTO | COCCI | KA | RBF | RF | LGV | WD |
|---|---|---|---|---|---|---|---|---|---|---|---|---|---|
| Hepatomegaly | – | + | – | ± | – | – | + | – | + | +[i] | + | – | – |
| Thigh tenderness | – | – | + | – | – | – | – | – | – | – | – | – | – |
| Epididymo-orchitis, epidymal nodules | – | – | – | – | – | – | – | – | – | +[j] | + | – | – |
| Arthritis, joint effusion | – | – | + | – | – | – | + | + | – | +[i] | + | – | + |
| Skin hyperpigmentation | – | – | – | – | – | – | +[k] | – | + | – | – | – | + |

*Abbreviations:* BRU, brucellosis; COCCI, coccidiomycosis; EHR-ANA, ehrlichosis, anaplasmosis; HISTO, histoplasmosis; KA, kala-azar (visceral leishmaniasis); LEPTO, leptospirosis; LGV, lymphogranuloma venereum; RBF, rat-bite fever (*S minus, S moniliformis*); RF, relapsing fever (*Borellia recurrentis*); TRICH, trichinosis; WD, Whipple's disease.

+, Usually present; ±, may be present; –, usually not present.

\* When presenting as an FUO.

[a] Pulse temperature deficit.

[b] If mixed malarial infection.

[c] Conjunctival nodules.

[d] Peripheral hypopigmented "histoplasmosis spots."

[e] Retinal hemorrhages.

[f] Cytoid bodies.

[g] If SBE.

[h] If myocarditis.

[i] *Streptobacillus moniliformis.*

[j] *Streptobacillus minus.*

[k] If Addison's disease.

Table 8
Common focused infectious disease causes of FUO: clues from initial laboratory tests*

| Laboratory tests | SBE | Abscess | CNS TB | Renal TB | Miliary TB | Typhoid | CMV | EBV | HIV | CSD | TOXO |
|---|---|---|---|---|---|---|---|---|---|---|---|
| **CBC** | | | | | | | | | | | |
| Leukocytosis | + | + | − | − | − | − | − | − | − | − | − |
| Leukopenia | − | − | − | − | + | + | + | + | + | − | − |
| Lymphopenia (relative) | − | − | − | − | + | + | + | + | + | − | − |
| Atypical lymphocytes[a] | − | − | ± | ± | + | − | + | + | − | − | + |
| Monocytosis | + | − | − | ± | + | − | − | − | − | − | − |
| Thrombocytosis | + | + | − | − | − | − | − | − | − | − | − |
| Thrombocytopenia | − | − | − | − | + | − | + | + | + | − | − |
| **ESR** | | | | | | | | | | | |
| Highly elevated (>100 mm/h) | + | + | − | − | − | − | − | − | − | − | − |
| **RF** | | | | | | | | | | | |
| ↑ RF | + | − | − | − | − | − | − | − | − | − | − |
| Cryoglobulins + Cryoglobulins | + | − | − | − | − | − | − | ± | ± | − | ± |
| **SPEP** | | | | | | | | | | | |
| Polyclonal gammopathy | − | − | − | − | − | − | − | − | + | − | − |
| **LFTs** | | | | | | | | | | | |
| ↑ SGOT/SGPT | − | − | − | − | + | ± | + | + | − | − | ± |
| ↑ alkaline phosphatase | − | +[b] | − | − | + | − | − | − | − | − | − |

*Abbreviations:* Abscess, intra-abdominal, pelvic; CBC, complete blood count; CMV, cytomegalovirus; CSD, cat-scratch disease (*Bartonella*); EBV, Epstein-Barr virus; ESR, erythrocyte sedimentation rate; HIV, human immunodeficiency virus; KA, kala-azar (visceral leishmaniasis); LFTs, liver function tests; RF, rheumatoid factors; SBE, subacute bacterial endocarditis; SGOT, serum glutamic-oxaloacetic transaminase; SGPT, serum glutamic-pyruvic transaminase; SPEP, serum protein electrophoresis; TB, tuberculosis; TOXO, toxoplasmosis; Typhoid, typhoid, enteric fever.

+, Usually present; ±, may be present; −, usually not present.

* When presenting as an FUO.

[a] Reactive, not abnormal lymphocytes.

[b] Liver abscess.

Table 9
Uncommon and rare infectious disease causes of FUO: initial laboratory tests*

| Laboratory tests | EHR-ANA | LEPTO | BRU | Q Fever | TRICH | Malaria | HISTO | COCCI | KA | RBF | RF | LGV | WD |
|---|---|---|---|---|---|---|---|---|---|---|---|---|---|
| **CBC** | | | | | | | | | | | | | |
| Leukocytosis | – | + | – | – | – | – | – | – | – | + | + | – | – |
| Leukopenia | + | – | – | – | – | – | + | – | – | – | + | – | + |
| Lymphopenia (relative) | + | – | + | – | – | + | – | – | – | – | – | – | + |
| Atypical lymphocytes[a] | ± | – | + | – | – | + | – | – | – | – | – | – | – |
| Monocytosis | – | – | + | – | – | + | ± | – | + | – | – | – | – |
| Eosinophilia | – | – | – | – | + | – | – | + | – | – | – | – | – |
| Thrombocytosis | – | – | – | – | – | – | – | – | – | – | – | – | – |
| Thrombocytopenia | + | + | – | – | – | + | +[b] | – | – | – | – | – | – |
| **ESR** | | | | | | | | | | | | | |
| Highly elevated (>100 mm/h) | – | – | +[c] | +[c] | – | – | – | – | – | – | – | – | – |
| Subnormal (~0 mm/h) | – | – | – | – | + | – | – | – | – | – | – | – | – |
| **Rheumatoid factor** | | | | | | | | | | | | | |
| ↑ Rheumatoid factor | – | – | – | – | – | – | – | – | – | – | – | – | – |
| **Cryoglobulins** | | | | | | | | | | | | | |
| + Cryoglobulins | – | – | – | – | – | + | ± | ± | + | – | – | – | – |
| **SPEP** | | | | | | | | | | | | | |
| Polyclonal gammopathy | + | – | – | – | – | + | – | – | + | + | – | + | – |

| | | | | | | | | | | |
|---|---|---|---|---|---|---|---|---|---|---|
| **LFTs** | | | | | | | | | | |
| ↑ SGOT, SGPT | ± | + | + | + | − | + | + | + | + | + |
| ↑ Alkaline phosphatase | − | + | + | − | − | + | + | − | − | − |
| **LDH** | | | | | | | | | | |
| ↑ LDH | − | − | − | − | + | − | − | − | + | − |
| **CPK** | | | | | | | | | | |
| ↑ CPK | − | + | + | + | − | − | − | − | − | − |

*Abbreviations:* BRU, brucellosis; CBC, complete blood count; COCCI, coccidiomycosis; CPK, creatine phosphokinase; EHR-ANA, ehrlichosis, anaplasmosis; HISTO, histoplasmosis; ESR, erythrocyte sedimentation rate; KA, kala-azar (visceral leishmaniasis); LDH, lactate dehydrogenase; LEPTO, leptospirosis; LFTs, liver function tests; LGV, lymphogranuloma venereum; RBF, rat-bite fever (*S minus*, *S moniliformis*); RF, relapsing fever (*B recurrentis*); SGOT, serum glutamic-oxaloacetic transaminase; SGPT, serum glutamic-pyruvic transaminase; SPEP, serum protein electrophoresis; TRICH, trichinosis; WD, Whipple's disease.

+, Usually present; ±, may be present; −, usually not present.

* When presenting as an FUO.

[a] Reactive, not abnormal lymphocytes.

[b] If disseminated.

[c] If PVE, SBE.

Table 10
Common infectious disease causes of FUO: clinical summaries*

| Infectious disease | | |
|---|---|---|
| SBE | History | Night sweats; weight loss; arthralgias; heart murmur; recent dental or surgical (below waist) or urologic procedure; recent or unexplained LUQ pain; back pain; recent or unexplained CVA |
| | Physical findings | Roth's spots, conjunctival hemorrhages, heart murmur, splinter hemorrhages, Osler's nodes, Janeway lesions, splenomegaly, spinal tenderness, joint pain or effusion, microscopic hematuria |
| | Laboratory tests | Leukocytosis, monocytosis, thrombocytopenia, ↑ ESR, ↑ RF |
| Abscess | History | Previous gastrointestinal or genitourinary or pelvic infection or invasive or surgical procedure, night sweats, chills, weight loss |
| | Physical findings | Trapezoidal tenderness (subdiaphragmatic abscess); hepatomegaly (if large liver abscess) |
| | Laboratory tests | Leukocytosis, thrombocytosis, ↑ ESR, + CT/MRI or gallium/indium scans, aspirate abscess |
| CNS TB | History | Previous TB, headache or mental status changes |
| | Physical findings | Morning temperature spikes, relative bradycardia, abducens palsy (CN VI) |
| | Laboratory tests | Cerebrospinal fluid: lymphocytic pleocytosis (<500 WBC/mm³); + RBCs; ↑ protein; ↓ glucose; ↑ lactic acid; + AFB smear or culture |
| Renal TB | History | Previous TB, night sweats, weight loss |
| | Physical findings | Morning temperature spikes, epididymo-orchitis or nodule |
| | Laboratory tests | Microscopic hematuria (not gross hematuria); urine pH <5.5' + CT/MRI or gallium/indium scans' + PPD + AFB smear or culture of urine |
| Miliary TB | History | Previous TB or exposure, immunosuppressive disorder or drugs, night sweats, weight loss with intact appetite |
| | Physical findings | Morning temperature spikes, choroid tubercles, hepatomegaly, splenomegaly, generalized adenopathy |
| | Laboratory test | Leukopenia, lymphopenia, thrombocytopenia, ↑ LFTs, + CT/MRI or gallium/indium scans, – PPD/anergic, + AFB smear or culture of liver or bone marrow |
| Typhoid, enteric fever | History | Recent contaminated food or water exposure, recent foreign travel, headache or mental status changes, night sweats, weight loss |
| | Physical findings | Morning temperature spikes, relative bradycardia, splenomegaly, hepatomegaly |
| | Laboratory tests | Leukopenia, lymphopenia, eosinopenia, ↑ LFTs, +CT/MRI, or gallium-indium scans, + IgM titers, + blood, urine, stool, or BM cultures |

| | | |
|---|---|---|
| CMV | History | Recent body secretion exposure, blood transfusions |
| | Physical findings | Chorioretinitis; cytoid bodies (cotton wool spots); retinal hemorrhages; palatal petechiae; adenopathy; splenomegaly |
| | Laboratory tests | Leukopenia, lymphopenia, atypical lymphocytes, ↑ LFTs, +CT/MRI or gallium-indium scans, ↑ IgM titers, + PCR |
| EBV | History | Recent body secretion exposure |
| | Physical findings | Palatal petechiae, adenopathy, splenomegaly |
| | Laboratory tests | Leukopenia, lymphopenia, atypical lymphocytes, ↑ LFTs, + PCR, +CT/MRI or gallium/indium scans, ↑ IgM VCA titers |
| HIV | History | Recent body secretion contact, IVDA, blood transfusions, headache or mental status changes, weight loss, night sweats, skin or nail changes, severe oral or rectal lesions |
| | Physical findings | Cytoid bodies (cotton wool spots), adenopathy |
| | Laboratory tests | Leukopenia, lymphopenia, thrombocytopenia, SPEP: polyclonal gammopathy, + CT/MRI or gallium-indium scans +HIV serology/↑ viral load |
| CSD | History | Recent kitten, cat licking, or scratch exposure; headaches or mental status changes |
| | Physical findings | Chorioretinitis; cytoid bodies (cotton wool spots); retinal hemorrhages; optic neuritis (with "macular star") adenopathy; splenomegaly, Roth's spots |
| | Laboratory tests | ↑ IgM *B henselae* titers, + BCs, node biopsy + CT/MRI or gallium-indium scans, ↑ IgM *B henselae* titers, + BCs, node biopsy |
| TOXO | History | Recent cat or undercooked meat exposure |
| | Physical findings | Vitreitis ("headlight in the fog"); Roth's spots; chorioretinitis (unilateral); adenopathy; splenomegaly |
| | Laboratory tests | Atypical lymphocytes, ↑ LFTs, + CT/MRI or gallium/indium scans, ↑ IgM titers, node biopsy |

*Abbreviations:* Abscess, intra-abdominal, pelvic; CMV, cytomegalovirus; CSD, cat-scratch disease (*Bartonella henselae*); CT, computer tomography; CVA, cerebrovascular accident; EBV, Epstein-Barr virus; ESR, erythrocyte sedimentation rate; HIV, human immunodeficiency virus; KA, kala-azar (visceral leishmaniasis); LFT, liver function tests; LUQ, left upper quadrant; MRI, magnetic resonance image; PCR, polymerase chain reaction; PPD, purified protein derivative (tuberculin); RF, rheumatoid factor; SBE, subacute bacterial endocarditis; SPEP, serum protein electrophoresis; TB, tuberculosis; TOXO, toxoplasmosis; typhoid, typhoid/enteric fever.

+, Usually present; ±, may be present; −, usually not present.

* When presenting as an FUO.

Table 11
Uncommon and rare infectious disease causes of FUO: clinical summaries*

| Infectious disease | | |
|---|---|---|
| Ehrlichiosis/anaplasmosis | History | Recent insect exposure, headache, myalgias |
| | Physical findings | Relative bradycardia, camelback fever curve, splenomegaly |
| | Laboratory tests | Leukopenia, lymphopenia, thrombocytopenia, ↑ LFTs, SPEP: polyclonal gammopathy, ↑ IgM titers, WBC inclusions (morula) |
| Leptospirosis | History | Recent contaminated water or rodent exposure, sleep disturbances, headache or mental status changes, sore throat, myalgias |
| | Physical findings | Relative bradycardia, conjunctival suffusion, abdominal wall tenderness, hepatomegaly |
| | Laboratory tests | Leukocytosis, thrombocytopenia, ↑ LFTs, ↑ CPK, ↑ IgM titers, abnormal UA, urine culture |
| Brucellosis | History | Recent animal exposure, contaminated milk or cheese exposure, sleep disturbances, headache or mental status changes, sore throat, myalgias, arthralgias, back pain |
| | Physical findings | Relative bradycardia, adenopathy, splenomegaly, thigh tenderness, spinal tenderness, arthritis, unusual affect |
| | Laboratory tests | Atypical lymphocytes, ↑ LFTs, ↑ IgM titers, + blood cultures |
| Q fever | History | Recent parturient cat or animal exposure, night sweats, chills, headache or mental status changes, heart murmur or prosthetic heart valve |
| | Physical findings | Relative bradycardia; heart murmur (if SBE); splenomegaly |
| | Laboratory tests | ↑ LFTs, ↑ phase I/II titers, + PCR |
| Trichinosis | History | Recent rare or raw meat ingestion or exposures, headache, myalgias |
| | Physical findings | Conjunctival suffusion, abdominal wall muscle tenderness, muscle tenderness |
| | Laboratory tests | ↑ CPK, eosinophilia, ↓ ESR, ↑ IgM BF titers |
| Malaria | History | Recent or frequent foreign travel, mosquito exposure, blood transfusion, headache |
| | Physical findings | Relative bradycardia H labialis, splenomegaly |
| | Laboratory tests | Lymphopenia, eosinophilia, atypical lymphocytes, thrombocytopenia, ↑ LFTs, ↑ LDH, SPEP: polyclonal gangliopathy, RBCs malarial inclusions |
| Histoplasmosis | History | Histoplasmosis exposure, night sweats, weight loss |
| | Physical findings | Uveitis, tongue ulcer, adenopathy, splenomegaly, hepatomegaly |
| | Laboratory tests | Leukopenia, thrombocytopenia, ↑ LFTs, + CT/MRI or gallium/indium scans, ↑ phase I/II titers, + fungal smear or culture of biopsy specimen |

| | | |
|---|---|---|
| **Coccidiomycosis** | History | Coccidiomycosis exposure, headaches, arthralgias, night sweats, weight loss |
| | Physical findings | Chorioretinitis, uveitis, spinal tenderness, arthritis, E nodosa |
| | Laboratory tests | Eosinophilia, ↑ IgM titers, + CT/MRI or gallium/indium scans, + fungal smear or culture of biopsy specimen |
| **Kala-azar** | History | Foreign travel or insect exposure, night sweats, weight loss, skin darkening |
| | Physical findings | Double quotidian fever, long eyelashes, adenopathy, hepatomegaly, splenomegaly, hyperpigmented skin |
| | Laboratory tests | ↑ LFTs, SPEP: polyclonal gammopathy, + CT/MRI or gallium/indium scans, stained biopsy specimen of liver, spleen, BM for intracellular amastigotes |
| **RBF** | History | Recent rodent exposure; contaminated or unpasteurized milk exposure (Haverhill fever); headaches; arthralgias; rash |
| | Physical findings | Conjunctival suffusion; heart murmur (if SBE); adenopathy; splenomegaly; hepatomegaly; arthritis |
| | Laboratory tests | Stained blood smear (S minus); blood culture (S moniliformis); + VDRL (S minus) |
| **RF** | History | Recent rodent exposure, chills, rash, sleep disturbances, tongue tenderness, headaches or mental confusion, arthralgias, myalgias |
| | Physical findings | Conjunctival suffusion, adenopathy, hepatomegaly, splenomegaly, jaundice, epididymo-orchitis or nodule |
| | Laboratory tests | B recurrentis in stained blood smears |
| **LGV** | History | STD exposure; headache; arthralgias; back pain (lower) |
| | Physical findings | Uveitis, adenopathy |
| | Laboratory tests | SPEP: polyclonal gammopathy; highly ↑ C trachomatis $L_{1-3}$ titers; node biopsy (stellate necrosis) |
| **Whipple's disease** | History | Headache or mental status changes; diarrhea; arthralgias; weight loss; skin darkening |
| | Physical findings | Heart murmur (if SBE); hyperpigmented skin; adenopathy; arthritis; edema |
| | Laboratory tests | Lymphopenia; + fecal occult blood; HLA B 27 +; tissue biopsy (PAS + stain of biopsy of small intestine or PCR of heart (if SBE) |

*Abbreviations:* BF, bentonite flocculation; CPK, creatine phosphokinase; CT, computer tomography; ESR, erythrocyte sedimentation rate; LDH, lactate dehydrogenase; LFTs, liver function tests; MRI, magnetic resonance image; PAS, periodic acid–Schiff; PCR, polymerase chain reaction; RBC, red blood cells; RBF, rat-bite fever; RF, rheumatoid factor; SBE, subacute bacterial endocarditis; SPEP, serum protein electrophoresis; STD, sexually transmitted disease; VDRL, Venereal Disease Research Laboratories; WBC, white blood cell.

* When presenting as an FUO.

Table 12
Common, uncommon, and rare rheumatic causes of FUO: focused rheumatic disorders history*

| Historical clues | SLE | LORA | Adult Still's disease | PAN | TA | Takayasu's arteritis | Kikuchi's disease | FMF | Sarcoidosis |
|---|---|---|---|---|---|---|---|---|---|
| Headache | – | – | – | – | + | + | – | – | ± |
| Dry eyes | – | – | – | – | – | – | – | – | + |
| Watery eyes | – | – | – | + | – | – | – | – | – |
| Eye pain or visual disturbances | ±[a] | – | + | – | + | +[a] | – | – | + |
| Transient facial edema | – | – | – | – | – | + | – | – | – |
| Neck pain | – | – | – | – | – | – | ± | – | – |
| Jaw pain or claudication | – | – | – | – | + | – | – | – | – |
| Nasal stuffiness | – | – | – | – | – | – | – | – | + |
| Tongue tenderness | – | – | – | – | + | – | – | – | + |
| Dry cough or chest pain | + | – | – | – | – | – | – | – | + |
| Abdominal pain | ± | – | ± | + | – | – | – | + | – |
| Myalgias, arthralgias | ± | + | + | – | + | – | – | + | ± |

*Abbreviations:* FMF, familial Mediterranean fever; LORA, late-onset rheumatoid arthritis; SLE, systemic lupus erythematous; PAN, periarteritis nodosa; TA, temporal arteritis.

+, Usually present; ±, may be present; –, usually not present.

* When presenting as an FUO.

[a] Amaurosis fugax.

Table 13
Common, uncommon, and rare rheumatic causes of FUO: focused rheumatic disease physical examination*

| Physical examination clues | SLE | LORA | Adult Still's disease | PAN | TA | Takayasu's arteritis | Kikuchi's disease | FMF | Sarcoidosis |
|---|---|---|---|---|---|---|---|---|---|
| Fever pattern | | | | | | | | | |
| Morning temperature spike | – | – | – | + | – | – | – | – | – |
| Double quotidian fever | – | – | + | – | – | – | – | – | – |
| Cranial nerve palsies (CN III, IV, VI) | + | – | – | + | – | – | – | – | + |
| External eyes | | | | | | | | | |
| Lacrimal gland enlargement | – | ± | – | – | + | – | – | – | + |
| Episcleritis | ± | + | + | + | – | – | – | – | – |
| Scleritis | – | + | + | – | – | – | – | – | – |
| Iritis | + | – | – | – | – | – | – | – | + |
| Band keratopathy | – | – | + | – | – | – | – | – | + |
| Conjunctivitis | + | – | + | – | – | – | – | – | +[a] |
| Dry eyes | – | – | – | – | – | – | – | – | + |
| Watery eyes | – | – | – | + | – | – | – | – | – |
| Argyll-Robertson or Adie's pupils | – | – | – | – | – | – | – | – | + |
| Fundi | | | | | | | | | |
| Uveitis | + | ± | + | – | – | – | – | – | + |
| Cytoid bodies | + | – | + | + | – | – | – | – | – |

(continued on next page)

Table 13 (continued)

| Physical examination clues | SLE | LORA | Adult Still's disease | PAN | TA | Takayasu's arteritis | Kikuchi's disease | FMF | Sarcoidosis |
|---|---|---|---|---|---|---|---|---|---|
| "Candlewax drippings" | – | – | – | – | – | – | – | – | + |
| Roth's spots | + | – | – | ± | ± | ± | – | – | – |
| Adenopathy | | | | | | | | | |
| Parotid enlargement | – | – | – | – | – | – | – | – | + |
| Regional or localized | – | – | – | – | – | – | + | – | + |
| Generalized lymphadenopathy | + | – | + | – | – | – | – | – | + |
| Splenomegaly | + | – | + | – | – | – | – | – | + |
| Heart murmur | ±[b] | – | – | – | – | – | – | – | – |
| Epididymo-orchitis, epididymal nodule | + | – | – | + | – | – | – | + | ± |
| Tender fingertips | + | – | – | – | – | – | – | – | – |
| Arthritis, joint effusion | + | + | + | + | – | – | – | ± | ± |

Abbreviations: FMF, familial Mediterranean fever; LORA, late-onset rheumatoid arthritis; PAN, periarteritis nodosa, microscopic polyangiitis; SLE, systemic lupus erythematous; TA, temporal arteritis.

+, Usually present; ±, may be present; –, usually not present

* When presenting as an FUO.

a Conjunctival nodules.

b If Libman-Sacks vegetations present.

Table 14
Common, uncommon, and rare rheumatic causes of FUO: rheumatic disorders laboratory tests*

| Rheumatic tests | SLE | LORA | Adult Still's disease | PAN | TA | Takayasu's arteritis | Kikuchi's disease | FMF | Sarcoidosis |
|---|---|---|---|---|---|---|---|---|---|
| **CBC** | | | | | | | | | |
| Leukocytosis | − | − | + | + | − | − | − | + | − |
| Leukopenia | + | − | − | − | − | − | − | − | + |
| Lymphopenia (relative) | + | + | − | − | − | − | − | − | + |
| Monocytosis | + | ± | − | + | + | − | − | − | ± |
| Eosinophilia | − | − | − | + | + | − | − | − | ± |
| Thrombocytosis | − | ± | − | + | − | − | − | + | − |
| Thrombocytopenia | − | − | − | − | − | − | − | − | − |
| **ESR** | | | | | | | | | |
| Highly elevated (>100 mm/h) | + | + | + | + | + | + | + | ± | − |
| **LFTs** | | | | | | | | | |
| ↑ SGOT, SGPT | − | − | + | ± | − | − | − | − | − |
| ↑ Alkaline phosphatase | − | − | + | + | + | − | − | − | ± |
| **SPEP** | | | | | | | | | |
| Polyclonal gammopathy | + | − | − | ± | − | − | − | − | + |
| ↑ ANA | + | ± | − | − | − | − | − | − | − |
| Cryoglobulins | | | | | | | | | |
| + Cryoglobulins | ± | − | − | − | − | − | − | − | − |
| ↑ ACE | − | − | − | − | − | − | − | − | + |
| Ferritin | | | | | | | | | |
| ↑ Ferritin | + | − | + | − | − | − | − | − | − |

*Abbreviations:* ACE, angiotensin-converting enzyme; ANA, antinuclear antibodies; CBC, complete blood count; ESR, erythrocyte sedimentation rate; FMF, familial Mediterranean fever; LFTs, liver function tests; LORA, late-onset rheumatoid arthritis; PAN, periarteritis nodosa, microscopic polyangiitis; SGOT, serum glutamic-oxaloacetic transaminase; SGPT, serum glutamic-pyruvic transaminase; SLE, systemic lupus erythematous; SPEP, serum protein electrophoresis; TA, temporal arteritis.

+, Usually present; ±, may be present; −, usually not present.

* When presenting as an FUO.

Table 15
Common, uncommon, and rare rheumatic causes of FUO: clinical summaries*

| Rheumatic disorder | Clinical summaries | Other tests | CT/MRI scans of organ involved | Tissue biopsy |
|---|---|---|---|---|
| SLE | History clues: photosensitivity, alopecia, eye symptoms, seizures, headache or mental confusion, sore throat, arthralgias, chest or abdominal pain, tender fingertips, rash, testicular pain, acalculous cholecystitis<br>Physical clues: alopecia; oral ulcers; scleritis; iritis; uveitis; Roth's spots; cytoid bodies (cotton wool spots); heart murmur (if Libman-Sacks endocarditis); Osler's nodes adenopathy; splenomegaly; epididymo-orchitis<br>Laboratory clues: leukopenia, relative lymphopenia, monocytosis, ↑ ferritin, ↑ ANA, cryoglobulins, ↓ complement, thrombocytopenia. SPEP: polyclonal gammopathy, proteinuria | DsDNA<br>Anti-SM<br>APA | Chest, abdomen | Lymph node |

| Disease | Clues | | | |
|---|---|---|---|---|
| Adult Still's disease | History clues: eye symptoms; sore throat; truncal rash (evanescent); arthralgias<br>Physical clues: conjunctival suffusion; double quotidian fever; uveitis; arthritis (late); if rash, dermatographia (Köbner's phenomenon), adenopathy, splenomegaly<br>Laboratory clues: marked ↑ WBC count, ↑ ESR, ↑ alkaline phosphatase, ↑ ferritin | NA | NA | NA |
| PAN | History clues: hearing loss, watery eyes, acalculous cholecystitis, hypertension<br>Physical clues: morning temperature spikes; watery eyes; episcleritis; cytoid bodies (cotton wool spots); optic neuritis (with "macular star"); Roth's spots; cranial nerve palsies; mononeuritis multiplex<br>Laboratory clues: eosinophilia, ↑ ESR, ↑ alkaline phosphatase. SPEP: polyclonal gammopathy | NA | Intra-abdominal angiography | Involved artery<br>Sural nerve |

(continued on next page)

Table 15 (*continued*)

| Rheumatic disorder | Clinical summaries | Other tests | CT/MRI scans of organ involved | Tissue biopsy |
|---|---|---|---|---|
| TA | History clues: depression, amaurosis fugax, headaches, eye pain, myalgias, jaw pain<br>Physical clues: scalp nodules; temporal artery tenderness; episcleritis; optic disc pallor; cytoid bodies (cotton wool spots); cranial nerve palsies<br>Laboratory clues: monocytosis; ↑ ESR (PMR-TA); ↑ alkaline phosphatase (TA) | NA | Temporal arteries | Temporal artery<br>Bone marrow |
| Takayasu's arteritis | History clues: headaches; amaurosis fugax early or severe HT; pain with arm movements over head; TIAs; arthralgias; night sweats; weight loss; rash; facial edema (transient); claudication<br>Physical clues: unequal pulses; bruits over affected arteries (subclavian, carotid, aorta, renal)<br>Laboratory clues: ↑ ESR | NA | Aorta, aortic arch, great vessels | Involved artery |
| Kikuchi's disease | History clues: neck swelling<br>Physical clues: cervical adenopathy<br>Laboratory clues: ↑ ESR | NA | Cervical nodes | Lymph node (eosinophilic adenopathy) |
| FMF | History clues: + FMH, abdominal-joint pain, rash, testicular pain<br>Physical clues: serositis; peritonitis with attacks; hepatomegaly (with amyloidosis); rash; arthritis; epididymo-orchitis or nodule<br>Laboratory clues: leukocytosis; ↑ fibrinogen; proteinuria (with renal amyloidosis) | Colchicine response<br>+ MEFV gene | Chest, abdomen, pelvis (to exclude other disorders) | NA |

| Sarcoidosis | History clues: headache or mental status changes, eye symptoms, stuffy nose, polyphagia, deafness, skin lesions or rash, SOB, ↑ central-peripheral neuropathy, arthritis, ↑ urinary output<br><br>Physical clues: violaceous skin plagues (lupus pernio) on face; facial nerve palsy (CN VII); deafness; basal keratopathy; Argyll-Robertson or Adie's pupils; iritis with keratitic precipitates ("mutton fat" deposits); lacrimal gland enlargement; keratoconjunctivitis sicca; conjunctival nodules; "candlewax drippings"; parotid enlargement; hepatomegaly; E nodosum<br><br>Laboratory clues: leukopenia, relative lymphopenia, monocytosis, eosinophilia, RF, hypercalciuria, hypercalcemia. SPEP: polyclonal gammopathy, anergic | • ↑ ACE<br>• PFTs<br>• ↓ $DL_{CO}$ | Gallium-indium scan (head-neck: "panda sign") | Conjunctival nodule<br>Lymph node<br>Lung |

*Abbreviations:* ACE, angiotensin-converting enzyme; Anti-SM, anti-Smith autoantibodies; APA, antiphospholipid antibody; BM, bone marrow; CCP, cyclic citrillated peptide; Dlco, carbon monoxide diffusing capacity; DsDNA, double stranding; ESR, erythrocyte sedimentation rate; FMF, familial Mediterranean fever; LB, liver biopsy; LORA, late-onset rheumatoid arthritis; N, lymph node; NA, not applicable; PAN, periarteritis nodosa/microscopic polyangiitis; PFTs, pulmonary function tests; PMR, polymyalgia rheumatica; RF, rheumatoid factor; SLE, systemic lupus erythematous; SOB, shortness of breath; SPEP, serum protein electrophoresis; TA, temporal arteritis; TIA, transient ischemic attack; WBC, white blood count.

+, Usually present; ±, may be present; −, usually not present.

* When presenting as an FUO.

Table 16
Common, uncommon, and rare neoplastic causes of FUO: focused neoplastic disorders historical clues, physical examination, and laboratory tests*

| Diagnostic clues | Lymphomas (HL-NHL) | Renal cell cancer | Hepatoma/liver metastases | CNS neoplasms/metastases | Preleukemias (AML) | CML[a] | CLL[b] | Atrial myxomas |
|---|---|---|---|---|---|---|---|---|
| Historical clues | | | | | | | | |
| Decreased appetite, weight loss | + | − | ± | − | ± | + | + | − |
| Night sweats | + | ± | ± | − | ± | + | + | − |
| Pruritus (post hot shower or bath) | + | − | − | − | − | + | + | − |
| Headache or mental status changes | ± | − | − | + | ± | ± | ± | − |
| Early satiety | + | − | − | − | − | + | ± | − |
| Abdominal fullness ± pain | ± | − | + | − | − | + | − | − |
| Physical examination clues | | | | | | | | |
| Relative bradycardia | ± | − | − | ± | − | − | − | − |
| Cranial nerve palsies | ± | − | − | ± | − | − | − | − |
| Sternal tenderness | − | − | − | − | ± | − | − | − |
| Fundi | | | | | | | | |
| Roth's spots | − | − | − | − | − | − | − | ± |
| Cytoid bodies | − | − | − | − | − | − | − | ± |
| Heart murmur | − | − | − | − | − | − | − | + |
| Localized adenopathy | ±[c] | − | − | − | − | − | − | − |
| Generalized adenopathy | ±[d] | − | ± | − | ± | ± | + | − |
| Splenomegaly | ± | − | + | − | ± | + | + | − |
| Hepatic bruit | − | − | − | − | − | − | − | − |
| Epididymo-orchitis or epididymal nodule | + | − | − | − | − | − | − | − |
| Splinter hemorrhages | − | − | − | − | − | − | − | + |

**Laboratory tests**

| Laboratory tests | | | | | | | | |
|---|---|---|---|---|---|---|---|---|
| **ESR** | | | | | | | | |
| Highly elevated (>100 mm/h) | + | + | ± | + | ± | + | + | + |
| **GGT** | | | | | | | | |
| ↑ GGT | − | + | + | − | + | − | − | − |
| **LFTs** | | | | | | | | |
| ↑ Alkaline phosphatase | ± | + | + | − | + | − | − | − |
| **SPEP** | | | | | | | | |
| ↑ $\alpha_1/\alpha_2$ globulins | + | − | − | − | − | − | − | − |
| Polyclonal gammopathy | ± | − | − | − | − | − | − | + |
| **Ferritin** | | | | | | | | |
| Highly elevated (≥ 2 x N) | + | + | ± | + | ± | + | + | − |
| **LDH** | | | | | | | | |
| ↑ LDH | + | − | − | ± | − | ++ | ++ | − |
| + Coombs test | + | − | − | − | − | ++ | ++ | − |
| **Cold agglutinins** | | | | | | | | |
| ↑ Cold agglutinins | ± | − | − | − | − | + | + | − |
| + Cryoglobulins | − | − | − | − | − | ++ | ++ | − |
| ↑ $B_{12}$ | − | − | − | − | − | + | + | + |
| ↓ $B_{12}$/folate | + | − | − | − | − | − | − | − |

*Abbreviations:* AML, acute myelogenous leukemia; CLL, chronic lymphocytic leukemia; CML, chronic myelogenous leukemia; ESR, erythrocyte sedimentation rate; GGT, γ-glutamyltransferase; HL, Hodgkin's lymphoma; LDH, lactate dehydrogenase; LFTs, liver function tests; N, normal; NHL, non-Hodgkin's lymphoma; SPEP, serum protein electrophoresis.

+, Usually present; ±, may be present; −, usually not present.

* When presenting as an FUO.
[a] With blast transformation.
[b] With Richter's transformation.
[c] HL.
[d] NHL.

Table 17
Common, uncommon, and rare neoplastic causes of FUO: clinical summaries*

| Neoplastic FUO causes | Clinical summaries | Special tests | CT/MRI/PET scans | Gallium, indium, or PET scans | Tissue biopsy |
|---|---|---|---|---|---|
| Lymphomas (HL-NHL) | History clues: treatment for HL; primary immune deficiencies; posttransplant immunosuppressive; HIV; high hectic or septic fever (Pel-Ebstein in some); night sweats; weight loss; pruritus; malabsorption symptoms (NHL); bone pain (NHL) Physical clues: regional adenopathy (HL); hepatomegaly; splenomegaly Laboratory clues: relative lymphopenia; monocytosis; eosinophilia; basophilia; thrombocytosis; thrombocytopenia (if ITP); ↑ alkaline phosphatase. SPEP: ↑ $\alpha_1\alpha_2$ globulins or hypogammaglobulinemia, ↑ ferritin, + cryoglobulins | ↑ cold agglutinins ↑ LAP ↑ haptoglobin ↑ $B_{12}$ level microglobulin ↑ $\alpha_1$-antitrypsin + Coombs test ↓ $B_{12}$ level[a] ↓ folate ↑ uric acid ↑ LDH | Chest/abdomen/pelvis + CT/MRI or gallium-indium scans: localized or contiguous nodes with HL; extranodal disease (ie, lung, liver, BM with NHL) | + | Lymph node Bone marrow NHL: (cytogenetic/phenotyping); HL: (Reed Sternberg cells [ie, large binucleated B-lymphocytes with clear halo "owl eyes"]) |
| Hypernephroma (renal cell carcinoma) | History clues: von Hippel-Lindau disease, adult polycystic kidney disease, excessive phenacetin use, flank pain, hematuria Physical clues: flank mass, left hydrocele Laboratory clues: gross/microscopic hematuria, ↑ alkaline phosphatase | + Urine cytology ↑ GGT ↑ calcium | Abdomen | + | Renal biopsy |

| Cause | Diagnostic clues | | | | |
|---|---|---|---|---|---|
| Hepatoma, liver metastases | History clues: $\alpha_1$-antitrypsin deficiency, cirrhosis<br>Physical clues: ↑ ESR, hepatomegaly, liver bruit<br>Laboratory clues: polycythemia, ↑ alkaline phosphatase | Polycythemia<br>↑ alpha-fetoprotein<br>↑ GGT<br>+ HBV/HCV serology<br>↑ calcium<br>↓ FBS<br>↓ folate levels | Abdomen | + | Liver biopsy |
| CNS neoplasms, metastases | History clues: headache or mental status changes, seizures<br>Physical clues: cranial nerve abnormalities, papilledema<br>Laboratory clues: CSF: highly ↑ protein, + RBCs | CSF cytology | Head | NA | Brain lesion |
| Preleukemia (AML) | History clues: night sweats, weight loss<br>Physical clues: sternal tenderness<br>Laboratory clues: metamyelocytes, nucleated or teardrop RBCs, ↑ ESR, ↑ LDH, ↑ ferritin | ↑ uric acid | NA | – | Bone marrow |
| CML (with blast transformation) | History clues: night sweats, weight loss, pruritus, bleeding, bone pain, abdominal fullness<br>Physical clues: retinal hemorrhage, adenopathy, splenomegaly, sternal tenderness<br>Laboratory clues: leukocytosis, eosinophilia, basophilia thrombocytopenia (if ITP)[b], thrombocytosis, ↑ ESR, ↑ LDH, ↑ ferritin, ↑ cold agglutinins | ↑ uric acid<br>↓ LAP<br>+ Philadelphia chromosome<br>↑ $B_{12}$ level<br>↑ LDH | NA | + | Bone marrow |

(continued on next page)

Table 17 (*continued*)

| Neoplastic FUO causes | Clinical summaries | Special tests | CT/MRI/PET scans | Gallium, indium, or PET scans | Tissue biopsy |
|---|---|---|---|---|---|
| CLL (with Richter's transformation) | History clues: night sweats, weight loss<br>Physical clues: adenopathy, splenomegaly<br>Laboratory clues: eosinophilia, basophilia, "smudge cells" in peripheral smear, ↑ ESR, SPEP: hypogammaglobulinemia, + Coombs test, ± cryoglobulins, | + Coombs test (AIHA)<br>↑ $B_{12}$ level<br>Urine immunoglobulins<br>↑ LDH | NA | + | Bone marrow |
| Atrial myxomas | History clues: heart murmur, weight loss<br>Physical clues: cytoid bodies (cotton wool spots), Roth's spots, heart murmur, splinter hemorrhages<br>Laboratory clues: ↑ ESR, SPEP: polyclonal gammopathy (vegetations on TTE/TEE with negative blood cultures) | TTE/TEE | NA | NA | Myocardial biopsy |

*Abbreviations:* AML, acute myelogenous leukemia; CEA, carcinoembryonic antigen; CLL, chronic lymphocytic leukemia; CML, chronic myelogenous leukemia; CNS, central nervous system; CSF, cerebrospinal fluid; ESR, erythrocyte sedimentation rate; GGT, glucose tolerance test; HL, Hodgkin's lymphoma; LAP, leukocyte alkaline phosphatase; LDH, lactate dehydrogenase; NHL, non-Hodgkin's lymphoma; RBCs, red blood cells; SPEP, serum protein electrophoresis; TTE-TEE, transthoracic-transesophageal echocardiogram.

+, Usually present; ±, may be present; −, usually not present.

\* When presenting as an FUO.

[a] $\beta_{12}$ is normal in HL, but may be ↓ in NHL; RF, rheumatoid factor.

[b] May be the first sign of blast transformation in CML; AIHA, autoimmune hemolytic anemia.

Table 18
Common, uncommon, and rare miscellaneous disorders causing FUO: focused miscellaneous disorders history, physical examination, and laboratory tests*

| Diagnostic clues | Alcoholic cirrhosis | Crohn's disease | Drug fever | Subacute thyroiditis | Cyclic neutropenia | DVTs | Hyper-IgD syndrome | Factitious fever | Schnitzler's syndrome |
|---|---|---|---|---|---|---|---|---|---|
| Historical clues | | | | | | | | | |
| On sensitizing medication | − | − | + | − | − | − | − | − | − |
| Hypercoagulable state/venous stasis | − | − | − | − | − | + | − | − | − |
| Arthralgias/joint pain | − | − | − | − | + | − | + | − | + |
| Sore throat | − | − | − | + | − | − | + | − | − |
| Thyroid/autoimmune disease | − | − | − | ± | − | − | − | − | − |
| Chronic alcoholism | + | − | − | − | − | − | − | − | − |
| Intermittent urticaria | − | − | − | − | − | − | + | − | + |
| Abdominal pain | − | ± | − | − | − | − | − | − | + |
| Diarrhea | − | − | − | − | − | − | + | − | − |
| Physical examination clues | | | | | | | | | |
| Relative bradycardia[a] | − | − | + | − | − | − | − | + | − |
| Clinically well appearing | − | − | + | + | +[b] | − | +[b] | + | +[b] |
| Fundi | | | | | | | | | |
| Episcleritis[c] | − | + | − | − | − | − | − | − | − |
| Choroiditis | − | + | − | − | − | − | − | − | − |
| Oral ulcers | − | − | − | − | − | − | + | − | − |
| Neck or angle of jaw tenderness | − | − | − | + | − | − | − | − | − |
| Adenopathy | − | − | − | − | − | − | +[d] | − | − |

(continued on next page)

Table 18 (*continued*)

| Diagnostic clues | Alcoholic cirrhosis | Crohn's disease | Drug fever | Subacute thyroiditis | Cyclic neutropenia | DVTs | Hyper-IgD syndrome | Factitious fever | Schnitzler's syndrome |
|---|---|---|---|---|---|---|---|---|---|
| Splenomegaly | ± | −[c] | − | − | − | − | + | − | − |
| Hepatomegaly | ± | − | − | − | − | − | + | − | − |
| Laboratory clues | | | | | | | | | |
| CBC | | | | | | | | | |
| Leukocytosis | − | ± | + | ± | − | ± | − | − | − |
| Leukopenia | − | − | − | − | +[b] | − | − | − | − |
| Lymphocytosis | − | − | + | − | − | − | − | − | − |
| Lymphopenia (relative) | + | − | − | − | − | − | − | − | − |
| Eosinophilia | − | − | ± | − | ±[b] | − | − | − | − |
| Atypical lymphocytes | − | − | + | − | − | − | − | − | − |
| Thrombocytosis | − | − | − | − | − | − | − | − | − |
| Thrombocytopenia | + | − | − | − | − | − | − | − | − |
| LFTs | | | | | | | | | |
| ↑ SGOT/SGPT | + | ± | + | − | − | − | − | − | − |
| ↑ Alkaline phosphatase | ± | − | − | + | − | − | − | − | − |
| ESR | | | | | | | | | |
| Elevated (≥2 x n) | − | + | + | + | − | ± | + | − | + |
| FSP | | | | | | | | | |
| Highly elevated | − | − | − | − | − | + | − | − | − |
| SPEP | | | | | | | | | |
| Monoclonal IgM/IgD spike | − | − | − | − | − | − | +[e] | − | + |
| Polyclonal gammopathy | + | − | − | − | − | − | − | − | − |

Thyroiditis tests
  ↑ TPO titers
  ↑ ATG titers
Urine
  Temperature less than rectal temperature
  ↑ urine mevalonic acid, neoptermin levels
Tissue biopsy
  Thyroid
  Ileum
  Liver
+ Doppler ultrasound (LE)

---

*Abbreviations:* ATG, antithyroglobulins; CBC, complete blood count; $C_3/CH_{50}$, serum complement; DVTs, deep vein thrombosis; ESR, erythrocyte sedimentation rate; FSP, fibrin split products; LE, lower extremity; LFTs, liver function tests; n, =normal; SGOT, serum glutamic-oxaloacetic transaminase; SGPT, serum glutamic-pyruvic transaminase; SPEP, serum protein electrophoresis; TPO, antithyroid peroxidase.

+, Usually present; ±, may be present; −, usually not present

* When presenting as an FUO.
a Pulse-temperature deficit.
b May be persistent during fever, attacks.
c Presents with Crohn's disease, but not ulcerative colitis.
d Cervical adenopathy.
e ↑ IgD.

Table 19
Common infectious disease causes of FUO: focused infectious disease diagnostic tests*

| Infectious disease | Stained blood smears | Special blood cultures ($\uparrow CO_2$/6 weeks) | TTE/TEE | Intra-abdominal pelvic CT/MRI[a] | Gallium/Indium scans[a] | Specific $\uparrow$IgM titers | CSF | AFB culture | DX aspirate-biopsy |
|---|---|---|---|---|---|---|---|---|---|
| SBE | − | + | + | − | − | +[b] | − | − | − |
| Abscess | − | − | − | + | + | − | − | − | + |
| CNS TB | − | − | − | − | − | − | + | + | − |
| Renal TB | − | − | − | + | + | − | − | + | − |
| Miliary TB | − | − | − | + | + | − | − | +[c] | +[c] |
| Typhoid | − | − | − | + | + | + | − | − | +[d] |
| CMV | − | − | − | ± | ± | + | − | − | + |
| EBV | − | − | − | + | + | + | − | − | + |
| HIV | − | − | − | − | − | +[e] | − | − | − |
| CSD | − | + | +[f] | + | + | + | − | − | + |
| TOXO | − | − | − | + | + | + | − | − | + |

Abbreviations: Abscess, intra-abdominal or pelvic; CMV, cytomegalovirus; CNS, central nervous system; CSD, cat-scratch disease (B henselae); CSF, cerebrospinal fluid; CT, computer tomography; EBV, Epstein-Barr virus; HIV, human immunodeficiency virus; KA, kala-azar (visceral leishmaniasis); MRI, magnetic resonance imaging; SBE, subacute bacterial endocarditis; TB, tuberculosis; TTE-TEE, transthoracic-transesophageal echocardiogram; TOXO, toxoplasmosis; Typhoid, typhoid or enteric fever.

+, Usually present; ±, may be present; −, usually not present.

* When presenting as an FUO.

[a] If not already done as part of initial FUO diagnostic tests.

[b] For culture-negative SBE pathogens (Q fever, brucellosis, and so forth).

[c] AFB smear or culture of liver, lymph nodes, or bone marrow.

[d] Blood, urine, stool, liver, or bone marrow.

[e] HIV serology or viral load.

[f] If SBE.

Table 20
Uncommon and rare infectious disease causes of FUO: further focused infectious disease diagnostic tests*

| Infectious disease | Stained blood smears | Special blood cultures (↑$CO_2$/6 wk) | TTE/TEE | Intra-ABD/ pelvic CT/MRI[a] | Gallium/indium scans[a] | Specific ↑IgM titers | CSF | AFB culture | Dx aspirate-biopsy |
|---|---|---|---|---|---|---|---|---|---|
| EHR-ANA | + | − | − | − | − | + | − | − | − |
| LEPTO | − | +[b] | − | + | + | + | − | − | − |
| BRU | − | +[b] | +[b] | − | − | +[c] | − | − | + |
| Q Fever | − | − | +[b] | + | + | +[c] | − | − | + |
| TRICH | − | − | − | − | + | + | − | − | + |
| Malaria | +[d] | − | − | + | + | − | − | − | − |
| HISTO | +[d] | +[b] | +[b] | + | + | +[c] | − | − | +[e] |
| COCCI | − | − | − | + | + | + | −[f] | − | +[e] |
| KA | − | − | − | + | + | + | − | − | +[e] |
| RBF | +[g] | − | − | − | − | − | − | − | +[h] |
| RF | + | − | − | − | + | − | − | − | +[e] |
| LGV | − | − | +[b] | + | + | +[i] | − | − | +[j] |
| WD | − | +[b] | +[b] | + | − | − | +[k] | − | +[k] |

*Abbreviations:* BRU, brucellosis; COCCI, coccidiomycosis; CT, computer tomography; EHR-ANA, ehrlichiosis-anaplasmosis; HISTO, histoplasmosis; KA, kala-azar (visceral leishmaniasis); LEPTO, leptospirosis; LGV, lymphogranuloma venereum; MRI, magnetic resonance tomography; RBF, rat-bite fever (*S moniliformis, S minus*); RF, relapsing fever (*B recurrentis*); TRICH, trichinosis; WD, Whipple's disease.

+, Usually present; ±, may be present; −, usually not present.

* When presenting as an FUO.

[a] If not already done as part of initial FUO diagnostic tests.

[b] If heart murmur or signs of SBE.

[c] ↑ phase I-II titers.

[d] With HIV only.

[e] Liver, spleen, node, muscle, or bone marrow.

[f] With CNS abnormalities.

[g] *S moniliformis*.

[h] *S minus*.

[i] Highly ↑ IgG *C trachomatis* $L_{1-3}$ titers diagnostic.

[j] Lymph node.

[k] PCR or PAS + stain of small intestine, nodes, or heart valve.

Table 21
Diagnostic tests for selected uncommon infectious disease causes of FUO*

| Obscure causes of FUOs | Tests that may provide clues | Diagnostic findings |
|---|---|---|
| Infected pacemaker wire or generator | Indium scan or PET scan | ↑ Uptake of wire, generator |
| Aortitis (infective) | Intermittently or persistently + BCs | |
| | PET scan | ↑ Uptake in aorta |
| Infected aortic aneurysm or graft or infected AV graft | Indium scan or PET scan | ↑ Uptake in graft, aneurysm |
| | CT/MRI scan of aneurysm/graft | Graft, aneurysm periluminal thickening or collection |
| Chronic sinusitis | Head CT/MRI | Mucosal thickening, air fluid level |
| Relapsing mastoiditis | Head CT/MRI | Abnormal mastoid |
| Periapical dental abscess | Panorex radiograph of jaws | Periapical collection |
| | Gallium scan of jaws | ↑ Periapical uptake |
| Subacute vertebral osteomyelitis | Bone scan | ↑ Vertebral uptake |
| | CT/MRI of spine | Vertebral osteomyelitis |
| Chikungunya fever | CT/MRI of hands and feet | Small joint arthritis |
| | Gallium/indium scan | ↑ Uptake posterior cervical nodes |

*Abbreviations:* AV, arteriovenous; CT, computer tomography; MRI, magnetic resonance imaging; PET, positron emission tomography.
+, Usually present; ±, may be present; −, usually not present.
* When presenting as an FUO.

period. The Naprosyn test may use other nonsteroidal anti-inflammatory drugs, but experience with these drugs is limited. The Naprosyn test is very useful diagnostically, but if the differential diagnosis of an FUO is between a neoplastic and infectious disorder the Naprosyn test is unhelpful in differentiating neoplastic from noninfectious disorders (ie, rheumatic, inflammatory, or miscellaneous disorders) [32,33].

## Fever of unknown origin: definitive evaluation

Definitive diagnostic testing is done in the third or final phase of diagnostic FUO evaluation. In patients with an appropriate epidemiologic history, serologic tests for visceral leishmaniasis should be obtained. Most infectious, rheumatic-inflammatory, neoplastic, and miscellaneous disorders should be diagnosed after an initial and focused diagnostic FUO evaluation. The disorders not diagnosed to this point are uncommon causes of FUO and require special testing or tissue biopsy for diagnosis as guided by nonspecific laboratory test abnormalities and pertinent features of the focused FUO history and physical examination [1,14,15,34–38].

## Invasive diagnostic tests

### Liver biopsy

If there are signs and symptoms in a presenting FUO syndrome complex that suggest liver involvement, then liver biopsy may be diagnostically helpful. Liver biopsy is most useful in granulomatous hepatitis where the differential diagnosis may be useful in differentiating granulomas caused by infections, rheumatic-inflammatory disorders, or neoplastic causes. A liver biopsy may be useful in diagnosing suspected miliary tuberculosis as a cause of FUO [4,39].

### Lymph node biopsy

Lymph node biopsy is most useful to diagnose lymphomas. Anterior cervical, axillary, or inguinal nodes should not be biopsied if at all possible because the pathology is invariably reported as "nonspecific/reactive cannot rule out lymphoma." The preferred nodes to biopsy are the posterior cervical, epitrochlear, or supraclavicular nodes. Lymph node pathology is diagnostic with lymphoma, lymphogranuloma venereum, toxoplasmosis, and Kikuchi's arteritis. Granulomas in lymph node biopsies may represent a granulomatous disorder (eg, tuberculosis, sarcoidosis) and lymphoma [40,41].

### Bone marrow biopsy

Bone marrow biopsy, as with liver biopsy, may be helpful diagnostically with disorders that are associated with bone marrow abnormalities. Bone marrow biopsy is of importance in diagnosing various neoplastic disorders (eg, preleukemia, multiple myeloma when other tests are negative). Bone marrow biopsy is also useful in detecting intracellular infectious pathogens associated with FUO (eg, disseminated histoplasmosis). Bone marrow biopsy is also useful diagnostically in cases of suspected miliary tuberculosis. Bone marrow biopsy is also helpful in a variety of miscellaneous disorders not usually associated with abnormal bone marrow findings (eg, temporal arteritis) [42–44].

*Exploratory laparotomy*

With the advent of sophisticated serologic tests and imaging and various imaging modalities, the necessity for exploratory laparotomy has been largely eliminated. Because the initial work-up of the FUO patient includes abdominal and pelvic CT and MRI scanning and total body gallium-indium scanning, exploratory laparotomy is useful primarily to obtain lymph node or organ biopsies that are otherwise unobtainable. Blind exploratory laparotomy has a low diagnostic yield. The clinical syndromic presentation and the pattern of physical and laboratory abnormalities determines the pattern of organ involvement, which should guide the surgeon to the appropriate tissue when doing an exploratory laparotomy [45,46].

**Fever of unknown origin: approach to undiagnosed and recurrent disorders after a focused evaluation**

Even some rare disorders may be potentially diagnosed during the initial and focused FUO evaluation. The serum protein electrophoresis may suggest otherwise unsuspected sarcoidosis, hyperimmunoglobulinemia D syndrome, or Schnitzler's syndrome. The serum protein electrophoresis with increase in IgD accompanied by a decrease in IgA should suggest hyperimmunoglobulinemia D syndrome. Schnitzler's syndrome is suggested by a monoclonal increase in IgM antibodies. Polyclonal gammopathy seen on the serum protein electrophoresis should suggest previously undiagnosed causes of FUO including sarcoidosis, lymphogranuloma venereum, or atrial myxoma (if heart murmur was missed). The ESR may be helpful in indicating trichinosis. Patients with trichinosis presenting as an FUO may no longer have eosinophilia. There are no causes of FUO with polymyositis that are associated with a subnormal ESR rate approaching 0 mm/h.

Highly elevated ESR rate accompanied by elevated fibrin split products should prompt further specific testing for deep vein thrombosis and small pulmonary emboli. Isolated cervical adenopathy not previously diagnosed during the initial or focused phases of FUO evaluation should raise the possibility of toxoplasmosis, Kikuchi's disease, or pseudolymphoma. Further specific diagnostic testing and tissue biopsy can be done to diagnose definitively each of these entities. In patients with an appropriate reason and zoonotic contact history, serologic tests may be sent for brucellosis, Q fever, and leptospirosis. When presenting as FUOs, both Q fever and to a lesser extent brucellosis may present as "culture-negative endocarditis." If rodent or rat bite exposure is present, then relapsing fever and rat-bite fever may be diagnosed by blood smear or culture. Symptoms referable to the great vessels in a patient with vasculitis should suggest the possibility of Takayasu's arteritis for testing with a positron emission tomography scan evaluation. Familial Mediterranean fever is suggested by migratory recurrence serositis in patients of Mediterranean descent. Appropriate genetic studies may be sent to confirm the diagnosis of familial Mediterranean fever [47,48].

A head CT reveals obscure chronic sinusitis; relapsing mastoiditis; apical dental abscesses; and primary, metastatic, and central nervous system neoplasms. There may be abnormalities on the head CT and MRI to suggest tuberculous meningitis or hypothalamic abnormalities. Serologic tests for histoplasmosis and coccidiomycosis should be obtained if the presenting syndrome complex and exposure history to these endemic mycoses indicates the diagnostic possibility.

Two diagnoses that are not readily diagnosable during the initial and focused FUO evaluation are Whipple's disease and factitious fever. Whipple's disease is a particularly difficult diagnosis because intestinal biopsy is required for confirmation for a tissue diagnosis and specific serologic tests must be ordered to confirm the diagnosis. Whipple's disease should be considered as a cause of FUO in patients with prolonged fever, mental status changes, arthritis symptoms, and diarrhea or malabsorption. Whipple's disease may also present as true culture-negative endocarditis. Whipple's disease may be diagnosed by demonstrating periodic acid–Schiff positive material in macrophages in small intestinal biopsies. Polymerase chain reaction may be used to diagnose Whipple's disease in tissue samples of the small intestine or heart valve (if the valve was replaced because of endocarditis).

Even a focused diagnostic FUO work-up can miss certain rare causes of FUO. Cervical carcinoma and colon carcinoma may be missed during the FUO evaluation. If FUO patients have persistent fever and no other diagnosis, then these diagnoses should be considered in the appropriate patient setting and diagnosis confirmed by endoscopy or biopsy of the cervix.

Factitious fever is rare cause of FUO. It occurs most commonly in young adults, usually in medical personnel. Factitious fever may be suspected during the initial or focused phases of FUO evaluation on the basis of negative history, physical, and nonspecific laboratory findings. If these FUO evaluations are a noncontribution, then factitious fever should be suspected in the proper clinical context. Factitious fever may be diagnosed by comparing rectal and oral temperatures with temperature of urine. Urine reflects the core temperature of the individual and in patients with factitious fever should be normal, or the temperature obtained from other sites is elevated by one means or another. Patients with factitious fever are inventive and have many ways to alter temperature recordings. An obvious clue to the factitious fever is a pulse-temperature deficit or relative bradycardia. In such patients, the rectal temperature should be taken under direct observation as should the urinary specimen collection to avoid maneuvers that alter temperatures [1,10,14,15,48].

The three-tiered focused diagnostic approach diagnoses all but the most unusual causes of FUO. The only disorders missed by focused FUO evaluation are very rare entities. After a focused FUO diagnostic approach, however, there are no more than half a dozen obscure disorders that may be pursued depending on the patient's age, ethnicity, and so forth, or for example the periodic fever syndromes. The phased diagnostic approach eliminates "shotgun testing" and undue reliance on laboratory testing at the expense of an FUO-relevant and detailed history and physical examination. Clinicians are often unaware of the diagnostic significance of certain physical findings in evaluating FUO patients. The significance of nonspecific laboratory tests is enhanced when considered together to increase diagnostic specificity. Although abnormalities are nonspecific, most entities responsible for FUO have several abnormalities, the significance of which taken together may point to the diagnosis. Laboratory tests should not be excessive; rather, they should be focused and comprehensive in the category dealing with differential diagnostic possibilities. A complete and detailed history and physical examination not relevant to FUO evaluation is unhelpful. Clinicians should endeavor to become more familiar with the causes of FUO that are not readily diagnosable by tests and that have subtle or uncommon findings that may be the only clues to diagnosis [47–50].

## Summary

FUOs usually are limited by their progression and are self-terminating or are terminated with effective therapy. Some causes of FUO are prone to recurrence. In the main, recurrent FUOs are most often caused by rheumatic-inflammatory etiologies. Patients with infectious FUOs usually resolve with or without therapy in less than a year. Neoplastic disorders usually present themselves in less than 1 year but some disorders may recur episodically over a prolonged period of time (eg, preleukemias, myeloproliferative disorders). Some infectious diseases are prone to recur (eg, relapsing fever). As a general rule, the longer that an FUO remains undiagnosed, the less likely it is caused by an infectious etiology [49,50].

Using a focused diagnostic approach a three-tiered system leaves very few disorders undiagnosed. Most of the common causes of FUO are diagnosed during the initial FUO evaluation. The focused FUO evaluation should be able to diagnose less common and obscure disorders associated with prolonged and perplexing fevers. The objective of the focused diagnostic evaluation is to prompt the clinician to order specific diagnostic tests to rule out or confirm various causes of FUO in the differential diagnosis based on the clinical syndromic presentation. Definitive FUO evaluation should be diagnostic for nearly all infectious, rheumatic-inflammatory, neoplastic, and miscellaneous causes of FUO. Some causes of FUO remain obscure even after such a focused and relevant FUO work-up. Clinicians faced with obscure causes of FUO that remain undiagnosed should consult the FUO literature to evaluate systemically each of these very rare diagnostic possibilities [14,15,28].

## References

[1] Keefer CS, Leard SE. Prolonged and perplexing fevers. Boston: Little, Brown; 1955.
[2] Petersdorf RG, Beeson PB. Fever of unexplained origin: report on 100 cases. Medicine (Baltimore) 1961;40:1–30.
[3] Petersdorf RF. Fever of unknown origin: an old friend revisited. Arch Intern Med 1992;152: 21–2.
[4] Knockaert DC, Vanneste LJ, Vannester SB, et al. Fever of unknown origin in the 1980s: an update of the diagnostic spectrum. Arch Intern Med 1992;152:51–5.
[5] Tumulty PA. Topics in clinical medicine. The patient with fever of undetermined origin. Johns Hopkins Med J 1967;120:95–106.
[6] Jacoby GA, Swartz MN. Fever of undetermined origin. N Engl J Med 1973;289:1407–10.
[7] Ergonul O, Willke A, Azap A, et al. Revised definition of fever of unknown origin: limitations and opportunities. J Infect 2005;50:1–5.
[8] Brusch JL, Weinstein L. Fever of unknown origin. Med Clin North Am 1988;72:1247–61.
[9] Cunha BA. Diagnostic significance of nonspecific laboratory abnormalities in infectious diseases. In: Gorbach SL, Bartlett JG, Blacklow NE, editors. Infectious diseases. 3rd edition. Philadelphia: Lippincott, Williams and Wilkins; 2004. p. 158–65.
[10] Murray HW, editor. Fever of unknown origin: fever of undetermined origin. Mount Kisco (NY): Informa Healthcare; 1983.
[11] Cunha BA. Fever of unknown origin. Infect Dis Clin North Am 1996;10:111–28.
[12] Cunha BA. Fever of unknown origin. In: Gorbach SL, Bartlett JG, Blacklow NE, editors. Infectious diseases. 3rd edition. Philadelphia: Lippincott, Williams & Wilkins; 2005. p. 1568–77.
[13] Cunha BA, editor. FUO: fever of unknown origin. New York: Informa Healthcare; 2007.
[14] Esposito AL. Planning and proceeding with the diagnostic evaluation. In: Murray HW, editor. Fever of undetermined origin. Mount Kisco (NY): Future Publishing; 1983. p. 141–55.
[15] Cunha BA. Fever of unknown origin: a focused diagnostic approach. In: Cunha BA, editor. Fever of unknown origin. New York: Informa Healthcare; 2007. p. 9–16.
[16] Tumulty PA. Obtaining the history: the effective clinician. Philadelphia: WB Saunders; 1973. p. 17–28.
[17] Tumulty PA. The physical examination: the effective clinician. Philadelphia: WB Saunders; 1973. p. 51–98.
[18] Orient JM. Sapira's art & science of bedside diagnosis. 3rd edition. Philadelphia: Lippincott, Williams & Wilkins; 2005.
[19] Tumulty PA. The history and physical examination. In: Murray HW, editor. FUO of undetermined origin. Mount Kisco (NY): Futura Publishing; 1983. p. 141–55.
[20] Tumulty PA, editor. The patient with fever of unknown origin (FUO): the effective clinician. Philadelphia: WB Saunders; 1973. p. 137–70.
[21] Gorbach SL, Bartlett JG, Blacklow NE, editors. Infectious diseases. 3rd edition. Philadelphia: Lippincott Williams & Wilkins; 2005.
[22] Kasper DL, Fauci AS, Longo DL, et al, editors. Harrison's principles of internal medicine. 16th edition. New York: Mc-Graw-Hill; 2005.

[23] Gold DH, Weingeist TA, editors. Color atlas of the eye in systemic disease. Philadelphia: Lippincott Williams & Wilkins; 2001.

[24] Quillen DA, Blodi BA. Clinical retina. Chicago: AMA Press; 2002.

[25] Schneiderman PI, Grossman ME. A clinician's guide to dermatologic differential diagnosis. London: Informa Healthcare; 2006.

[26] Wallach J. Interpretation of diagnostic tests. 7th edition. Philadelphia: Lippincott Williams & Wilkins; 2000.

[27] Cunha BA. Nonspecific tests in the diagnosis of fever of unknown origin. In: Cunha BA, editor. Fever of unknown origin. New York: Informa Healthcare; 2007.

[28] Bleeker-Rovers CP, Vos FJ, de Kleijn EM, et al. A prospective multicenter study on fever of unknown origin: the yield of a structured diagnostic protocol. Medicine (Baltimore) 2007;86: 26–38.

[29] Woodward TE. The fever pattern as diagnostic aid. In: Mackowiak PA, editor. Fever: basic mechanisms and management. 2nd edition. Philadelphia: Lippincott-Raven; 1997. p. 215–35.

[30] Cunha BA. The diagnostic significance of fever curves. Infect Dis Clin North Am 1996;10: 33–44.

[31] Cunha BA. Diagnostic significance of relative bradycardia. Infectious Disease Practice 1997; 21:38–40.

[32] Chang JC. How to differentiate neoplastic fever from infectious fever in patients with cancer: usefulness of the Naproxen test. Heart Lung 1987;16:122–7.

[33] Reme P, Cunha BA. NSAIDs and the Naprosyn test in fever of unknown origins. Infectious Disease Practice 2000;24:32.

[34] Purnendu S, Louria DB. Non-invasive and invasive diagnostic procedures and laboratory methods. In: Henry W Murray, editor. FUO of undetermined origin. Mount Kisco (NY): Futura Publishing Company; 1983.

[35] Kosmin AR, Lorber B. Specific tests in the diagnosis of fever of unknown origin. In: Cunha BA, editor. Fever of unknown origin. New York: Informa Healthcare; 2007. p. 159–208.

[36] Trivedi Y, Yung E, Katz DS. Imaging in fever of unknown origin. In: Cunha BA, editor. Fever of unknown origin. New York: Informa Healthcare; 2007. p. 209–28.

[37] Meller J, Sahlmann CO, Scheel AK. 18F-FDG PET and PET/CT in fever of unknown origin. J Nucl Med 2007;48:35–45.

[38] Rijinders AJ, Bleeker-Rovers CP, Vos FJ, et al. A prospective multi-center study of the value of FDG-PET as part of a structured diagnostic protocol in patients with fever of unknown origin. Eur J Nucl Med Mol Imaging 2007;34:694–703.

[39] Holtz T, Moseley RH, Scheiman JM. Liver biopsy in fever of unknown origin: a reappraisal. J Clin Gastroenterol 1993;17:29–32.

[40] Sinclair S, Beckman E, Ellman L. Biopsy of enlarged superficial lymph nodes. JAMA 1974; 228:602–3.

[41] Dorfman RF, Remington JS. Value of lymph node biopsy in the diagnosis of acute acquired toxoplasmosis. N Engl J Med 1973;289:878–81.

[42] Pease GL. Granulomatous lesions in bone marrow. Blood 1956;11:720–34.

[43] Ellman L. Bone marrow biopsy in the evaluation of lymphoma, carcinoma and granulomatous disorders. Am J Med 1976;60:1–7.

[44] Enos WF, Pierre RV, Rosenblatt JE. Giant cell arteritis detected by bone marrow biopsy. Mayo Clin Proc 1981;56:381–3.

[45] Arch-Ferrer JE, Velazquez-Fernandez D, Sierra-Madero J, et al. Laparoscopic approach to fever of unknown origin. Surg Endosc 2003;17:494–7.

[46] Tanaka PY, Hadad DJ, Barletti SC, et al. Bone marrow biopsy in the diagnoses of infectious and non-infectious causes in patients with advanced HIV infection. J Infect 2007;54: 362–6.

[47] Wolff SM, Fauci AS, Dale DC. Unusual etiologies of fever and their evaluation. Annu Rev Med 1975;26:277–81.

[48] Molavi A, Weinstein L. Persistent perplexing pyrexia: some comments on etiology and diagnosis. Med Clin North Am 1970;54:379–96.
[49] Knockaert DC, Dujardin KS, Bobbaers HJ. Long-term follow up of patients with undiagnosed fever of unknown origin. Arch Intern Med 1996;156:618–20.
[50] Knockaert DC. Recurrent fever of unknown origin. In: Cunha BA, editor. Fever of unknown origin. New York: Informa Healthcare; 2007. p. 133–50.

ELSEVIER
SAUNDERS

INFECTIOUS
DISEASE CLINICS
OF NORTH AMERICA

Infect Dis Clin N Am 21 (2007) 1189–1211

# Recurrent Fevers of Unknown Origin

## Daniel C. Knockaert, MD, PhD

*Division of General Internal Medicine, Gasthuisberg University Hospital,
Herestraat 49, B-3000 Leuven, Belgium*

Fever of unknown origin (FUO), as defined by Petersdorf and Beeson [1] in 1961, is a rather rare clinical syndrome well known as one of the major diagnostic challenges of internal medicine. In the last two decades several modifications have been proposed for the criteria of FUO and subpopulations of FUO have also been defined [2–5]. Many clinicians and even investigators, however, continue to use the term FUO loosely for acute fever without a source or prolonged fever without adequate initial work-up. An update of criteria of a syndrome is warranted as the practice of medicine evolves but with respect for the original intentions of the definition [4]. Petersdorf and Beeson [1] defined FUO as a clinical syndrome of prolonged fever ($>3$ weeks) to exclude transient self-limited illnesses, which are mostly viral or undiagnosed infections. The 1 week in hospital investigation criterion was introduced to include the difficult perplexing fevers that escaped an appropriate intelligent first diagnostic work-up. Duration of initial investigation is not the matter, yet the required investigations, which may change over time as insights and practice of medicine evolve [4,5]. Petersdorf indeed mentioned in his original paper the studies that must be performed in the first week of in-hospital investigation, much less than what is proposed nowadays, and performed in 1 or 2 outpatient visits [4,5]. The range of fever (38.3°C) was intended to exclude habitual hyperthermia, but even low-grade fever meets the intention of this Petersdorf criterion on condition that signs of inflammation (increased erythrocyte sedimentation rate, C-reactive protein level) are present [4].

Subpopulations, such as HIV-associated FUO, neutropenic FUO, and nosocomial FUO, are caused by another spectrum of diseases than classic FUO (ie, more infections, [hematologic] malignancies, and drug-induced cases). These subsets of patients require another approach, namely early empiric anti-infective therapy (antibiotics, antiviral, antifungals) because these

*E-mail address:* daniel.knockaert@uz.kuleuven.ac.be

patients are more at risk for rapid deterioration as a result of their immune dysfunction [2,4].

Recurrent or episodic FUO is probably the most intriguing and most difficult to diagnose subtype of FUO. Few literature data, however, are available on this entity. The paper of Reimann and Mc Closkey [6] was published in 1974, and the author's own study pertains to patients seen in the 1980s [7]. An update of the spectrum can be found in two very recent French series that emphasize the importance of the hereditary fever syndromes, but these studies lack methodologic strictness [8,9]. The author defined recurrent FUO as classic FUO with a least two episodes of fever with fever-free intervals of at least 2 weeks and seeming remission of the causative disease as characterized by normalization of the signs of inflammation [7]. This symptom-free period may vary from weeks to years and this interval of at least 2 weeks was suggested because it allows excluding those diseases that recur because of interruption or tapering of an inadequate empiric therapy. Some authors use an interval between two episodes of only 48 hours, but the author finds this too short [9,10]. Patients remain prepared to undergo additional investigations as long as fever persists and regression of symptoms during 1 or 2 days does not reassure them or the involved physician. After a week or more, however, patients become more reluctant for further investigations and physicians start doubting the value of further testing. A watchful waiting outpatient follow-up is then greatly appreciated [7,11].

The term "periodic fever" is not used because this latter term has sometimes been used for familial Mediterranean fever (FMF), which is designated as "maladie périodique" (periodic disease) in the French-language based literature. Periodic fever has also been considered as a distinct clinical entity in the 1940s with a specific periodicity of 20 or 21 days, being a multiple of the biblical holy number of 7, or multiples of these numbers [6,7,12]. When fever was the prominent symptom the periodic disease was called "periodic fever" and diagnosis was mainly based on analysis of the temperature chart [12]. This entity survived in the medical literature through the early 1970s but it is no longer withheld.

## Epidemiologic features

Recurrent FUO represents between 18% and 42% of the cases in large series of patients with FUO [5,7–9,13–15]. All these data are from tertiary care centers and these centers probably see more patients with recurrent FUO because these patients mostly want a second opinion when their initially unexplained fever recurs.

A recurrent fever pattern is a strong independent predictor of not establishing the diagnosis in FUO [5,7,10]. The author was able to establish a final diagnosis in only 49% of 45 patients with recurrent FUO versus 82% final diagnoses in 154 cases with continuous fever in his first series [14]. In his second study these figures were respectively 52% of 105 episodic cases versus 74% of 185 classic cases [15]. de Kleijn and colleagues [10] established a final diagnosis in 50% of 56 recurrent FUO and in 80% of 111 patients with continuous fever. Bleeker-Roovers and colleagues [5] established a final diagnosis in 24% of 25 patients with recurrent fever and in 69% of 48 patients with continuous fever in a new study from the same Dutch center. Quite a lot of patients with recurrent FUO have very prolonged disease duration, even up to several years. It is well known from the classic FUO literature that the chance of establishing a diagnosis in cases with fever lasting longer than 6 months is low. In the large series of 347 patients with FUO lasting more than 6 months, referred to the US National Institutes of Health, a cause could be identified in only 54% of the cases [16]. In a German study of 85 patients with recurrent fever for more than 6 months, 40% remained unexplained [17].

## Mechanisms and causes of recurrent fevers of unknown origin

A first episode of recurrent FUO with a short interval is frequently caused by relapse of a partially treated disorder, mostly a deep-seated infection, such as osteomyelitis, spondylitis, endocarditis, and so forth. Another mechanism is renewed exposure to antigens, other substances, crystals, or necrotic tissue. Extrinsic allergic alveolitis or hypersensitivity pneumonitis is caused by inhalational allergens; metal fume fever is caused by inhalation of freshly formed metallic particles. Necrosis leads to phagocytosis with subsequent secretion of pyrogenic cytokines. This is the mechanism of recurrent FUO in some cases of neoplastic recurrent FUO, of pulmonary embolism, and hemolytic anemia.

Drug fever is caused by different mechanisms. The recurrent pattern occurs in cases of repeated intake of medications, such as quinine for nocturnal leg cramps, cimetidine for dyspepsia, and so forth. Another example is nitrofurantoin fever in patients who repeatedly undergo urologic procedures and receive nitrofurantoin prophylactically for a couple of days.

Recurrent FUO may also be caused by diseases with a known course of spontaneous remission and flare-up. Still's disease is the most common of these entities. This is also the case for relapsing polychondritis and mastocytosis, Behçet's disease, and the familial autoinflammatory syndromes [13].

The causes of recurrent FUO are classified into four major diagnostic categories, similar to those of classic FUO. The so called "big three" categories (infections, tumors, and systemic inflammatory diseases [SIDs]) account for 50% to 70% of the diagnoses in classic FUO, but for only 20% to 30% of the causes in recurrent FUO (Table 1). The miscellaneous group represents about 25% of the cases and in this category the "little three" (drug fever, factitious fever, and habitual hyperthermia) should always be excluded before starting an investigation for the whole array of exotic causes of

Table 1
Causes of recurrent FUO in reported series

| Reference | 7 | 8 | 9 |
|---|---|---|---|
| N | 45 | 87 | 95 |
| Infection | 4 (9%) | 10 (11.5%) | 4 (4%) |
| Tumor | 2 (5%) | 13 (15%) | 14 (15%) |
| SID | 5 (11%) | 8 (9.2%) | 17 (18%) |
| Miscellaneous | 11 (25%) | 17 (20%) | 19 (20%) |
| FMF | 2 | 11 | 12 |
| Undiagnosed | 23 (52%) | 39 (45%) | 41 (43%) |

Figures rearranged according to the proposed classification of causes.
*Abbreviations:* FMF, familial Mediterranean fever; SID, systemic inflammatory diseases.

recurrent FUO. About 50% remain unexplained. In a review of the literature of FUO from 1961 to 1991, 55 different conditions were identified that met the criteria of recurrent FUO and 33 belonged to the miscellaneous category [7]. In a renewed search, up to April 2005, 70 different disorders could be identified of which 40 belonged to the miscellaneous category [13]. Several reported cases of so-called "recurrent FUO" represent examples of partially treated infectious or inflammatory conditions. An unexpected recurrent course with spontaneous remissions has been reported, however, for such diseases as giant cell arteritis and tuberculosis [8,9,18,19].

*Infections*

Only a limited number of infections give rise to a pattern of recurrent fever, although exceptions to this rule continue to be reported. Even tuberculosis cannot be omitted from the list of causes of recurrent FUO [8,9,18]. Most infections that present as so-called "recurrent FUO" are partially treated mostly deep-seated infections in patients who get antibiotics before referral to the hospital or who have been treated in hospital during a too short period. Typical examples are osteomyelitis, particularly spondylitis; endocarditis; infective aortic aneurysm; septic jugular or subclavian vein thrombosis; infected vascular prosthesis; and hidden, deep-seated abscesses (abdominal, mediastinal, gluteal, retroperitoneal). In the present CT and ultrasonography era, abscesses are much rarer because they are easily detected by these routine imaging techniques [5,15]. Septic jugular or subclavian vein thrombosis should be looked for in case of recurrent FUO in patients who have been recently hospitalized and who received central venous lines. Less experienced physicians continue to search for bacterial endocarditis in these cases because blood cultures remain continuously positive, a finding that suggests an intravascular focus.

The classic bacterial diseases that cause recurrent FUO are prostatitis, cholangitis, and otitis media-mastoiditis. The mechanism is intermittent seeding of bacteria from these silent foci with spontaneous resolution of the fever even without antibiotic treatment. Many patients have dental and sinus abnormalities as focus, but these findings are rarely the cause of FUO, be it classic or recurrent [14]. A very unusual recently reported hidden focus is bronchoesophageal fistula [20].

A few unusual bacterial infections should be looked for in selected cases. Brucellosis may cause an undulating fever that mostly does not meet the criterion of recurrence. The fever may fluctuate with episodes of less elevated temperature but seldom normalization of the temperature. Persistent *Yersinia* infection is considered as cause of recurrent FUO by some investigators but the final proof is difficult to yield [5,10]. The diagnosis is based on specialized serologic tests and the specificity of these tests is a matter of debate [4,7]. Leptospirosis is traditionally mentioned as a cause of FUO, but this is mostly a short-lived infection that may present with a biphasic pattern but the interval between the infectious and immunologic phase is too short to meet the criteria of recurrent FUO. Rat-bite fever is caused by infection with *Spirillum minor* or *Streptobacillus moniliformis* and it is easily suspected by the history of contact with rats. Melioidosis is a granulomatous, bacterial, infection caused by *Burkholderia pseudomallei*, endemic in Southeast Asia, which may cause repeated bouts of fever during years. It may remain silent for years and become symptomatic years after leaving the endemic area [21]. Whipple's disease has in the past been included in the miscellaneous group but it is an infection caused by *Tropheryma whippelii*. It is one of the most difficult diagnoses in the field of FUO.

*Borrelia recurrentis* is transmitted by either fleas or ticks. It causes a distinct recurrent fever pattern, with short fever-free intervals. Travel history must be the clue to the diagnosis because it occurs only in well-described geographic areas [22]. Q fever is a very contagious disease transmitted not only by cattle, sheep, and goats but also by cats. It is rare in Western Europe but a common disease in Spain, North Africa, and Turkey.

Toxoplasmosis may cause repeated bouts of fever and waxing and waning enlargement of lymph nodes. The interval of fever-free periods in case of nonfalciparum *Plasmodium* sp, such as *P vivax* and *P ovale*, is mostly too short, but here again travel history is one of the diagnostic clues. Trypanosomiasis is another tropical cause of recurrent FUO.

Except for some members of the herpes group, viral infections should not be looked for in case of recurrent FUO. Viral infections, however, may be a trigger for the so-called "macrophage activation syndrome" or hematophagocytic lymphohistiocytosis, a nonmalignant, yet potentially fatal immune dysregulation syndrome [23]. All members of the herpes virus group are notorious causes of FUO in HIV-associated, nosocomial, and neutropenic FUO. Herpes simplex and herpes zoster reactivate also in immunocompetent individuals but not as unexplained fever, although an unusual 13-year history of recurrent-persistent Epstein-Barr virus infection has been reported in a child without immune deficiency [24]. Human herpes virus 8, also known as "Kaposi's sarcoma–associated herpes virus," has been reported as cause of episodic fever preceding the development of

Kaposi sarcoma with 1 year [25]. Human herpes virus 6 and human herpes virus 8 are suspected to play a role in some of the atypical histiocytic or lymphocytic proliferative disorders, such as Rosai-Dorfman disease and the multicentric plasmablastic subtype of Castleman disease, respectively [26,27].

*Tumors*

Tumors cause recurrent fever by intermittent necrosis with subsequent phagocytosis and cytokine production. In case of colon carcinoma recurrent infection in the ulcerated mucosa also plays a role. In the past, cancer of the liver and the kidneys were typical examples but nowadays these tumors are readily detected by ultrasonography and CT scan [14,28]. Colon carcinoma is a classic neoplastic cause of recurrent FUO, although the so-called "relapsing Pel-Ebstein fever pattern" of Hodgkin's and non-Hodgkin's lymphoma is better known [14,29]. Most physicians, however, consider spontaneous remission of fever and regression of enlarged lymph nodes as proof of infectious origin. Relapse weeks or even months later and subsequent diagnosis of lymphoma comes as a big surprise. Angioimmunoblastic lymphadenopathy and malignant histiocytosis have also been reported to present with a recurrent FUO pattern [7,13,30]. Schnitzler syndrome is mostly included in the miscellaneous group, but a malignant course is now reported in 20% of the cases [9,31,32]. It is a very rare condition but it should be known by FUO experts because intermittent fever is a cardinal feature. It was the cause in 3 of 95 patients in a recent study [9]. It is a prototype of disease that escapes the diagnosis because one has never heard of it. The typical features are chronic urticaria, episodic fever, monoclonal IgM gammopathy, bone pain, and bone densification on radiographs. It has a very slow chronic course and most patients are erroneously treated with cytostatic drugs [31,32].

Cardiac myxoma is a classic yet very rare cause of episodic FUO and one of the reasons to consider echocardiography in the diagnostic evaluation. It is a benign tumor of endocardial origin that may cause fever by silent distal embolization or by production of interleukin (IL)-6 by the tumor itself [7,33].

*Systemic inflammatory diseases*

A whole array of inflammatory diseases, designated as rheumatic diseases, vasculitides, multisystem diseases, connective tissue diseases, collagen vascular diseases, and autoimmune diseases, have been grouped in the FUO literature as noninfectious inflammatory diseases by de Kleijn and colleagues [10]. The author prefers the term "systemic inflammatory diseases" because it cannot be proved that these diseases are indeed not infectious. The author defines SIDs as inflammatory syndromes of unknown origin with constitutional symptoms, signs of inflammation, and involvement of at least two organ systems [34]. Several of these diseases are truly rare diseases unfamiliar to most physicians, so that the delay in diagnosis exceeds years. A typical example is relapsing polychondritis. Diagnostic delay is also frequently caused by an atypical presentation, which does not allow a diagnosis because the internationally defined criteria are not met. Quite a lot of these patients get repeated empiric treatment with nonsteroidal anti-inflammatory drugs (NSAIDs) or corticosteroids, which suppress more typical manifestations and prevent the diagnostic signs to manifest. For some SIDs, such as Still's disease, Behçet's disease, and relapsing polychondritis, a seemingly spontaneous remission and relapse months or even years later is typical. In contrast, a recurrent course with spontaneous remissions is very unusual for such diseases as giant cell arteritis and ankylosing spondylitis [7,19]. Understandably, this recurrent FUO pattern then prevents the diagnostician from considering these etiologies.

Adult-onset Still's disease is by far the most common SID, with a classic course of recurrent FUO [35,36]. It causes episodic, mostly very high fever with major constitutional symptoms with varying asymptomatic intervals of even more than 1 year. There is no single true specific feature or diagnostic test and too many physicians establish too easily this diagnosis in the case of recurrent FUO [4,7]. The author considers this diagnosis only in patients younger than 40 years of age, although numerous case reports of so-called adult-onset Still's disease in older patients can be found in the literature. Diagnosis of adult-onset Still's disease requires exclusion of other diseases and it is only definite after a prolonged follow-up, although classic full-blown cases are easily diagnosed at the first encounter. Typical features are a very high fever up to $41°C$; sore throat without signs of pharyngitis; an evanescent, macular, salmon-colored rash during the time of fever; and more frequently arthralgia than arthritis. Diffuse lymphadenopathy and splenomegaly may suggest lymphoma, and pleuritis and pericarditis are present in 20% to 40% of the cases. An unexpected finding, which delayed diagnosis, was neutrophil meningitis in four cases [37]. Conspicuous laboratory features are markedly elevated erythrocyte sedimentation rate ($>150$ mm/h) or C-reactive protein value; neutrophil leukocytosis greater than $15.10^9$ cells/L; and spectacularly elevated ferritin levels ($>10,000$ pg/L) [36]. Patients with adult-onset Still's disease are more at risk for NSAID-induced acute liver damage and even liver failure.

Behçet's disease is a SID with a tendency of recurrence and spontaneous remission. Recurrent aphthous stomatitis, genital ulcerations, and uveitis are the typical manifestations, which when present as a triad, allowing immediate diagnosis. Its prevalence is high along the ancient Silk Road (the eastern Mediterranean littoral, particularly Turkey, over the Middle East to Japan) but very low in the United States and Western countries [38]. Thrombophlebitis is common and aneurysm of the peripheral arteries and pulmonary arteries is a dreaded complication. It is a well known cause of recurrent FUO in the ethnic groups at risk for that disease, yet very rare in a white population, although 5 of 95 cases in the recent French series were ascribed to Behçet's disease [9,39].

Relapsing polychondritis is an extremely rare SID with a fluctuating course, as suggested by its name. The diagnosis is easily missed in the early phase. It is characterized by bouts of fever and inflammation resulting in destruction of the cartilaginous tissues throughout the body, such as the external auricular, nasal and laryngotracheal cartilage, the joints, the sclera, heart valves, and inner ear. It is another example of a diagnosis one never has heard of and is not looked for [40].

Crohn's disease is included as granulomatous disease in the SID category together with sarcoidosis by several authors. The author considers Crohn's disease as a gastrointestinal condition, not a SID, because abdominal symptoms predominate the clinical picture in nearly all patients. Nevertheless it was an unexpected cause of recurrent FUO in 4 of 45 patients because the lack of abdominal complaints and normal bowel habits were the reason why bowel investigations were not ordered initially [7].

*Miscellaneous*

The miscellaneous category is the most important one, both in number and types of diseases. In contrast to classic FUO, which is mostly caused by an unusual presentation of common, well-known diseases, recurrent FUO is frequently caused by rare exotic diseases. The list of miscellaneous disorders contains several diseases with exotic names many physicians have never heard of (Box 1). The "little three" causes of classic FUO (drug fever, factitious fever, and habitual hyperthermia) should always be considered in case of recurrent FUO. Drug fever caused by intermittent intake of drugs and factitious fever are too frequently forgotten in clinical practice, whereas habitual hyperthermia resurges as cause for referral in the present chronic fatigue syndrome era [7,15,41,42].

Factitious fever is caused by either manipulation of the thermometer or self-injection of contaminated material. It characteristically occurs in young women who are frequently allied with health professions, although it has also been reported in elderly patients [7]. It was the cause in 9% of 343 cases evaluated at the US National Institutes of Health [42]. Unusual fever patterns with very high or very brief spikes, lack of diurnal variation, rapid defervescence without diaphoresis, lack of so-called "pulse-temperature differential," a long history of fever, and good physical appearance all point to factitious fever. An impressive discrepancy between the fever chart and the laboratory findings is an important clue for fraudulent fever. The presence of a mixed bacterial flora in blood cultures suggests self-inoculation of saliva or fecal or other material rather than a focus in the gastrointestinal or genitourinary tract when abdominal symptoms are absent in case of recurrent FUO [13,42].

Habitual hyperthermia, which displays some overlap with chronic fatigue syndrome and fibromyalgia, was the reason for Petersdorf and Beeson [1] to

**Box 1. Miscellaneous conditions reported as cause of recurrent FUO**

- "Little three"
  - Drug fever
  - Factitious fever
  - Habitual hyperthermia
- Hypersensitivity pneumonitis
- Metal fume fever
- Lung embolism
- Familial autoinflammatory syndromes and hereditary periodic fever syndromes
  - Familial Mediterranean fever
  - Hyper IgD syndrome
  - Cryopyrin-associated periodic syndromes
    - Muckle-Wells syndrome (urticaria, deafness, and amyloidosis)
    - Familial cold urticaria (familial cold autoinflammatory syndrome)
    - Neonatal onset multisystem inflammatory disease or chronic infantile neurologic, cutaneous, and articular syndrome
  - Tumor necrosis factor receptor-1–associated periodic syndrome (familial Hibernian fever)
- Lymphoproliferative-histiocytic disorders
  - Castleman disease
  - Kikuchi-Fujimoto disease
  - Inflammatory pseudotumor of lymph nodes
  - Erdheim-Chester disease
  - Rosai-Dorfman disease
- Large granular lymphocyte syndrome
- Macrophage activation syndrome (hemophagocytic syndrome)
- Cyclic neutropenia
- Periodic fever, aphthous stomatitis, pharyngitis (cervical) adenitis
- Mastocytosis
- Gout
- Pseudogout
- Hemolytic anemia
- Addison's disease
- Aortoenteric fistula
- Brewer's yeast ingestion
- Cholesterol embolism

- Chronic fatigue syndrome
- Crohn's disease
- Fabry's disease
- Gaucher's disease
- Hypothalamic hypopituitarism
- Hypertriglyceridemia
- Idiopathic granulomatosis
- Klippel-Trénaunay syndrome
- Milk protein allergy
- Poikilothermia
- Polymer fume fever
- Rathke's cleft cyst
- Seizures

introduce the cutoff value of 38.3°C as a criterion of FUO. This entity is poorly known and in the author's center it is an increasing reason for referral of so-called "recurrent FUO." The main complaint is fever, particularly after physical or intellectual exertion. Laboratory tests and radiographs all are normal and spontaneous resolution mostly ensues, yet sometimes only after years. Several patients are suspected of manipulating the thermometer because temperature may be normal in hospital where they rest but when returning home and assuming normal physical activities they experience the typical exertion-related rise in body temperature.

Hypersensitivity pneumonitis or extrinsic allergic alveolitis may cause episodic FUO when exposure to inhaled allergens is intermittent. Diagnosis is easily missed when systemic symptoms, such as fever, overshadow the respiratory manifestations. Farmer's lung, pigeon breeder's lung, and bird fancier's lung are known even for many medical students but cases are initially confused with a viral or bacterial lung infection that resolves quickly during hospital admission or with an empiric antibiotic treatment. The presence of fine rales on lung auscultation despite a normal chest film is an important but easily overlooked clue. It should always be considered when symptoms subside spontaneously during hospital admission and recur after discharge. It is an immune complex reaction to a continuously expanding list of inhaled antigens, be it at home (birds, indoor molds, contaminated humidifiers); in the workplace (farmers, mushroom-workers, swimming pool lifeguards, bakers, woodworkers, bird and fowl breeders and handlers); or elsewhere (sauna). Over 300 causes of hypersensitivity pneumonitis have been reported.

Metal fume fever is another typical respiratory episodic disease resulting from the inhalation of a variety of small freshly formed metallic oxide particles released during welding. Symptoms typically resolve 24 to 48 hours. It is easily recognized by occupational medicine physicians but overlooked by most others who consider it as a transient respiratory tract infection. The pathogenesis is probably not immunologic but an inflammatory response caused by direct toxic effect of the particles.

Venous thromboembolism may cause recurrent FUO but it is rarely considered as a reason because few physicians know that high fever up to 40°C may be caused by this condition. All these respiratory conditions are the reason why there is a low threshold for ordering lung function tests and particularly carbon monoxide diffusion capacity measurement in recurrent FUO. Screening with D-dimer level determination makes no sense in patients with signs of inflammation.

The hereditary periodic fever syndromes have received much attention in the medical literature of the last decade and they have been regrouped as familial autoinflammatory syndromes The term "autoinflammatory," and not autoimmune, has been proposed because autoantibodies or antigen-specific T cells, the effectors of the adaptive immune system, do not play a role in the pathogenesis [43–46]. FMF is the most common worldwide and best known familial autoinflammatory syndrome [47,48]. Muckle-Wells syndrome, reported in 1962, has been included in the cryopyrin-associated periodic syndromes [49–51]. Familial Hibernian fever, originally described in 1982 in an Irish family, has been renamed tumor necrosis factor (TNF)-receptor-1–associated periodic syndrome (TRAPS) and hyperimmunoglobulinemia D syndrome has been reported from the Netherlands in 1984 [43,52–58]. These rare syndromes were until recently only known by a few specialists and they have probably been overlooked in the past. With exception of FMF, however, even in patients from or originating from North and Western Europe they remain rare. In the author's experience with more than 500 cases of FUO, only one case of hyperimmunoglobulinemia D syndrome was found but several cases of FMF were found. In the two French series of recurrent FUO, 29 (16%) of 182 cases were caused by hereditary autoinflammatory syndromes. Twenty three of the 29 cases were FMF, 3 were TRAPS, 2 were hyperimmunoglobulinemia D syndrome, and 1 was a cryopyrin-associated periodic syndrome [8,9]. Typical features of these hereditary syndromes are lifelong, spontaneously resolving periods of fever, with onset in the early years of life, inflammation, cutaneous, serosal, abdominal, synovial, and musculoskeletal symptoms [43]. Distinguishing and rather specific clinical characteristics allow those few physicians familiar with these syndromes to establish early the diagnosis on a clinical basis [4,43,45]. Genetic analysis, performed in specialized laboratories, may yield the final proof [51,54,56,57]. Vaccination, minor trauma, surgery, or stress may provoke an attack. This can be explained by the current insights in the innate immunity, which consists of nonselective pattern-recognition surface receptors, such as Toll-like receptors and an intracellular protein cascade system consisting of a whole complex of interacting proteins, called the inflammasome. Activation of the inflammasome results in liberation of cytokines, such as IL-1, and mutations of genes that code for proteins of the inflammasome result in defective inhibition or inappropriate activation of the inflammatory intracellular cascade and release of IL-1 after the aforementioned minor stimuli [45,46]. FMF and cryopyrin-associated periodic syndromes can be considered inflammophilia syndromes, a name that refers to the hereditary thrombophilia syndromes, caused by mutations of components of the coagulation cascade that results in unexpected thrombosis.

FMF is by far the most common hereditary periodic fever syndrome worldwide. It is an autosomal-recessive disorder, very prevalent in Jews, Turks, Arabs, Armenians, and less common in other populations of the Mediterranean [43,47,48]. The most prominent feature of FMF is short (1–3 days), spontaneously resolving attacks of fever, mostly starting before the age of 20 years. Diagnosis is frequently missed during childhood in case of low frequency of attacks because these episodes are considered transitory viral infections. Impressive abdominal pain, caused by serositis, frequently leads to exploratory laparoscopy. Many clinicians know this type of serositis but pleural and pericardial serositis and synovitis, frequently confined to one large joint, is less well known. Erysipelas-like rash of the distal lower limbs, orchitis, and meningitis are rare clinical manifestations [47,48]. The genetic basis is a mutation of the MEFV gene on the short arm of chromosome 16 that encodes for a protein, named pyrin or marenostrin, a component of the inflammasome [44,45]. It's so-called "N-terminal PYD domain" is shared with other proteins of the inflammasome. That particular protein is predominantly expressed in myeloid cells, such as neutrophils and monocytes. Numerous mutations of the MEFV gene have already been identified and the list continues to grow [45,47,48]. AA-type amyloidosis is a dreaded complication with a variable prevalence in different genetic populations. Colchicine is the first-line treatment and essential in the prevention of amyloidosis. Anakinra, recombinant IL-1 receptor antagonist, is a new therapeutic option in refractory cases.

Hyperimmunoglobulinemia D syndrome is an autosomal-recessive disorder, initially described in the Netherlands in 1984 by Van der meer and colleagues [55,58]. Most cases originate from Western Europe, particularly the Netherlands and France. The international registry (www.HIDS.NET) is updated by the Nijmegen Periodic Fever Research Group and contained information on 203 cases in February 2005. The genetic basis is mutation in the gene encoding for mevalonate kinase, an enzyme that follows the well-known 3-hydroxy-methylglutanyl-coenzyme A reductase of the isoprenoid pathway with cholesterol, ubiquinone, and other substances as end product [55,56]. This gene is located on the long arm of chromosome 12. It is not known how mevalonate kinase deficiency leads to inflammation and fever and the relation of this mutation to the characteristically elevated IgD level is unclear. Most patients develop fever episodes in the first year of life and abdominal symptoms and (cervical) lymphadenopathy are nearly always present. The attacks are also rather short but last a little bit longer than in FMF, 3 to 5 days or more. Hepatosplenomegaly, erythematous macules and plaques, arthritis of large joints, and oral or vaginal painful aphthous ulcers are occasionally present. IgD levels are elevated in most cases and the same holds true for IgA, but the height of IgD level does not correlate with disease severity. No effective treatment is available but provisional data from a trial with simvastatin, a 3-hydroxy-methylglutanyl-coenzyme A reductase inhibitor, were encouraging [59].

Muckle-Wells syndrome, described in 1962 as "urticaria, deafness and amyloidosis: a new heredofamilial syndrome" is now grouped with familial cold autoinflammatory syndrome and neonatal-onset multisystemic inflammatory disease, also known as chronic infantile neurologic, cutaneous, and articular syndrome, as cryopyrin-associated periodic syndromes. These three autosomal-dominant hereditary syndromes reflect actually a spectrum of cryopyrinopathies, ranging from the most severe, neonatal-onset multisystemic inflammatory disease or chronic infantile neurologic, cutaneous, and articular syndrome to Muckle-Wells syndrome and familial cold autoinflammatory syndrome, the mildest form [49–51]. The latter, also described as familial cold urticaria, is characterized by very short bouts of fever, joint inflammation, and urticaria-like rash, typically induced by exposure to mild cold (eg, cool breezes of air-conditioned rooms). Conjunctivitis is a typical symptom and the attacks resolve spontaneously within 24 to 48 hours. The typical distinguishing feature of Muckle-Wells syndrome is progressive neural deafness, occurring later in life. Neonatal-onset multisystemic inflammatory disease or chronic infantile neurologic, cutaneous, and articular syndrome is a pediatric disease, characterized by very early onset, severe joint malformation, hearing loss, chronic aseptic meningitis, and mental retardation. These three clinically defined syndromes are caused by mutations of the same gene [44,49–51,60] variously named the $CIAS_1$ gene (cold-induced autoinflammatory syndrome 1), NALP3, and PYFAF1 gene, located on the long arm of chromosome 1. It encodes a protein known as "cryopyrin" or NALP3 that is predominantly expressed in myeloid cells and chondrocytes. It's N-terminal PYD domain is similar to that of marenostrin (pyrin) of FMF. It is part of the NALP3 inflammasone and it has a role in inflammation by activating caspase 1, an IL-1 converting enzyme [51,60]. The new insights in the pathogenesis have resulted in a new therapeutic approach, anakinra (IL-1 receptor antagonist), shown to be effective in Muckle-Wells syndrome and in familial cold autoinflammatory syndrome [50,60].

TRAPS was originally described in 1982 as "familial Hibernian fever" in an Irish family [52]. It is an autosomal-dominant disorder caused by mutations in the gene of TNF-receptor type 1 (TNFRSF-1A), located on the short arm of chromosome 12, probably resulting in defective shedding of the receptor [53,54]. In contrast with the other hereditary autoinflammatory syndromes, the attacks of fever last several weeks instead of days. The age of onset is also variable. Periorbital edema, centrifugal migratory erysipelas-like painful skin lesions, mainly on distal upper limbs, and testicular pain are the distinguishing features. Amyloidosis occurs rather commonly. Etanercept, recombinant soluble TNF receptor, is a logical therapeutic approach and found to be an effective treatment [53,57].

Gaucher's disease and Fabry's disease are also hereditary diseases that occasionally manifest as episodic FUO. This presentation is very unusual for these lysosomal storage diseases that present mostly as infiltrative disorders with organomegaly and organ dysfunction and not as inflammatory conditions [7,61–63].

Another number of diseases of the long list of miscellaneous causes are grouped as nonspecific reactive lymphoproliferative or histiocytic disorders. They mostly present as pseudotumor or lymphadenopathy and they are probably autoimmune or infectious triggered conditions. Included in this group are Castleman disease [27,64], Kikuchi-Fujimoto disease [65,66], Rosai-Dorfman disease [26], inflammatory pseudotumor of lymph nodes [67,68], and Erdheim-Chester disease [69,70]. A few other diseases resemble these entities clinically at first glance, but the author does not classify them in this group. Angio immunoblastic lymphadenopathy, Schnitzler syndrome, and large granular lymphocyte lymphocytosis are rather considered as malignant and not as reactive lymphoid proliferation in many cases [30,32,71,72]. The macrophage activation syndrome, formerly described as hematophagocytic lymphohistiocytosis, may cause episodic fever but the course is mostly pseudomalignant fulminant, requiring early aggressive empiric treatment with corticosteroids and immunosuppressive drugs [23,73–75].

Castleman disease is a lymphoproliferative disorder that presents in a localized or unicentric and a multicentric form with three histologic variants: (1) a hyaline vascular, (2) a plasma cell, and (3) a mixed type [27,64]. These subtypes each have a different clinical presentation, prognosis, and treatment. Fever and constitutional symptoms are rarely present in the hyaline vascular type in contrast to the other histologic variants. The localized type can be cured by surgical resection, whereas the multicentric form mostly requires treatment with corticosteroids and occasionally chemotherapy. Increased IL-6 production, possibly linked to human herpes virus 8 infection, might play a role in the inflammatory response.

Kikuchi-Fujimoto disease is a histiocytic necrotizing lymphadenitis first described in Japan in 1972 [65]. It mainly affects young females. Cervical lymph nodes are typically involved and axillary nodes occasionally. It is common in Japan and other Asian countries and less well known in western countries but it is reported from all over the world. Cat-scratch disease, systemic lupus erythematodes, and lymphoma, is the main differential diagnosis, which can be made by appropriate immunologic tests, serology for *Bartonella henselae*, and the presence of a granuloma. It is a benign self-limiting disease with a low but definite risk of recurrence of about 3% to 5%. Hydroxychloroquine has been reported to be effective in a few cases [66].

Inflammatory pseudotumor of lymph nodes resembles histologically plasma cell granuloma, a benign extranodal mesenchymal proliferation [67,68]. Inflammatory pseudotumor of lymph nodes presents as FUO when located in "hidden" lymph node sites, such as the mediastinum, the mesentery, or retroperitoneum [7,68,76]. Only experienced pathologists recognize it as a distinct entity based on the presence of a mixture of lymphocytic, plasmocytic, histiocytic, and myofibroblastic cells [68]. Surgical resection frequently leads to cure experience. NSAIDs suffice in some cases to suppress fever and inflammation, although corticosteroids may be needed [67].

Rosai-Dorfman disease, known as "sinus histiocytosis with massive lymphadenopathy," is another reactive lymph node disease of unknown, probably infectious origin. Diagnosis is easily established by appropriate immunohistochemical studies. Many patients experience spontaneous remission but more intensive therapeutic approaches with surgery, radiotherapy, or chemotherapy may be needed in case of vital organ compression [26,77].

Erdheim-Chester disease is a non–Langerhans cell histiocytosis presenting as an infiltrative process that may affect numerous organs. Mediastinal and retroperitoneal localization may be difficult to diagnose, although the "coated aorta" aspect caused by periaortic fibrosis is very specific [69,70]. The lack of plasma cells and presence of many foamy histiocytes allows the differential diagnosis with retroperitoneal fibrosis in case of perirenal localization.

All these lymphoproliferative-histiocytic disorders are gallium and fluorodeoxyglucose avid and hence easily detected in hidden areas, such as the mediastinum and abdomen, by nuclear medicine techniques [67,76]. The definite diagnosis mostly requires the opinion of an experienced pathologist and many cases are classified as nonspecific reactive abnormalities or, regrettably, as neoplastic [68].

Box 1 summarizes the so-called miscellaneous cases of recurrent FUO that came to the author's attention by careful study of the literature on FUO since 1961 [4,7,13]. In an initial study on recurrent FUO, a number of older entities were included of which the existence as a separate entity has been questioned in the meantime [7]. Omitted from this list are etiocholanolone fever and periodic fever. The same holds true for granulomatous hepatitis, which is not a disease but a distinct histologic reaction caused by numerous well-defined infectious, neoplastic, and other conditions [4,78]. The author doubts the existence of fever attributed solely to cirrhosis and to alcoholic hepatitis [4,79]. Fever ascribed to alcoholic hepatitis is mostly caused by concomitant infection, alcohol withdrawal symptoms per se, or seizure-associated hyperthermia. Periodic fever, aphthous stomatitis, pharyngitis, adenitis, also named Marshall's syndrome, is a pediatric disease that resembles cyclic neutropenia. It may occur in adolescents but onset in adults has not been reported [80,81]. Central fever supposed to be caused by a lesion of the thermoregulation center is a misnomer that persists in the literature. So-called "central fever" in case of sarcoidosis, hemorrhage, stroke, trauma, and so forth is a classic fever caused by release of pyrogenic cytokines in the central nervous system. Lesions of the thermo-regulation area of the brainstem cause poikilothermia with episodes of hypothermia and, very rarely, episodes of hyperthermia depending on the temperature of the environment [82].

## Diagnostic strategy

### General principles

The diagnostic strategy in case of recurrent FUO is different from classic FUO. The spectrum of causative disorders is different with much less infec-tions and tumors, the diseases most clinicians fear. More than 50% of the cases remain unexplained and patients with recurrent FUO remain in good health despite repeated episodes of fever [7,11]. When patients and re-ferring colleagues are informed of this, they mostly accept a watchful wait-ing strategy. This strategy permits the underlying disease to reveal itself during follow-up or to resolve definitely. Starting a FUO investigation in an asymptomatic phase is never indicated and patients should be asked to present when a new episode starts. Periodic reassessment with complete physical examination and a few routine laboratory tests is indicated but re-peating extensive diagnostic rounds makes little sense. Renewed investiga-tion should be directed by new clues, which should be carefully evaluated. It is traditional to look for possible clues, but most cases of prolonged fever become FUO because the clues, when present, are misleading [4,5,10]. Clues are valuable when they fit in a complex that allows diagnosis by pattern rec-ognition, the typical diagnostic approach of the experienced clinician. No single disease or group of diseases arises as common cause. This means that the pretest probability for most of the possible causative disorders is low and ordering multiple diagnostic tests in patients at low risk for the tested conditions increases considerably the chance of false-positive results [4,5]. Data from previous investigations should be critically analyzed and the author was repeatedly able to establish the diagnosis on the spot by sim-ple pattern recognition. A typical example is Schnitzler syndrome: periodic fever, a rash that is described as urticaria, and a monoclonal peak on protein electrophoresis only requires the confirmation that the paraprotein is indeed an IgM to establish the diagnosis [31,32]. Lack of laboratory signs of inflam-mation during repeated symptomatic phases points to either habitual hyper-thermia or factitious fever. Seizures may cause fever without signs of inflammation, described in case reports, but this is only mentioned for the sake of completeness, [7,83]. In case of recurrent fever for more than 1 year, tests should be guided to the classic very prolonged recurrent FUOs, such as Still's disease, the hereditary periodic fever syndromes, and the atypical lymphoproliferative diseases.

## History

Particular attention should be paid to the ethnic origin, age at first episode of fever, and family history. These are the clues for the hereditary auto-inflammatory syndromes. Intermittent drug intake should be specifically and repeatedly asked for (eg, quinine for occasional nocturnal leg cramps). Occupation, hobbies, animals, and birds may point to exposure to inhalational antigens causing hypersensitivity pneumonitis, such as pigeon's breeder's disease, farmer's lung, and so forth.

## Physical examination

The skin must be carefully inspected in search of the typical evanescent rash of Still's disease, whereas the urticaria of Schnitzler syndrome should not be overlooked. Lung auscultation may reveal the fine roles of hypersensitivity pneumonitis. In case of suspicion of factitious fever, temperature measurement should be supervised and in case of doubt, simultaneous body and urine temperature can solve the problem [84].

## Laboratory tests

Cultures should only be taken during a symptomatic phase and very few infectious serologic and immunologic tests are required in the standard laboratory battery of the classic FUO patient [4,5]. Serum ferritin levels should be measured routinely in case of recurrent FUO because a value above 10,000 µg/L is typical for the active phase of Still's disease and for macrophage activation syndrome [35,74]. Serum protein electrophoresis should be screened for the presence of a monoclonal spike, a clue for possible Schnitzler syndrome. Differential diagnosis of eosinophilia is broad but in case of recurrent FUO it suggests drug fever. Low white blood cell count suggests cyclic neutropenia, large granular lymphocyte lymphocytosis, or macrophage activation syndrome, and bone marrow biopsy is indicated in these cases [23,72,85]. Increased lactic dehydrogenase should raise suspicion not only of a neoplastic disease but also of a hemolytic crisis and pulmonary embolism. Elevated alkaline phosphatase value is an indication for ordering a bone scintigraphy that may yield the first clue to mastocytosis, Schnitzler syndrome, or Erdheim-Chester disease, all causes of bone densification on standard bone radiographs [32,70,86]. An increased D dimer value points to thromboembolic phenomenon, but this only holds true in cases without signs of inflammation and this test is not indicated in case of FUO.

Specialized serologic and immunologic tests must be requested with a specific diagnosis in mind. Undirected infectious serology has very poor predictive value because of the low prevalence of the screened disorders. Even for tests with high specificity, the rate of false-positive results remains high. This is the case for most viral serologic tests, and tests for *Yersinia* infection, Q fever, and so forth. IgD levels should routinely be determined in cases with multiple bouts of fever. Testing for cryoglobulins has little diagnostic value because this is frequently a nonspecific finding.

## Imaging studies

Chest radiograph and abdominal ultrasonography belong to the initial work-up of patients with prolonged fever, but they seldom reveal a diagnosis [4,5]. Echocardiography may reveal a myxoma.

Abdominal and chest spiral CT is warranted, mainly in search of neoplastic and nonspecific histiocytic or lymphoproliferative disorders. Lung function testing with measurement of lung diffusion capacity is a sensitive tool for lung involvement, such as lung embolism or hypersensitivity pneumonitis. Colonoscopy is an essential investigation because colon cancer and Crohn's disease are classic causes of recurrent FUO [7].

Based on experience with fluorodeoxyglucose positron emission tomography (FDG-PET) since 1996, the author now orders a fluorodeoxyglucose positron emission tomography in a symptomatic phase instead of CT scans and colonoscopy [76]. This is a sensitive total body screening technique, useful in the search for infections, neoplastic, atypical reactive lymphoproliferative and histiocytic disorders, inflammatory bowel disease, and other entities, such as Whipple's disease and even FMF. Fluorodeoxyglucose positron emission tomography is preferred to gallium because fluorodeoxyglucose positron emission tomography takes less time and allows a better assessment of the abdomen. It seldom yields the diagnosis but this total body investigation is a guidance for more specific delineation of abnormal areas with directed imaging techniques, such as ultrasonography, CT, MRI, endoscopy, and surgical procedures [4,76].

MRI is used to identify specific features of abnormalities detected by other techniques; total body MRI will perhaps replace nuclear medicine total body study but imaging time and costs preclude its use for that purpose.

## Genetic analysis

Genetic tests are indicated for atypical cases of familial autoinflammatory syndromes and they allow confirmation of the diagnosis in more than 90% of the cases of FMF [47,48]. Tests are rather widely available for FMF, at least in Europe, in contrast to genetic tests for the other hereditary periodic fever syndromes [51,56,57]. The advent of these tools brought a real breakthrough in the diagnostic approach of recurrent FUO in certain ethnic groups.

## Other tests

Invasive procedures, such as liver biopsy and exploratory laparotomy, may only be helpful when other features point to abdominal disease. Slight liver abnormalities are so common in FUO patients that this sole finding does not warrant liver biopsy [4,5].

## Therapeutic trials

Therapeutic trials make little or no sense and they have very poor if any diagnostic value in case of recurrent FUO because spontaneous resolution of fever is common and may coincide with the therapeutic trial. Trials with antibiotics have mostly been performed before referral and should not be repeated. Antituberculous drugs are nearly never indicated because tuberculosis does not give rise to recurrent FUO, although a single exception has been reported.

NSAIDs are more effective than paracetamol as an antipyretic drug and they may be useful as symptomatic treatment pending a definite diagnosis or spontaneous resolution of fever. Attention should be paid, however, to possible serious liver toxicity of NSAIDs in this clinical setting and particularly in case of possible Still's disease. The naproxen test is sometimes proposed on the assumption of a specific antipyretic activity in neoplastic fever, but it was shown that the accuracy of this test is too low in an unselected FUO population to be discriminative [87].

When corticosteroids have been given for symptomatic relief the dose should be rapidly tapered as soon as the illness subsides but a small percentage of patients require a continuous low dose of corticosteroids (eg, 4–6 mg prednisolone per day) for suppression of fever and debilitating general symptoms [7,11].

In the twenty-first century there is no longer room for empiric treatment with heparins. Appropriate imaging techniques, and particularly CT scan, are sensitive enough to exclude thromboembolic disease in case of suspicion of these rare causes of recurrent FUO.

## Summary

Recurrent FUO is mostly caused by rare diseases and many cases remain unexplained. The very limited literature data do not allow one to construct a diagnostic algorithm. A number of general principles should be kept in mind before starting the investigation for this rare subtype of FUO.

## References

[1] Petersdorf RB, Beeson PB. Fever of unexplained origin: report on 100 cases. Medicine 1961; 40:1–30.
[2] Durack DT, Street AC. Fever of unknown origin: reexamined and redefined. Curr Clin Top Infect Dis 1991;11:35–51.
[3] Bryan CS. Fever of unknown origin: the evolving definition. Arch Intern Med 2003;163(9): 1003–4.

[4] Knockaert DC, Vanderschueren S, Blockmans D. Fever of unknown origin in adults: 40 years on. J Intern Med 2003;253(3):263–75.

[5] Bleeker-Rovers CP, Bos FJ, de Kleijn EM, et al. A prospective multicenter study on fever of unknown origin: the yield of a structured diagnostic protocol. Medicine 2007;86(1): 26–38.

[6] Reimann HA, Mc Closkey RV. Periodic fever: diagnostic and therapeutic problems. JAMA 1974;228(13):1662–4.

[7] Knockaert DC, Vanneste LJ, Bobbaers HJ. Recurrent or episodic fever of unknown origin: review of 45 cases and survey of the literature. Medicine 1993;72(3):184–96.

[8] Vidal E. Fièvres récurrentes non génétiques. Rev Med Interne 2006;27(S3):S261–3.

[9] Hot A, Pérard L, Coppéré B, et al. Diagnostic étiologique des fièvres récurrente à l'âge adulte: a propos de 95 observations. Rev Med Interne 2006;27(S3):S289.

[10] de Kleijn EM, Vandenbroucke JP, Van Der Meer JWM. Fever of unknown origin (FUO). Medicine 1997;76(6):392–400.

[11] Knockaert DC, Dujardin KS, Bobbaers HJ. Long-term follow-up of patients with undiagnosed fever of unknown origin. Arch Intern Med 1996;156(6):618–20.

[12] Reimann HA. Periodic disease. Medicine 1951;30(3):219–45.

[13] Knockaert DC. Recurrent fever of unknown origin. In: Cunha BA, editor. Fever of unknown origin. New York: Information healthcare; 2007. p. 133–49.

[14] Knockaert DC, Vanneste LJ, Vanneste SB, et al. Fever of unknown origin in the 1980s. Arch Intern Med 1992;152(1):51–4.

[15] Vanderschueren S, Knockaert D, Adriaenssens T, et al. From prolonged febrile illness to fever of unknown origin. Arch Intern Med 2003;163(9):1033–41.

[16] Aduan RP, Fauci AS, Dale DC, et al. Prolonged fever of unknown origin (FUO): a prospective study of 347 patients. Clin Res 1978;26:558A.

[17] Winckelmann G, Lütke A, Löhner J. Uber 6 Monate besthendes rezidivierendes Fieber ungeklärter Ursache. Bericht über 85 Patienten. Deutsche Medizinische Wochenschrift 1982;107(26):1003–7.

[18] Collazos J, Guerra E, Mayo J, et al. Tuberculosis as a cause of recurrent fever of unknown origin. J Infect 2000;41(3):269–72.

[19] Rho JP, Montori VM, Bauer BA. 74-year-old women with intermittent fever, headache and stroke. Mayo Clin Proc 1998;73(1):73–6.

[20] Kaul DR, Orringer MB, Saint S, et al. The drenched doctor. N Engl J Med 2007;356(18): 1871–6.

[21] Scully RE. Case records of the Massachusetts general hospital. Case 40-1992. N Engl J Med 1992;327(15):1081–7.

[22] Dworkin MS, Schwan TG, Anderson DE. Tick-borne relapsing fever in North America. Med Clin North Am 2002;86(2):417–33.

[23] Grom AA. Macrophage activation syndrome and reactive hemophagocytic lymphohistiocytosis: the same entities? Curr Opin Rheumatol 2003;15(5):587–90.

[24] Lekstrom-Himes JA, Dale JK, Kingma DW, et al. Periodic illness associated with Epstein-Barr virus infection. Clin Infect Dis 1996;22(1):22–7.

[25] Dagna L, Broccolo F, Paties CT, et al. A relapsing inflammatory syndrome and active human herpesvirus 8 infection. N Engl J Med 2005;353(2):156–63.

[26] Sakai Y, Atsumi T, Itoh T, et al. Uveitis, pancarditis, haemophagocytosis, and abdominal masses. Lancet 2003;361(9360):834.

[27] Herrada J, Cabanillas F, Rice L, et al. The clinical behavior of localized and multicentric Castleman disease. Ann Intern Med 1998;128(8):657–62.

[28] Scully RE, Mark EJ, McNeely WF, et al. Case records of the Massachusetts general hospital. Case 2-1996. N Engl J Med 1996;334(3):176–82.

[29] Kaufmann Y, Many A, Rechavi G, et al. Brief report: lymphoma with recurrent cycles of spontaneous remission and relapse. Possible role of apoptosis. N Engl J Med 1995;332(8): 507–10.

[30] Dogan A, Attygalle AD, Kyriakou C. Angioimmunoblastic T-cell lymphoma. Br J Haematol 2003;121(5):681–91.
[31] Lautenschlager S, Itin PH. Des Schnitzler syndrome. Hautarzt 1993;44(12):781–4.
[32] Lipsker D, Veran Y, Grunenberger F, et al. The Schnitzler syndrome: four new cases and review of the literature. Medicine 2001;80(1):37–44.
[33] Pinede L, Duhaut P, Loire R. Clinical presentation of left atrial cardiac myxoma: a series of 112 consecutive cases. Medicine 2001;80(3):159–72.
[34] Knockaert DC. Systemic inflammatory diseases (SID's): what's in a name. Acta Clin Belg 2007;62(1):21–5.
[35] Fautrel B, Zing E, Golmard JL, et al. Proposal for a new set of classification criteria for adult-onset Still disease. Medicine 2002;81(3):94–200.
[36] Mert A, Ozaras R, Tabak F. Fever of unknown origin: a review of 20 patients with adult-onset Still's disease. Clin Rheumatol 2003;22(2):89–93.
[37] Blockmans DE, Knockaert DC, Bobbaers HJ. Still's disease can cause neutrophilic meningitis. Neurology 2000;54(5):1203–5.
[38] Sakane T, Takeno M, Suzuki N, et al. Behcet's disease. N Engl J Med 1999;341(17): 1284–91.
[39] Saltoglu N, Tasova Y, Midikli D, et al. Fever of unknown origin in Turkey: evaluation of 87 cases during a nine-year-period of study. J Infect 2004;48(1):81–5.
[40] Trentham DE, Le CH. Relapsing polychondritis. Ann Intern Med 1998;129(2):114–22.
[41] Johnson DH, Cunha BA. Drug fever. Infect Dis Clin North Am 1996;10(1):85–91.
[42] Aduan RA, Fauci AS, Dale DC, et al. Factitious fever and self-induced infection: a report of 32 cases and review of the literature. Ann Intern Med 1979;90(2):230–42.
[43] Drenth JPH, van der Meer JWM. Hereditary periodic fever. N Engl J Med 2001;345(24): 1748–57.
[44] Hull KM, Shoham N, Chae JJ, et al. The expanding spectrum of systemic autoinflammatory disorders and their rheumatic manifestations. Curr Opin Rheumatol 2003;15(1):61–9.
[45] Samuels J, Ozen S. Familial Mediterranean fever and the other autoinflammatory syndromes: evaluation of the patient with recurrent fever. Curr Opin Rheumatol 2006;18(1): 108–17.
[46] Drenth JPH, van der Meer JWM. The inflammasome: a linebacker of innate defense. N Engl J Med 2006;355(7):730–2.
[47] Ben-Chetrit E, Levy M. Familial Mediterranean fever. Lancet 1998;351(9103):659–64.
[48] Samuels J, Aksentijevich I, Torosyan Y, et al. Familial Mediterranean fever at the millennium. Clinical spectrum, ancient mutations, and a survey of 100 American referrals to the National Institutes of Health. Medicine 1998;77(4):268–97.
[49] Johnstone RF, Dolen WK, Hoffman HM. A large kindred with familial cold autoinflammatory syndrome. Ann Allergy Asthma Immunol 2003;90(2):233–7.
[50] Hawkins PN, Lachmann HJ, Aganna E, et al. Spectrum of clinical features in Muckle-Wells syndrome and response to Anakinra. Arthritis Rheum 2004;50(2):607–12.
[51] Dodé C, Le Dû N, Cuisset L, et al. New mutations of CIAS1 that are responsible for Muckle-Wells syndrome and familial cold urticaria: a novel mutation underlies both syndromes. Am J Hum Genet 2002;70(6):1498–506.
[52] Williamson LM, Hull D, Mehta R, et al. Familial Hibernian fever. Q J Med 1982;51(204): 469–80.
[53] Hull KM, Drewe E, Aksentijevich I, et al. The TNF receptor-associated periodic syndrome (TRAPS): emerging concepts of an autoinflammatory disorder. Medicine 2002;81(5): 349–68.
[54] Dodé C, André M, Bienvenu T, et al. The enlarging clinical, genetic, and population spectrum of tumor necrosis factor receptor-associated periodic syndrome. Arthritis Rheum 2002;46(8):2181–8.
[55] Drenth JPH, Haagsma CJ, van der Meer JWM. Hyperimmunoglobulinemia D and periodic fever syndrome: the clinical spectrum in a series of 50 patients. Medicine 1994;73(3):133–44.

[56] Simon A, Cuisset L, Vincent MF, et al. Molecular analysis of the mevalonate kinase gene in a cohort of patients with the hyper-IgD and periodic fever syndrome: its application as a diagnostic tool. Ann Intern Med 2001;135(5):338–43.

[57] Simon A, Van Deuren M, Tighe PJ, et al. Genetic analysis as a valuable key to diagnosis and treatment of periodic fever. Arch Intern Med 2001;161(20):2491–3.

[58] van der Meer JW, Vossen JM, Radl J, et al. Hyperimmunoglobulinaemia D and periodic fever: a new syndrome. Lancet 1984;ii:1084–90.

[59] Simon A, Drewe E, van der Meer JWM, et al. Simvastatin treatment for inflammatory attacks of the hyperimmunoglobulinemia D and periodic fever syndrome. Clin Pharmacol Ther 2004;75(5):476–83.

[60] Hoffman HM, Rosengren S, Boyle DL, et al. Prevention of cold-associated acute inflammation in familial cold autoinflammatory syndrome by interleukin-1 receptor antagonist. Lancet 2004;364(9447):1779–85.

[61] Yosipovitch Z, Katz K. Bone crisis in Gaucher disease: an update. Isr J Med Sci 1990;26(10): 593–5.

[62] Brady RO, Schiffmann R. Clinical features of and recent advances in therapy for Fabry disease. JAMA 2000;284(21):2771–5.

[63] Desnick RJ, Brady R, Barranger J, et al. Fabry disease, an under-recognized multisystemic disorder: expert recommendations for diagnosis, management, and enzyme replacement therapy. Ann Intern Med 2003;138(4):338–46.

[64] Lachmann HJ, Gilbertson JA, Gillmore JD, et al. Unicentric Castleman's disease complicated by systemic AA amyloidosis: a curable disease. Q J Med 2002;95(4):211–8.

[65] Parappil A, Rifaath A, Doi SAR, et al. Pyrexia of unknown origin: Kikuchi-Fujimoto disease. Clin Infect Dis 2004;39(1):138–43.

[66] Rezai K, Kuchipudi S, Chundi V, et al. Kikuchi-Fujimoto disease: hydroxychloroquine as a treatment. Clin Infect Dis 2004;39(12):e124–6.

[67] Knockaert DC, Schuermans A, Vlayen J, et al. Fever of unknown origin due to inflammatory pseudotumour of lymph nodes. Acta Clin Belg 1998;53(6):367–70.

[68] Moran CA, Suster S, Abbondanzo SL. Inflammatory pseudotumor of lymph nodes: a study of 25 cases with emphasis on morphological heterogeneity. Hum Pathol 1997;28(3):332–8.

[69] Oliveira L, Moraes MF, Oliveira P, et al. A train driver with painful legs. Lancet 1999; 353(9169):2034.

[70] Veyssier-Belot C, Cacoub P, Caparros-Lefebvre D, et al. Erdheim-Chester disease: clinical and radiological characteristics of 59 cases. Medicine 1996;75(3):157–69.

[71] Scott CS, Richards SJ, Sivakumaran M, et al. Transient and persistent expansions of large granular lymphocytes (LGL) and NK-associated (Nka) cells: the Yorkshire Leukaemia Group Study. Br J Haematol 1993;83(3):504–15.

[72] Lamy T, Loughran TP Jr. Clinical features of large granular lymphocyte leukaemia. Semin Hematol 2003;40(3):185–95.

[73] Reiner AP, Spivak J. Hematophagic histiocytosis: a report of 23 patients and a review of the literature. Medicine 1988;67(6):369–88.

[74] Imashuku S. Differential diagnosis of hemophagocytic syndrome: underlying disorders and selection of the most effective treatment. Int J Hematol 1997;66(2):135–51.

[75] Ramanan AV, Schneider R. Macrophage activation syndrome. What's in a name!. J Rheumatol 2003;30(12):2513–6.

[76] Blockmans D, Knockaert D, Maes A, et al. Clinical value of [18F]fluoro-deoxyglucose positron emission tomography for patients with fever of unknown origin. Clin Infect Dis 2001;32(2):191–6.

[77] Pulsoni A, Anghel G, Falcucci P, et al. Treatment of sinus histiocytosis with massive lymphadenopathy (Rosai-Dorfman Disease): report of a case and literature review. Am J Hematol 2002;69(1):67–71.

[78] Knockaert DC, Vanderschueren S, Blockmans DE. Diagnostic strategy in systemic inflammatory diseases. Acta Clin Belg 2007;62(1):26–35.

[79] Singh N, Yu VL, Wagener MM, et al. Cirrhotic fever in the 1990s: a prospective study with clinical implications. Clin Infect Dis 1997;24(6):1135–8.

[80] Long SS. Syndrome of periodic fever, aphthous stomatitis, pharyngitis, and adenitis (PFAPA). What it isn't. What is it? J Pediatr 1999;135(1):1–5.

[81] Thomas KT, Feder HM, Lawton AR, et al. Periodic fever syndrome in children. J Pediatr 1999;135(1):15–21.

[82] MacKenzie MA, Hermus RM, Wollersheim HC, et al. Poikilothermia in man: pathophysiology and clinical implication. Medicine 1991;70(4):257–68.

[83] Boeve BF, Wijdickx FM, Benarroch EE. Paroxysmal sympathetic storms (diencephalic seizures) after severe diffuse axonal head injury. Mayo Clin Proc 1998;73(2):148–52.

[84] Murray HW, Tuazon CU, Guerrero IC, et al. Urinary temperature: a clue to early diagnosis of factitious fever. N Engl J Med 1977;296(1):23–4.

[85] Dale DC, Bolyard AA, Aprikyan A. Cyclic neutropenia. Semin Hematol 2002;39(2):89–94.

[86] Lopez-Gomez M, Garcia JDM, Jimenez-Alonso J, et al. Systemic mast cell disease as a cause of fever of unknown origin. Eur J Intern Med 1993;4(2):171–5.

[87] Vanderschueren S, Knockaert DC, Peetermans WE, et al. Lack of value of the naproxen test in the differential diagnosis of prolonged febrile illnesses. Am J Med 2003;115(7):572–5.

INFECTIOUS
DISEASE CLINICS
OF NORTH AMERICA

Infect Dis Clin N Am 21 (2007) 1213–1220

# Fever of Unknown Origin: Is There a Role for Empiric Therapy?

Charles S. Bryan, MD*, Divya Ahuja, MD

*Department of Medicine, University of South Carolina School of Medicine,
Two Medical Park, Suite 502, Columbia, SC 29203, USA*

*Fever in its varied forms is still with us … but it is of equal importance to know that the way has been opened, and that the united efforts of many workers in many lands are day by day disarming this great enemy of the race.* William Osler, 1896 [1].

To the question posed in the title to this article, the short answer is no. Set aside those cases in which findings strongly suggest a presumptive diagnosis, such as vegetations found on echocardiography; caseating granulomas in biopsy specimens; travel to an area where certain infections, such as malaria, are endemic; or clinical features that point to adult-onset Still's disease. Set aside those cases in which impaired host defenses predispose to infections by more-or-less predictable pathogens, such as advanced AIDS and chemotherapy-induced granulocytopenia. In the remaining cases of classic community-acquired fever of unknown origin (FUO), if by FUO one means prolonged FUO ($\geq 3$ weeks) with no diagnosis established after at least 1 week of intensive investigation (ie, cases that fulfill the modified Petersdorf-Beeson criteria [2–4]), continued observation while searching for a cause nearly always constitutes the best strategy. In 1963 Sheon and Van Ommen [5] wrote: "One cannot overemphasize the value of expectant management…. The use of antibiotics on an empiric basis in a patient with obscure fever may create as well as resolve diagnostic problems … the best management consists of striving to make a correct diagnosis." In 1983, Hurley [6] similarly concluded: "The patient with classic protracted fever of unknown origin requires a methodical approach, and precision is of utmost importance. Fortunately, such a patient is rarely desperately ill, so the physician has time to perform the evaluation." More recently, Mackowiak and Durack [7] state that with rare exception, "A fundamental principle in the management of

* Corresponding author.
*E-mail address:* cbryan@gw.mp.sc.edu (C.S. Bryan).

classic FUO is that therapy should be withheld, whenever possible, until the cause of fever has been determined, so that it can be tailored to a specific diagnosis." We agree.

Most infectious disease specialists rank high among their contributions to society their advocacy for curtailing indiscriminate use of antimicrobial agents. Schooled in the subtleties of diagnosis and engaged by their colleagues mainly in a consultative capacity, infectious disease specialists typically strive to temper the use of potent drugs for marginal indications. Relieved of the pressure to "do something now" at the first point of clinical encounter and given the advantage of "tincture of time," infectious disease specialists often recognize "mistakes" made by other physicians. One of the authors, while preparing a textbook of infectious diseases specifically for primary care physicians, asked 600 fellows of the Infectious Diseases Society of America to checkmark from a list of 23 diagnoses those in which they had determined that a mistake by a physician acting in a primary care capacity led to some combination of death, disability, or litigation [8]. Results are shown in Table 1. One should remember, however, Calvin Coolidge's admonition that "any fool can criticize, and most fools do." The authors are aware of no similar survey of mistakes made by infectious disease specialists. Many and perhaps most experienced infectious disease consultants can recall occasional cases of "true FUO" that they would manage differently had they the opportunity to do it over again. Consider the following two cases seen by one of the authors (CSB).

**Cases**

An elderly retired dentist was seen in 1975 (before the availability of transesophageal echocardiography and imaging studies based on CT and nuclear MRI) for prolonged FUO. Physical examination was unremarkable except for a systolic murmur. He continued to be febrile after 2 months of observation and studies that included liver and bone marrow biopsies. His fever seemed to respond to empiric therapy for cryptic military tuberculosis, only to recur. His fever then seemed to respond to empiric therapy for culture-negative endocarditis only to recur again. Laparotomy revealed Hodgkin's disease.

A 56-year-old woman was seen in 2007 for suspected endocarditis with acute aortic regurgitation. She gave a history of intermittent fever, chills, and malaise of 4 months' duration. Blood cultures were sterile. Endocarditis was confirmed at surgery, during which she underwent replacement of the aortic valve and drainage of an adjacent myocardial abscess. Cultures of the excised valve and material from the abscess were sterile. She was treated with a regimen currently recommended for culture-negative endocarditis that, however, was probably inadequate for *Bartonella henselae*, subsequently identified by polymerase chain reaction of the excised heart valve and confirmed by silver stain and by serology (IgG titer >1:512). At the

Table 1

Frequency of diseases in which mistakes made by primary care physicians resulted in serious consequences

| Condition | No. (%) of positive responses |
|---|---|
| Necrotizing soft tissue infection | 112 (64) |
| Spinal epidural abscess | 96 (55) |
| Sepsis syndrome | 95 (54) |
| Endocarditis | 94 (54) |
| Meningococcal disease | 89 (51) |
| Tuberculosis | 84 (48) |
| Herpes simplex encephalitis | 82 (47) |
| Antibiotic toxicity | 82 (47) |
| Pneumonia | 80 (46) |
| Pneumococcal meningitis | 80 (46) |
| Intra-abdominal sepsis | 59 (34) |
| AIDS-related problem | 58 (33) |
| Brain abscess | 58 (33) |
| Toxic shock syndrome | 58 (33) |
| Asplenia (failure to vaccinate) | 57 (33) |
| Rocky Mountain spotted fever | 54 (31) |
| Travel-related problems | 54 (31) |
| Acute epiglottitis | 35 (20) |
| Pelvic inflammatory disease | 32 (18) |
| Clostridial syndrome | 31 (18) |
| *Haemophilus influenzae* meningitis | 29 (17) |
| Sphenoid sinusitis | 22 (13) |
| Cavernous sinus thrombosis | 21 (12) |
| Miscellaneous | 32 (18) |

From a survey sent to 600 fellows of the Infectious Diseases Society of America. The survey instrument listed 23 diagnoses (shown here) and asked the recipients to checkmark those diagnoses in which, in their experience, mistakes made by a physician acting in a primary care capacity had led to death, disability, or litigation. The rate of the response to the survey was 30%. These data do not indicate the actual incidence of mistakes made by primary care physicians, which some data suggest is relatively low. Rather, they indicate pitfalls in diagnosis and disease management as seen from the perspective of infectious disease specialists, who are usually consulted on especially difficult cases.

*Data from* Bryan CS. Infectious disease emergencies. In: Bryan CS, editor. Infectious diseases in primary care. Philadelphia: WB Saunders; 2002. p. 111–52.

time of this writing, she is asymptomatic and receiving appropriate therapy for *Bartonella* endocarditis.

In the first case, early laparotomy would have been preferable to empiric therapy because, in retrospect, the Pel-Ebstein fever of Hodgkin's disease toyed with the consultant. In the second case, which probably represents the first case of *B henselae* endocarditis reported from South Carolina, closer attention to the history would have facilitated earlier diagnosis because the patient had been scratched and bitten by a feral kitten before the onset of symptoms. These cases illustrate the truism that, as one internal medicine resident put it, "The three most important principles in medicine are diagnosis, diagnosis, and diagnosis."

### The generally favorable prognosis of prolonged fever of unknown origin that defies diagnosis

Studies to date suggest that cases of FUO that defy precise diagnosis after intensive investigation and prolonged observation generally carry a favorable prognosis. Larson and colleagues [9], in whose series 12% of 105 cases of FUO persisted without a diagnosis on follow-up, divided such fevers into two categories: those that resolved over time and those that did not. Most patients in the former group, they concluded, had "an illness which best fits a self-limited prolonged viral infection," often with some combination of lymphadenopathy, splenomegaly, hepatomegaly, and abnormal liver function tests. Their five patients with prolonged or recurrent, undiagnosed FUO were all alive at the time of their publication. Knockaert and colleagues [10], in whose series 11% of 199 cases of FUO persisted without a diagnosis on follow-up for at least 5 years, determined the attributable mortality of undiagnosed FUO to be only 3.2%. These Belgian investigators also described 45 cases of "recurrent or episodic" FUO, defined as FUO meeting the Petersdorf-Beeson criteria but with fever-free intervals of at least 2 weeks' duration [11]. Only one death attributable to FUO occurred among the 23 patients for whom no final diagnosis was ever reached; the patient, who had refused readmission to the hospital, was suspected to have had temporal arteritis.

### Situations that sometimes call for empiric therapy of fever of unknown origin, and the case for symptomatic therapy

Cunha [12] in 1996 recommended empiric therapy for FUO in only four situations: (1) antibiotics for culture-negative endocarditis; (2) low-dose corticosteroids for presumed temporal arteritis; (3) antituberculous drugs for suspected military tuberculosis in elderly patients; and (4) naproxen for suspected neoplastic fever. These four conditions are briefly reviewed next after first addressing the advisability of symptomatic therapy with corticosteroids or nonsteroidal anti-inflammatory agents (NSAIDs) for FUO.

A small, anecdotal, and amorphous body of published literature suggests a limited role for corticosteroids and NSAIDs for symptomatic therapy of FUO. Larson and colleagues [9] reported that anti-inflammatory drugs were only transiently successful, if at all, in those patients whose fevers resolved spontaneously and without a diagnosis. Two patients with febrile illnesses lasting 7 years or more, however, were concluded to have a steroid-responsive form of focal hepatitis. Larson and colleagues [9] referred to "apparently similar patients" with benign but chronic, steroid-responsive

FUO described in a personal communication by R.P. Aduan and D.C. Dale of the National Institutes of Health. Unfortunately, a MEDLINE search reveals no papers on FUO by either of these investigators. Larson and colleagues [9] also described cases resembling temporal arteritis, polymyalgia rheumatica, vasculitis, or adult-onset Still's disease that responded to steroids but for which no definitive diagnosis was reached. Knockaert and colleagues [10] reported that, among their 18 patients with prolonged undiagnosed FUO, four were treated with steroids and six with NSAIDs. They concluded that NSAIDs usually sufficed for symptomatic patients. Similarly, among their 21 surviving patients with "recurrent or episodic" FUO for whom no diagnosis was reached, seven received intermittent short-term therapy with NSAIDs or corticosteroids. There is probably a limited role for cautious use of NSAIDs or corticosteroids in symptomatic patients who are well-informed of the potential pitfalls of such therapy. As Larson and colleagues [9] put it, "There is no substitute for observing the patient, talking to him, and thinking about him," a process that involves "going over the patient again and again, repeating the history and physical examination, reviewing the chart, discussing the problem with colleagues to glean new ideas, and spending time in quiet contemplation of the clinical enigma."

## Culture-negative endocarditis

Although data published through the years indicate that up to 31% of cases of infective endocarditis have sterile blood cultures, more recent studies suggest that only about 5% of cases are culture-negative when defined by strict criteria, sometimes backed by transesophageal echocardiography. Apart from cases in injecting drug users, optimum management remains controversial. Albrich and colleagues [13] have recently published a structured approach to diagnosis and management along with an extremely useful algorithm. Infectious disease consultants would do well to keep their paper and also the paper by Broqui and Raoult [14] on endocarditis caused by rare and fastidious microorganisms on file, because the distribution of recognized causes of culture-negative endocarditis seems to be changing. Application of polymerase chain reaction to excised heart valves can be of great value in cases that require surgical intervention [15,16]. There is general agreement that a regimen for empiric therapy should be appropriate for enterococci, nutrient-variant streptococci, and fastidious gram-negative bacilli of the HACEK group. To that end, an appropriate regimen consists of penicillin or ampicillin plus gentamicin or streptomycin plus ceftriaxone [17,18].

## Cryptic disseminated tuberculosis

Current guidelines from the Centers for Disease Control and Prevention support the use of drugs for strongly suspected culture-negative pulmonary tuberculosis [19]. These guidelines are largely silent, however, on the issue of when to treat suspected disseminated tuberculosis. This diagnosis should be suspected especially in elderly patients, who may present with an afebrile wasting illness [20]; in febrile patients with HIV-AIDS; in patients with rheumatoid arthritis treated with corticosteroids, methotrexate, or infliximab [21]; and in recipients of solid organ transplants [22]. There are no clear guidelines on what constitutes an adequate duration of a therapeutic trial in this situation. Because the bacillary populations of the individual lesions are substantially lower than those encountered in cavitary pulmonary tuberculosis, however, a response usually becomes apparent within 2 months unless the disease is caused by a multidrug-resistant strain. Patients should be informed of the potential for adverse reactions including hepatitis from isoniazid, optic neuritis from ethambutol, and drug interactions from rifamycin derivatives.

*Temporal arteritis (giant cell arteritis)*

Management of suspected temporal arteritis, an important cause of FUO in elderly persons sometimes complicated by blindness or cerebrovascular accident, is discussed elsewhere in this issue. Suspected visual impairment mandates immediate therapy with corticosteroids, because treatment after the onset of loss of visual acuity or central visual field defects rarely restores these deficits, and then only when corticosteroids are begun within 4 days of the onset of visual symptoms [23]. Temporal artery biopsy remains highly desirable and should be performed within 2 weeks from starting corticosteroids despite reports that characteristic changes are sometimes found when biopsies are delayed for longer periods [24]. Some data suggest that the addition of low-dose aspirin to a corticosteroid regimen lowers the incidence of intracranial ischemic events [25].

*The naproxen test for differentiating between neoplastic and other causes of fever of unknown origin*

Brief mention should be made of the naproxen test, because it was included among the indications for empiric therapy in Cunha's review [12] published in 1996. The naproxen test dates to a 1984 report by Chang and Gross to the effect that naproxen, a NSAID, induced a prompt, complete, and sustained lysis of fever in 14 of 15 cases of fever caused by neoplasm but in none of five cases of fever caused by infection [26]. More recently, Vandeerschuren and colleagues [27] concluded the naproxen test to be only 55% sensitive and 62% specific for neoplastic FUO. In retrospect, earlier investigators did not use tight criteria for FUO and may have had selection bias toward cases likely to be of neoplastic etiology. Moreover, there is no good theoretical explanation as to why NSAIDs should uniquely lyse fever caused by neoplasms and not fever from other causes [28].

## Summary

The practice of medicine revolves around three questions: (1) What is wrong with the patient? (2) What can I do for the patient? (3) What will be the likely outcome? The advice of Celsus (25 BC–AD 50) that "better a doubtful remedy than none at all" generally rings true for acute life-threatening illnesses but seldom holds for cases of prolonged FUO ($\geq 3$ weeks) that satisfy the modified Petersdorf-Beeson criteria. Patients with prolonged FUO and for whom no diagnosis is reached after months and years of intense observation generally have a favorable prognosis. Empiric therapy should be used only in carefully defined circumstances, with the patient's informed consent, and with the physician's commitment to keep searching for an etiology.

## References

[1] Osler W. The study of the fevers of the South. JAMA 1896;26:999–1004.
[2] Petersdorf RG, Beeson PB. Fever of unexplained origin: report on 100 cases. Medicine (Baltimore) 1961;40:1–30.
[3] Durack DT, Street AC. Fever of unknown origin: reexamined and redefined. In: Remington JS, Swartz MN, editors. Current clinical topics in infectious diseases, vol. 3. Boston: Blackwell Science; 1991. p. 35–51.
[4] Bryan CS. Fever of unknown origin: the evolving definition. Arch Intern Med 2003;163:1003–4.
[5] Sheon RP, Van Ommen RA. Fever of obscure origin. Am J Med 1963;34:486–99.
[6] Hurley DL. Fever in adults: what to do when the cause is not obvious. Postgrad Med 1983;74:232–44.
[7] Mackowiak PA, Durack DT. Fever of unknown origin. In: Mandell GL, Bennett JE, Dolin R, editors. Principles and practice of infectious diseases. 6th edition. Philadelphia: Elsevier Churchill Livingstone; 2005. p. 718–29.
[8] Bryan CS. Infectious disease emergencies. In: Bryan CS, editor. Infectious diseases in primary care. Philadelphia: W.B. Saunders Company; 2002. p. 111–52.
[9] Larson EB, Featherstone HJ, Petersdorf FG. Fever of undetermined origin: diagnosis and follow-up of 105 cases, 1970–1980. Medicine (Baltimore) 1982;61:269–92.
[10] Knockaert DC, Dujardin KS, Bobbaers HJ. Long-term follow-up of patients with undiagnosed fever of unknown origin. Arch Intern Med 1996;156:618–20.
[11] Knockaert DC, Vanneste LJ, Bobbaers HJ. Recurrent or episodic fever of unknown origin: review of 45 cases and survey of the literature. Medicine (Baltimore) 1993;72:184–96.
[12] Cunha BA. Fever of unknown origin. Infect Dis Clin North Am 1996;10:111–27.
[13] Albrich WC, Kraft C, Fisk T, et al. A mechanic with a bad valve: blood-culture-negative endocarditis. Lancet Infect Dis 2004;4:777–84.
[14] Broqui P, Raoult D. Endocarditis due to rare and fastidious bacteria. Clin Microbiol Rev 2001;14:177–207.
[15] Qin X, Urdahl KB. PCR and sequencing of independent genetic targets for the diagnosis of culture negative bacterial endocarditis. Diagn Microbiol Infect Dis 2001;40:145–9.
[16] Khulordava I, Miller G, Haas D, et al. Identification of the bacterial etiology of culture-negative endocarditis by amplification and sequencing of a small ribosomal RNA gene. Diagn Microbiol Infect Dis 2003;46:9–11.
[17] Fowler VG, Scheld WM, Bayer AS. Endocarditis and intravascular infections. In: Mandell GL, Bennett JE, Dolin R, editors. Principles and practice of infectious diseases. 6th edition. Philadelphia: Churchill Livingstone; 2005. p. 975–1022.

[18] Moreillon P. Endocarditis and endarteritis. In: Cohen J, Powderly WG, editors. Cohen and Powderly: infectious diseases, vol. 1. 2nd edition. St. Louis: Mosby; 2004. p. 653–68.

[19] American Thoracic Society, CDC, and Infectious Diseases Society of America. Treatment of tuberculosis. MMWR Morb Mortal Wkly Rep 2003;52(No. RR-11):1–77.

[20] Ozbay B, Uzan K. Extrapulmonary tuberculosis in high prevalence of tuberculosis and low prevalence of HIV. Clin Chest Med 2002;23:351–4.

[21] Mayordomo L, Marenco JL, Gomez-Mateos J, et al. Pulmonary miliary tuberculosis in a patient with anti-TNF-alpha treatment. Scand J Rheumatol 2002;31:44–5.

[22] Korner MM, Hirata N, Tenderich G, et al. Tuberculosis in heart transplant recipients. Chest 1997;111:365–9.

[23] Hayreh SS, Zimmerman B, Kardon RH. Visual improvement with corticosteroid therapy in giant cell arteritis: report of a large study and review of literature. Acta Ophthalmol Scand 2002;80:353–67.

[24] Ah Kine D, Tijani SO, Parums DV, et al. Effects of prior steroid treatment on temporal artery biopsy findings in giant cell arteritis. Br J Ophthalmol 2002;86:530–2.

[25] Nesher G, Berkun Y, Mates M, et al. Low-dose aspirin and prevention of cranial ischemic complications in giant cell arteritis. Arthritis Rheum 2004;50:1332–7.

[26] Chang JC, Gross HM. Utility of naproxen in the differential diagnosis of fever of undetermined origin in patients with cancer. Am J Med 1984;76:597–603.

[27] Vanderschueren S, Knockaert DC, Peetermans WE, et al. Lack of value of the naproxen test in the differential diagnosis of prolonged fever. Am J Med 2003;115:572–5.

[28] Plaisance KI, Mackowiak PA. Antipyretic fever: physiologic rationale, diagnostic implications, and clinical consequences. Arch Intern Med 2000;160:449–56.

**ELSEVIER
SAUNDERS**

INFECTIOUS
DISEASE CLINICS
OF NORTH AMERICA

Infect Dis Clin N Am 21 (2007) 1221–1231

# Index

*Note:* Page numbers of article titles are in **boldface** type.

*id.theclinics.com*

# Moving?

## Make sure your subscription moves with you!

To notify us of your new address, find your **Clinics Account Number** (located on your mailing label above your name), and contact customer service at:

**E-mail: elspcs@elsevier.com**

**800-654-2452 (subscribers in the U.S. & Canada)**
**407-345-4000 (subscribers outside of the U.S. & Canada)**

**Fax number: 407-363-9661**

**Elsevier Periodicals Customer Service**
6277 Sea Harbor Drive
Orlando, FL 32887-4800

*To ensure uninterrupted delivery of your subscription, please notify us at least 4 weeks in advance of move.

# United States Postal Service

## Statement of Ownership, Management, and Circulation
### (All Periodicals Publications Except Requestor Publications)

| 1. Publication Title | 2. Publication Number | 3. Filing Date |
|---|---|---|
| Infectious Disease Clinics of North America | 0 0 1 - 5 5 6 | 9/14/07 |

| 4. Issue Frequency | 5. Number of Issues Published Annually | 6. Annual Subscription Price |
|---|---|---|
| Mar, Jun, Sep, Dec | 4 | $184.00 |

7. Complete Mailing Address of Known Office of Publication (Not printer) (Street, city, county, state, and ZIP+4)

Elsevier Inc.
360 Park Avenue South
New York, NY 10010-1710

Contact Person
Stephen Bushing

Telephone (Include area code)
215-239-3688

8. Complete Mailing Address of Headquarters or General Business Office of Publisher (Not printer)

Elsevier Inc., 360 Park Avenue South, New York, NY 10010-1710

9. Full Names and Complete Mailing Addresses of Publisher, Editor, and Managing Editor (Do not leave blank)

Publisher (Name and complete mailing address)

John Schrefer, Elsevier, Inc., 1600 John F. Kennedy Blvd. Suite 1800, Philadelphia, PA 19103-2899

Editor (Name and complete mailing address)

Barbara Cohen-Kligerman, Elsevier, Inc., 1600 John F. Kennedy Blvd. Suite 1800, Philadelphia, PA 19103-2899

Managing Editor (Name and complete mailing address)

Catherine Bewick, Elsevier, Inc., 1600 John F. Kennedy Blvd. Suite 1800, Philadelphia, PA 19103-2899

10. Owner (Do not leave blank. If the publication is owned by a corporation, give the name and address of the corporation immediately followed by the names and addresses of all stockholders owning or holding 1 percent or more of the total amount of stock. If not owned by a corporation, give the names and addresses of the individual owners. If owned by a partnership or other unincorporated firm, give its name and address as well as those of each individual owner. If the publication is published by a nonprofit organization, give its name and address.)

| Full Name | Complete Mailing Address |
|---|---|
| Wholly owned subsidiary of | 4520 East-West Highway |
| Reed/Elsevier, US holdings | Bethesda, MD 20814 |

11. Known Bondholders, Mortgagees, and Other Security Holders Owning or Holding 1 Percent or More of Total Amount of Bonds, Mortgages, or Other Securities. If none, check box → ☐ None

| Full Name | Complete Mailing Address |
|---|---|
| N/A | |

12. Tax Status (For completion by nonprofit organizations authorized to mail at nonprofit rates) (Check one)
The purpose, function, and nonprofit status of this organization and the exempt status for federal income tax purposes:
☐ Has Not Changed During Preceding 12 Months
☐ Has Changed During Preceding 12 Months (Publisher must submit explanation of change with this statement)

PS Form 3526, September 2006 (Page 1 of 3 (Instructions Page 3)) PSN 7530-01-000-9931 PRIVACY NOTICE: See our Privacy policy in www.usps.com

| 13. Publication Title | | | 14. Issue Date for Circulation Data Below |
|---|---|---|---|
| Infectious Disease Clinics of North America | | | June 2007 |

| 15. Extent and Nature of Circulation | | Average No. Copies Each Issue During Preceding 12 Months | No. Copies of Single Issue Published Nearest to Filing Date |
|---|---|---|---|
| a. Total Number of Copies (Net press run) | | 2600 | 2500 |
| b. Paid Circulation (By Mail and Outside the Mail) | (1) Mailed Outside-County Paid Subscriptions Stated on PS Form 3541. (Include paid distribution above nominal rate, advertiser's proof copies, and exchange copies) | 1424 | 1291 |
| | (2) Mailed In-County Paid Subscriptions Stated on PS Form 3541 (Include paid distribution above nominal rate, advertiser's proof copies, and exchange copies) | | |
| | (3) Paid Distribution Outside the Mails Including Sales Through Dealers and Carriers, Street Vendors, Counter Sales, and Other Paid Distribution Outside USPS® | 465 | 420 |
| | (4) Paid Distribution by Other Classes Mailed Through the USPS (e.g. First-Class Mail®) | | |
| c. Total Paid Distribution (Sum of 15b (1), (2), (3), and (4)) | ▶ | 1889 | 1711 |
| d. Free or Nominal Rate Distribution (By Mail and Outside the Mail) | (1) Free or Nominal Rate Outside-County Copies Included on PS Form 3541 | 77 | 47 |
| | (2) Free or Nominal Rate In-County Copies Included on PS Form 3541 | | |
| | (3) Free or Nominal Rate Copies Mailed at Other Classes Through the USPS (e.g. First-Class Mail) | | |
| | (4) Free or Nominal Rate Distribution Outside the Mail (Carriers or other means) | | |
| e. Total Free or Nominal Rate Distribution (Sum of 15d (1), (2), (3) and (4)) | ▶ | 77 | 47 |
| f. Total Distribution (Sum of 15c and 15e) | ▶ | 1966 | 1758 |
| g. Copies not Distributed (See instructions to publishers #4 (page 83)) | ▶ | 634 | 742 |
| h. Total (Sum of 15f and g) | ▶ | 2600 | 2500 |
| i. Percent Paid (15c divided by 15f times 100) | | 96.08% | 97.33% |

16. Publication of Statement of Ownership
☐ If the publication is a general publication, publication of this statement is required. Will be printed in the December 2007 issue of this publication.     ☐ Publication not required

17. Signature and Title of Editor, Publisher, Business Manager, or Owner

*[signature]*     Date
Stephen Bushing – Executive Director of Subscription Services     September 14, 2007

I certify that all information furnished on this form is true and complete. I understand that anyone who furnishes false or misleading information on this form or who omits material or information requested on the form may be subject to criminal sanctions (including fines and imprisonment) and/or civil sanctions (including civil penalties).

PS Form 3526, September 2006 (Page 2 of 3)